HOW TO BE YOUR OWN

Herbal Pharmacist

Herbal Traditions, Expert Formulations

Herbs have a unique spirit on earth.
When used with respect and with wisdom in their whole form,
herbal combinations provide mankind
with the essential elements for survival, health,
and well being.

Linda Rector Page, N.D., Ph.D.

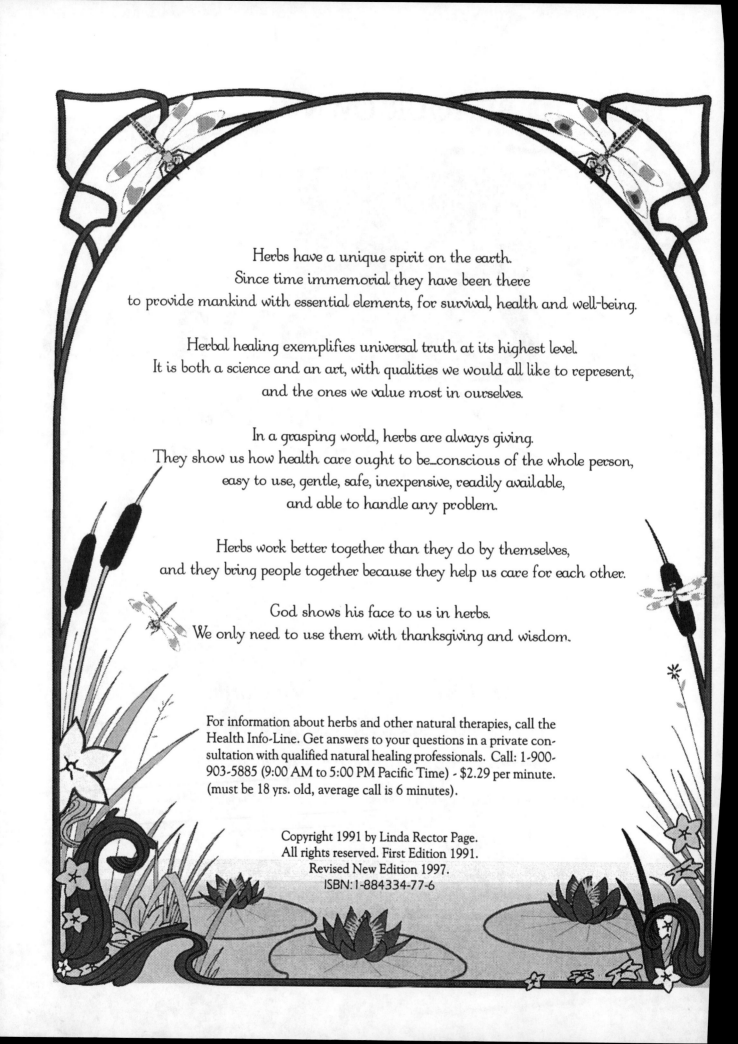

Herbs have a unique spirit on the earth.
Since time immemorial they have been there
to provide mankind with essential elements, for survival, health and well-being.

Herbal healing exemplifies universal truth at its highest level.
It is both a science and an art, with qualities we would all like to represent,
and the ones we value most in ourselves.

In a grasping world, herbs are always giving.
They show us how health care ought to be...conscious of the whole person,
easy to use, gentle, safe, inexpensive, readily available,
and able to handle any problem.

Herbs work better together than they do by themselves,
and they bring people together because they help us care for each other.

God shows his face to us in herbs.
We only need to use them with thanksgiving and wisdom.

For information about herbs and other natural therapies, call the
Health Info-Line. Get answers to your questions in a private consultation with qualified natural healing professionals. Call: 1-900-
903-5885 (9:00 AM to 5:00 PM Pacific Time) - $2.29 per minute.
(must be 18 yrs. old, average call is 6 minutes).

*H*ere's what some of America's expert herbalists say about
*H*ow To Be Your Own Herbal Pharmacist ....

"Well researched information that is amazingly easy to read and understand. Highly recommended for the medical profession as well as the lay person who is vitally interested in their own health care."
>Howard B. Peiper, co-author of the Pulitzer Prize nominated book,
>*Over 50 Looking 30 - The Secrets of Staying Young*

"Linda has gifted us with a book that is not only practical, well laid out and user friendly, but poetic and inspirational as well. I read this book not only for its eminently useful information, but for the gems of wisdom sprinkled throughout. *How To Be Your Own Herbal Pharmacist* presents perhaps better than any other herb book, the fundamentals of combining and formulating herbal compounds. Linda does an excellent job of taking this somewhat daunting subject, and presenting it in simple, easy-to-understand terms so that even the beginner herbalist can blend and formulate effective herbal formulas."
>Rosemary Gladstar
>Herbalist, Author, Educator

"This is a wonderful book...beautifully written in its clearly focused organization. It is easy to use and orientated to provide the reader with an opportunity to fully appreciate the power of herbal/natural medicine to support optimal health and well-being."
>Dr. Wayne Diamond, N.D.

"I highly recommend Linda Rector Page's *How To Be Your Own Herbal Pharmacist*. It is an easy to use, herbal pharmacology for the family. This valuable handy reference work is brimming with user-friendly herbal knowledge both informative and empowering to the reader."
>Janet Zand, OMD, LAc

"Primary health care will become informed self-care. The new *How To Be Your Own Herbal Pharmacist* brings practical, proven herbal information to the general public. Dr. Page teaches us to build herbal formulas rather than follow rigid prescriptions. As health conditions change, herbal support also must change. Centuries of ancient and modern herbal nutrition are conveniently arranged allowing a dynamic alchemy of plant healing to spring forth. A welcome resource for my clients and students."
>Edward Bauman, Ph.D.
>Director, Partners In Health Clinic & Nutrition
>Consultant Training Program, Cotati, CA.

How To Formulate Herbal Medicinals With This Book......

How To Be Your Own Herbal Pharmacist includes all forms of herbal medicinals; teas, broths, capsules, extracts, compresses, poultices, oils, syrups, ointments, liniments and baths. It addresses a wide range of ailments and conditions that can be improved and normalized through herbal combinations and techniques. Herbal remedies are appropriate for almost any necessity of life. It is simply a matter of knowing their properties, how they work together and how to use them correctly.

An effective herbal formula requires building on several levels. Careful consideration about what you want from a combination is the first step.

1️⃣ **Consider the following questions first:**
• Is the formula for short or long term use? or both?
• Is it for a chronic or acute problem?
• Is it a cleansing, rebuilding, maintenance, or disease preventive formula?
• Is it for an overall body system, such as the respiratory system? or for a specific area?
• Is it for symptomatic relief? or causal rebalance? or both?

2️⃣ **Then, turn to the appropriate page for your problem:**
Each page specifies effective herbs which you can use to build a medicinal formula for your condition. **Herbs listed in the top category section address the areas most relevant to improving or correcting the particular problem.** You can blend a compound for your needs by choosing from the desired properties and attributes of the herbs within these categories. **Bold print entries** indicate the most effective or most often used herbs.
Note: All of the herbs in each category are effective, but every person is an individual with a different body and different needs. Healing and response seem to accelerate when a person chooses for himself.

3️⃣ **Next, rank your chosen herbs in order of importance using the middle section.**
• Herbs in the primary category generally comprise about 50 to 60% of a complex formula, and about 75 to 80% of a simple formula. Choose two to four primary herbs.
• Herbs in the assisting/secondary category normally comprise about 30 to 35% of a complex formula, and about 15 to 20% of a simple formula. Choose two to four assisting herbs.
• Herbs in the transporter category act as carriers to put the herbal benefits into the body quickly and optimally. They comprise about 5 to 10% of a formula. Choose one to two transporter herbs.
• Other complementary herbs may be chosen to support your own individual desires and needs.
Note: If you have a complicated or long term problem, with many facets and needs, consider developing several compounds for the different requirements. More concentration and better focus on each area can be attained in this way.

4️⃣ **Decide on the herbal medium you want.**
Do you want a tea, an extract, a capsule formula or a topical preparation? You may have to adjust some of your chosen herbs so they will work with your chosen preparation medium. For example, use powdered herbs in a capsule or to make an extract. Seeds and highly fibrous herbs like horsetail work better in an extract. Use unpleasant tasting herbs in capsules instead of in a tea. Medicinal teas often have bitter tasting properties. You can add mint, lemon peel, spices, or sweet herb (stevia) to improve taste without harm to therapeutic activity.

5️⃣ **The last section on each page provides sample formulas to illustrate how an effective formula might look.** Two different medium choices are offered.

6️⃣ **Now blend your chosen herbs. "Parts" are a good common denominator for building a formula.**
For individual use, use one tablespoon as one part for powdered herbs for filling capsules. Use one handful as one part for cut herbs in a tea or bath blend. (See How To Make An Herbal Extract for quantity information for an extract). To make an herbal broth or drink, first combine the dry ingredients in a blender until ground. Then mix about 2 TBS. of the dry mix in 2 cups hot water. Let flavors bloom for 5 minutes before drinking. Herbal broths are rich in minerals, plant enzymes and amino acids. Add 1 teaspoon Bragg's Liquid Aminos to each drink for a flavor/nutrient boost if desired. Sip over a half hour period for best assimilation.

About the Author....

Linda Rector-Page has been working in the fields of nutrition and herbal medicine both professionally and as a personal lifestyle choice, since the early seventies. She is a certified Doctor of Naturopathy and Ph.D., with extensive experience in formulating herbal combinations. She received a Doctorate of Naturopathy from the Clayton College of Natural Health in 1988, and a Ph.D. in Nutritional Therapy from the American Holistic College of Nutrition in 1989. She is a member of both the American and California Naturopathic Medical Associations.

Linda opened and operated the "Rainbow Kitchen," a natural foods restaurant, then became a working partner in The Country Store Natural Foods store. She is also the founder and formulator of Crystal Star Herbal Nutrition, a manufacturer of over 250 premier herbal compounds. A major, cutting edge influence in the herbal medicine field, Crystal Star Herbal Nutrition products are carried by over twenty-five hundred natural food stores in the U.S. and around the world.

Linda has written four major, internationally distributed books about natural healing. and a Library Series of specialty books in the field. Today, she is the editor-in-chief of a national monthly, natural health newsletter, *The Natural Healing Report*. She has a weekly CBS News TV segment where she discusses a wide range of natural healing topics, and she hosts her own weekly, one-hour radio talk show program called "*The World of Healthy Healing.*" Linda also lectures around the country, contributes articles to national publications, is regularly featured on radio and television, and is an adjunct professor at Clayton College of Natural Health.

Continuous research in all aspects of the alternative healing world has been the cornerstone of success for her reference work *Healthy Healing* now in its tenth edition, with sales of almost a million books.

Cooking For Healthy Healing, now in its second revised edition, is a companion to Healthy Healing. It draws on both the recipes from the Rainbow Kitchen and the more defined, lifestyle approach that she has developed from her healing experience with diet and herbal remedies. This book contains thirty-three diet programs, and over 900 healthy recipes.

In *How To be Your Own Herbal Pharmacist*, Linda addresses the rising appeal of herbs and herbal healing in America. This book is designed for those wishing to take more definitive responsibility for their health through individually developed herbal combinations.

Another popular work is Linda's party reference book, *Party Lights*, written with restaurateur and chef Doug Vanderberg. *Party Lights* takes healthy cooking one step further by adding fun to a good diet.

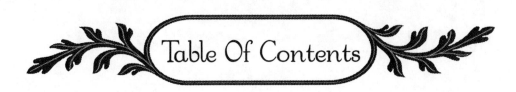

Table Of Contents

Section One

Herbal Healing Today — Pg. 3

  •Herbal remedies vs. drugs. Using herbs as part of today's health care.

  •How to use herbs correctly for disease treatment and nutrition improvement
  •Herbal Medicine Choices...Whole Herb Healing or Standardized Plant Extracts

  •Growing pesticide-free herbs   •Companion planting herbs   •A family medicine chest

Section Two

Formulating Herbal Remedies For Specific Body Areas & Needs — Pg. 30

Easy to follow, step-by-step charts for making your own individual herbal remedies.

  •Blood Purification   •Mucous Cleansing   •Colon Cleansing
  •Rebuilding System Health   •Maintaining a Clean Healthy System

  •Improving Body Chemistry   •Detoxifying the Liver & Organs
  •Rebuilding Immunity After Illness or Surgery   •Maintaining Strong Immunity with Enzymes

  •Accelerate Toxin Release   •Enzyme Therapy to Strengthen Cells, Organs & Deep Body Tissue
  •Rebuild Healthy New Blood & Immune Defenses

  •Accelerate Toxin Release   •Normalize Blood Composition & Deter Cancer Cell Proliferation
  •Rebuilding Clean Blood After Chemotherapy & Radiation

  •Bacterial, Staph & Strep Infections   •Fighting Viral Infections   •Beating Fungal Infections
  •Cold & Flu Infections   •Shortening or Preventing Colds   •Overcoming Flu
  •Overcoming Pneumonias, Bronchitis and Severe Respiratory Conditions

Section Three

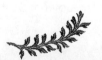

About This Book & Herbal Healing

How To Be Your Own Herbal Pharmacist is an herbal formulating reference for people at the beginning of a new concept in health and healing. It is a short, easy-to-use book for those wishing to take more responsibility for their own health with herbs.

Medical science is changing fast. Can the tradition of Herbal Healing fit in? In America, and indeed around the world, we are in a time of paradigm shift in the global approach to healing. As our world grows smaller, people are interacting more, and changing long-held beliefs. Herbal medicines are part of this larger picture, because they are worldwide, alive, big enough and intelligent enough to grow along with us.

Herbal medicines have been meeting people's health needs for thousands of years as a safe, effective, readily available means of healing. In fact, herbs have been used from the time of recorded history for every facet of life - disease prevention, healing, energy, creativity, work, love, birth, death, regeneration, meditation, survival, and more. We are just beginning to scratch the surface of their forgotten truth.

Today, Americans are rediscovering herbal healing with enthusiasm. Studies show that more than 75 per cent of American health care consumers use some form of alternative healing for their well-being. Herbal remedies have become enormously popular as natural complements to drugs and drugstore medicines.

Using herbs for healing brings us back to one of the basics of life. Herbs give you respect for the wonders of our planet. They are highly complex, intelligent plants.... living medicines.... one of the powers of the universe.

Many thinking people are coming to see the Earth as an intelligent being, evolving and growing. Mankind is also evolving and growing. Unfortunately pathogenic organisms that cause disease, are changing, too - often replicating at an enormous rate. Both organisms and diseases are becoming more virulent, and our immune defenses are becoming weaker.

The latest scientific drugs aren't the answer. All the advances made by modern medicine are hardly effective at all against chronic diseases or in disease prevention. In fact, many new drugs are becoming *less* effective against pathogens like powerful viruses, instead of more effective. Recent research shows that new antibiotics scarcely survive a year before the microbe they were designed to arrest, develops, mutates and grows stronger against them. **It's a good example of a non-living agent like a drug trying to control a living thing.**

I call today's allopathic medicine "heroic medicine" because it was developed largely in wartime for wartime emergencies. But this type of medicine often hits the body with a heavy hammer, preventing it from being able to rebuild against slow-growing, degenerative diseases. Nor can drugs help the body by stimulating its immune response. In fact, most drugs, and all surgeries, create body trauma along with their corrective benefits.

While we must be respectful of all ways of healing, until recently most of us didn't realize we have a choice. **Herbal medicines are products for problems.** They can be used in the first line of defense against disease. I find that except for emergency or life-threatening situations, herbs deserve a place in your primary care healing program.

Herbal knowledge is not difficult or esoteric, but it is extensive. Even though herbal remedies are still the primary means of health care in 80% of the world, much herbal knowledge in the general population has dropped away in 20th century America as medical advances and "letting the doctor do it" have become a way of life.

Yet, many people realize today that traditional medical methods can only go so far before major expense outweighs the value of the treatment or the insurance costs, and also that "the doctor can't always do it". The last decade of this century is becoming a turning point in traditional health treatment, as medical costs, and even reasonable medical insurance payments, go beyond the reach of most families. In addition, as orthodox medical treatment becomes more invasive, and less in touch with the patient, Americans are becoming more knowledgeable about, and more willing to take, a measure of responsibility for their own health. They are seeing that natural remedies work, often far better than drugs or surgery, with a minimum of side effects; consequently use of alternative therapies, vitamins, herbal and homeopathic remedies is increasing dramatically.

Immune strength is where natural complementary medicines, like herbs and homeopathic compounds are important. Each of us is so individual; our healing supports need to be able to work with us in our own way for permanent health. Herbal remedies work integrally with each person's body, involving the body's cooperation in its own healing. Each of us can draw from an herb's wonderful complexity the properties we need in order to heal.

Although herbs respond to scientific methods, they are much more than a scientific, or even a natural healing system. God seems to show us his face through herbs, allowing us to see them as a healing art, tools of metaphysical Nature as well as of Science. Herbs may be our only hope to bring the balance back between the healing forces and diseases. Their healing work goes on automatically, whether it is analyzed or not. Our bodies know how to use the body-balancing nutrients of herbs without our brains having to know why.

I have long believed that herbs are a path to the universe - an eye of the needle through which we can glimpse the wonders of creation and what it's really all about. Herbs can perhaps point out a path for us on how we might grow and change in a big world that is becoming a global village.

Herbs are without a doubt... UNIVERSAL. They do not discriminate, but embrace humans of all sorts and animals of all kinds, with their benefits. While it seems, on a day-to-day basis that we are hopelessly divided - in the end we are all one. Our hopes and dreams are the same. Herbs help us care for each other. Perhaps they are moving along the universal continuum with us.... always available for us, with a highly complex structure able to match our own increasing complexity of need.

We can count on the safety and efficacy of herbs in ways that the latest drug can never achieve. Therapeutic herbs have a unique spirit, with wide ranging properties, and far reaching possibilities for medicinal activity. Herbs are intricate, sophisticated plants, filled with long memory. They have intelligently adapted to the Earth's changes as we have, and over the millennia, they have always interacted with mankind. The tradition of herbal healing is so rich that it can adapt to today's requirements with the same strength and reliability that it addressed ancient ones.

Hundreds of herbs are regularly available today in many forms and at all quality levels. Worldwide communications and improved storage allow us to work with herbs from different countries and different harvests simultaneously, an advantage ages past did not enjoy. Medicinal properties and benefits can be dramatically different when herbs are used in combination. This book shows you how to work with the herbs available today and some of the applications they can address in combinations.

Herbs are all-encompassing and timeless, as nature itself is infinite and eternal. Like all great realities of nature, there is so much more than we shall ever know.

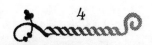

A Practical Guide For Using Herbs Safely

Herbal medicines have been meeting people's medical needs for thousands of years. Although today we think of herbs as natural drugs, they are really foods with medicinal qualities. Because they combine with our bodies as foods do, herbs are able to address both the symptoms and causes of a problem. As nourishment, herbs can offer the body nutrients it does not always receive, either because of poor diet, or environmental deficiencies in the soil and air. As medicine, herbs are system balancers that normalize the body so it can heal and regulate itself.

Herbs work like precision instruments in the body, not like sledge hammers.
Herbal medicines can be broad based for over all support, or specific to a particular problem.

Herbs provide a rich variety of healing agents, and most herbs, as edible plants, are as safe to take as foods. They have almost no side effects. Occasionally a mild allergy-type reaction may occur as it might occur to a food. This could happen because an herb has been adulterated with chemicals in the growing or storing process, or in rare cases, because incompatible herbs were used together. Or it may be just an individual adverse response to a certain plant. The key to avoiding an adverse reaction is moderation, both in formulation and in dosage. Anything taken to excess can cause negative side effects. Common sense, care, and intelligence are needed when using herbs for either food or medicine.

Two-thirds of the drugs on the American market today are based on medicinal plants.

But modern drugs are not herbs; they are chemicals. Even when a drug is derived from an herb, it is so refined, isolated and purified that only a chemical formula remains. Chemicals work on the body much differently than herbs do. As drugs, they cause many effects - only some of which are positive. Eli Lilly, a pharmaceutical manufacturer, once said "a drug isn't a drug unless it has side effects."

Herbs in their whole form are not drugs. Do not expect the activity or response of a drug, which normally treats only the symptoms of a problem. In general, you have to take more and more of a drug to continue therapeutic effects.

Herbal medicines work differently. Herbs are foundation nutrients, working through the glands, nourishing the body's most basic elements, such as the brain, glands and hormones. Results will seem to take much longer. But this fact only shows how herbs actually work, acting as support to control and reverse the cause of a problem, with more permanent effect. Even so, some improvement from herbal treatment can usually be felt in three to six days. Chronic or long standing problems take longer, but herbal remedies tend to work more quickly with each new infection, and cases of infections grow fewer and further between. A traditional rule of thumb is one month of healing for every year of the problem.

Balance is the key to using herbs for healing. Herbal combinations are not addictive, but they are powerful nutritional agents that should be used with care. Every person is different with different needs. It takes a little more attention and personal responsibility than mindlessly taking a prescription drug, but the extra care is worth far more in the results you can achieve for your well-being.

As with other natural therapies, there is sometimes a "healing crisis" in an herbal healing program. This is known as the "Law of Cure," and simply means that you seem to get worse before you get better. The body may eliminate toxic wastes heavily during the first stages of a cleansing therapy. This is particularly true in the traditional three to four day cleansing fast that many people use to begin a serious healing program. Temporary exacerbation of symptoms can range from mild to fairly severe, but usually precedes good results. Herbal therapy without a fast works more slowly and gently. Still, there is usually some weakness as disease poisons are released into the bloodstream to be flushed away. Strength shortly returns when this process is over. Watching this phenomenon allows you to observe your body at work healing itself..... an interesting experience indeed.

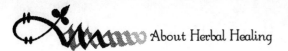

Herbs work better in combination than they do singly.
Like the notes of a symphony, herbs work better in harmony than standing alone.

There are several reasons why herbs work better in combination:

• Each formula contains two to five primary herbs for specific healing purposes. Since all body parts, and most disease symptoms, are interrelated, it is wise to have herbs which can affect each part of the problem. For example, in a prostate healing formula, there would be herbs to dissolve sediment, anti-inflammatory herbs, tissue-toning and strengthening herbs, and herbs with antibiotic properties.

• A combination of herbal nutrients encourages body balance rather than a large supply of one or two focused properties. A combination works to gently stimulate the body as a whole.

• A combination allows inclusion of herbs that can work at different stages of need. A good example of this is an athlete's formula, where there are herbs for short term energy, long range endurance, muscle tone, glycogen and glucose use, and reduction of lactic acid build-up.

• A combination of several herbs with similar properties increases the latitude of effectiveness, not only through a wider range of activity, but also reinforcing herbs that were picked too late or too early, or grew in adverse weather conditions.

• No two people, or their bodies, are alike. Good response is augmented by a combination of herbs.

• Certain herbs, such as capsicum, lobelia, sassafras, mandrake, tansy, Canada snake root, wormwood, woodruff, poke root, and rue are beneficial in small amounts and as catalysts, but should not be used alone.

Herbs work better when combined with a natural foods diet.

Everyone can benefit from an herbal formula, but results increase dramatically when fresh foods and whole grains form the basis of your diet. Subtle healing activity is more effective when it doesn't have to labor through excess waste material, mucous, or junk food accumulation. (Many congested people carry around 10 to 15 pounds of excess density.)

Interestingly enough, herbs themselves can help counter the problems of "civilization foods." They are rich in minerals and trace minerals, the basic elements missing or diminished in today's "quick-grow," over-sprayed, over-fertilized farming. Minerals and trace minerals are a basic element in food assimilation. Mineral-rich herbs provide not only the healing essences to support the body in overcoming disease, but also the foundation minerals that allow it to take them in!

Each person has its own&ìnique, wonderful body mechanism able to bring itself to its own balanced and healthy state. Herbs simply pave the way for the body to do its own work, by breaking up toxins, cleansing, lubricating, toning and nourishing. They work through the glands at the deepest levels of the body processes - at the cause, rather than the effect.

Herbs promote the elimination of waste matter and toxins from the system by simple
natural means. They support nature in its fight against disease.

Here's how to take herbs correctly for the most benefit:
Herbs are not like vitamins.

• Herbs are not isolated substances. Their value is in their wholeness and complexity, not their concentration.

Herbs should not be taken like vitamins.

• Vitamins are usually taken on a maintenance basis to shore up nutrient deficiencies. Except for some food-grown vitamins, vitamins are partitioned substances. They do not combine with the body in the same way as foods.

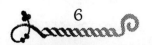

or herbs do, and excesses are normally flushed from the system. Herbs combine and work with the body's enzyme activity; they also contain food enzymes, and/or proteolytic enzymes themselves. They accumulate in and combine with the body.

- Taking herbs all the time for maintenance and nutrient replacement would be like eating large quantities of a certain food all the time. The body would tend to have imbalanced nourishment from nutrients that were not in that food. This is also true of multiple vitamins. They work best when strengthening a deficient or weak system, not as a continuing substitute for a good diet.

- However, certain very broad-spectrum "superfood" herbs like the green grasses, sea plants, algae and bee products, and adaptogen tonics like ginsengs can be taken for longer periods of body balancing.

- Vitamins work best when taken with food; it is not necessary to take herbal formulas with food.

- Unlike vitamins, herbs provide their own digestive enzymes for the body to take them in. In some cases, as in a formula for mental acuity, the herbs are more effective if taken when body pathways are clear, instead of concerned with food digestion.

Therapeutic herbs work best when used as needed.
Dosage should be reduced and discontinued as the problem improves.

Herbal effects can be quite specific; take the best formula for your particular goal at the right time - rather than all the time - for optimum results. In addition, rotating and alternating herbal combinations according to your changing health needs allows the body to remain most responsive to their effects. Reduce dosage as the problem improves. Allow the body to pick up its own work and bring its own vital forces into action. If you are taking an herbal remedy for more than a month, discontinue for one or two weeks between months to let your body adjust and maintain your personal balance.

Best results may be achieved by taking herbal capsule combinations in descending strength: 6 the first day, 5 the second day, 4 the third, 3 the fourth, 2 the fifth, and 2 the sixth for the first week. Rest on the 7th day. When a healing base is built in the body, decrease to the maintenance dose recommended for the formula. Most combinations should be taken no more than 6 days in a row.

Take only one or two herbal combinations at the same time. When working with herbs and natural healing methods, address your worst problem first. Take the herbal remedy for that problem - reducing dosage and alternating on and off weeks as necessary to allow the body to thoroughly use the herbal properties. One of the bonuses of a natural healing program is the frequent discovery that other conditions were really complications of the first problem, and often take care of themselves as the body comes into balance.

☙

Herb effectiveness usually goes by body weight, especially for children. Child dosage is as follows:

$1/2$ dose for children 10-14 years $1/4$ dose for children 2-6 years
$1/3$ dose for children 6-10 years $1/8$ dose for infants and babies

☙

Herbs are amazingly effective in strengthening the body's immune response. But the immune system is a fragile entity, and can be overwhelmed instead of stimulated. Even when a good healing program is working, and obvious improvement is being made, adding more of the medicinal agents in an effort to speed healing can aggravate symptoms. Even for serious health conditions, moderate amounts are the way to go, mega-doses are not. Much better results can be obtained by giving yourself more time and gentler treatment. It takes time to rebuild health.

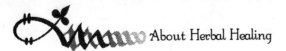

Your Herbal Medicine Choices

Whole-Herb Healing or Standardized Plant Constituents?

Clearly, American health care consumers are increasing their use of herbs as natural alternatives to drugs. Standardizing separate herbal constituents for potency is becoming popular today as herbal manufacturers enter drug-oriented health care markets.

But what is sacrificed when herbal constituents are "standardized."

It's a case of government regulations and orthodox medicine trying make herbal healing fit into a laboratory drug mold. Without question, Americans need safe, effective, alternative medicines. But this time the demand includes incredibly intricate, living medicines...medicines whose value lies in their complexity, and their ability to combine easily with the human body, not in their concentration or the potency of any one constituent. Standardization uses synthetic chemicals to peel away one or two so-called "active ingredients" out of dozens of constituents that make up a single herb. The result is an overly refined product that misses the full range of benefits offered by the natural herb.

As a naturopath and traditional herbalist, I believe that standardization short-changes the full spectrum of whole-herb healing. Throughout the ages, from all cultures and traditions, herbalists have effectively used whole herbs for whole bodies with immense success that rivals modern day allopathic medicine. **There is tremendous value in the knowledge gained through empirical observation and interpretive understanding of real people with real problems and natural solutions.** Yet, in the modern health care world, laboratory yardsticks are the only measurements science understands or governments approve. Herbal healing fell out of favor not because it was ineffective, or even because something better was discovered, but because scientific technology had little understanding of nature, and medical market economics had no incentive to investigate it, because no one can "patent a plant."

Standardizing a so-called "active ingredient" in a drug-like approach neglects one of the main benefits of whole herbs. As naturally concentrated foods, herbs have the unique ability to address a multiplicity of problems simultaneously. In most cases, the full medicinal value of herbs is in their internal complexity. Single herbs contain dozens of natural chemical constituents working synergistically. It's why an herb is rarely ever known for just a single function. The evolutionary development of each herb has created a whole essence: the natural herb in correct and balanced ratios with all its constituents. Many of the constituents within a whole herb are unknown - even to modern science - and internal chemical reactions within and among herbs are even less understood.

How can we integrate herbal healing into scientific methodology to make it available to everybody?

It's a question that's splitting herbal product providers apart. Standardization is seen by some companies, especially those whose main focus has been vitamins or other partitioned supplements, as a way for herb products to challenge the mainstream drug company monopoly, by measuring and assuring an "active constituent" of a plant for medicinal use. Standardization is also considered a way to deal with FDA regulations that require drug measureability, and FDA guidelines that require so-called "active" ingredients to be stated on product labels. As herb companies begin to educate the public about the health benefits of herbs, a way must be found to work with regulations that were never intended to deal with the complexities or broad-based effects of herbal healing.

Standardizing potency for only one or two extracted "active ingredients" for certain vested interests, attempts to use limited laboratory procedures to convince the AMA, the FDA and medical scientists of the value of herbal therapy. **We must not fall into the same wrong-headed, self-defeating pit that occurred forty years ago, when the regulations for standardization of drugs nearly killed all herbal medicine.**

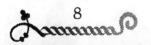

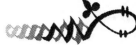

We can't let ourselves forget that the activity of herbs is due not only to their bio-chemical properties, but also to their unique, wholistic effects, and most importantly, to their interaction with the human body.

Herbs have rejuvenative qualities entirely missed by standardization. Yet, quality and consistency are a major concern in ascertaining herbal effectiveness. Somehow, herbalists and herbal product suppliers must integrate herbal traditions, ethical commitment, FDA regulations and consumer concerns.

Here's what we lose when we try to standardize a complex medicinal plant.

- **Standardization attempts to isolate "active constituents" for a very limited function.** For example, ginseng has become a popular ingredient in many herbal products. One laboratory test identified two of its 22 known constituents (called Rb1, and Rb2), in an attempt to isolate ginseng's functions as an anti-oxidant and for lowering cholesterol. Yet thousands of years of world-wide, well-documented experience show that ginseng has dozens of other actions that control disease and promote wellness, functions entirely missed by this test. Should we deny people the ultimate value and effectiveness of ginseng's activity simply because a laboratory hasn't tested for every one of its functions yet?

- **Standardization fails to take advantage of the synergistic power of herbs in combination.** Standardizing one constituent never works within an herbal combination because the whole balance of the compound is lost or changed. As a professional herbalist since 1978, I use combinations because, in most instances, they work more efficiently with multiple body functions. To make use of the full spectrum of healing possibilities, we combine ginseng, for example, with licorice. The resulting extract has synergistic benefits - exceptional body cleansing and nutrient assimilation support, and a significant role in balancing of body sugar levels - **significantly more than either of these herbs used alone.**

- **Only a combination of herbal nutrients encourages overall body balance.** Since all body parts, and most disease symptoms, are interrelated, it is wise to use a compound of herbs which can affect each part of the problem. For example, a prostate healing formula contains herbs that help dissolve sediment, herbs with anti-inflammatory and antibiotic properties, and herbs to tone and strengthen tissue. A "standardized" supply of one or two constituents in a drug-like dose is not intended for this wholistic purpose.

Indeed, a good herbal combination will contain much more than even the **primary** whole herbs. It will include **secondary herbs** to soothe and help the body repair itself; **catalysts and transporter herbs** to carry active constituents into the body for optimal absorption and utilization, and **complementary herbs** to address side effects related to the main problem and balance acid/alkaline levels.

The interaction of constituents within a single whole, non-standardized herb is much like the supportive roles that secondary herbs, or catalysts and transporters perform in effective herbal combinations.

How do we assure ourselves that the herbs we buy have the medicinal qualities we want? How can we know that the herbs in the products we buy will work? Are the herbs on the label in there? I believe the answer is two-fold. It is the method used by Crystal Star Herbal Nutrition for two decades to assure that their products will do the job.

The first part of the answer calls for the evidence of your senses and for common sense. Here are some checkpoints to use when buying medicinal herbs:

✓ Buy organically grown or wildcrafted (grown in their natural state) herbs whenever available. Buy fresh-dried, locally grown herbs whenever possible, to assure the shortest transportation time and freshest quality.

✓ When choosing unpackaged, loose herbs, rub a sample between your fingers, smell it and look at its color. Even in a dried state, the life and potency of an herb are easily evident.

✓ Buy the best herbs available. The experience and quality control methods at the growing/gathering/storage end of the herbal medicine chain are more costly, but they increase its healing abilities.

✓ When buying packaged herbs choose a product from a company that specializes in herbs. Herb companies live and breath herbs and generally are regarded as having the highest level of integrity. Be sure the product is tightly sealed and away from light and heat. Also, check the expiration date.

✓ Ask the supplement buyer at your local natural food store for the names of reputable herbal product manufacturers who have earned the trust of consumers for products that work.

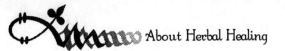

The second part of the answer involves what I have come to trust.

A wise man once said that trust could settle every problem in the world right now. But, we're not talking about blind trust, or pie-in-the-sky trust. We're talking about common sense trust. All of us have to trust experts every day, to advise and inform us about things we don't know. We don't have to become physicists to use products that come from physics research, or mechanics in order to drive a car. Nor do we have to become herbal experts to avail ourselves of herbal medicines.

In my experience that there are three things you can trust when you buy an herbal product in America today.

✓ You can trust the herb or herbal combination to do what its centuries old tradition says it will do.

✓ You can trust the vast majority of herbal product suppliers, most of whom are dedicated people, pledged to herbal excellence. In my opinion, their herbal knowledge and standards are worth more than chemical lab assays, many of which are incomplete, poorly done and expensive. A testimonial to this comes from a third party, non-profit lab that buys and tests health products for efficacy and quality. They have informed me that almost 100% of the traditional herbal products they review from open market samples contain what they say they contain.

✓ Finally, you can trust your natural food store. The typical herbal expert in a natural food store is in the job largely because of a commitment to the wonders of natural medicines, and a desire to share that commitment.

Just like you can't cheat an honest man, you can't cheat the honesty of herbs either. They will put out their truth no matter what. And to get the whole truth, I believe you have to use the whole herb. Here's why:

• The so-called "active constituent" of a plant is only a part of the whole. Herbs, as whole foods have complex properties that combine with the body's enzyme activity. When an isolated constituent is used, a powerful but imbalanced reaction takes place, similar to eating refined sugar or taking a drug.

• Standardizing one constituent for one plant denies the far greater benefits to be had from herbal combinations. Using a standardized herb is like using a "natural drug," with one property for one problem. Potentizing a single property only gives you part of the picture. And it does a disservice to the balance within the plant, and its ability to work with other herbs. The whole herb offers wide latitude to work with several aspects and stages of a problem, and also allows each person to draw what he or she needs from the complexity of the whole combination. Herbs are living medicines. Just like our own bodies, they work best in their natural balance.

• No lab test can even begin to quantify all that whole natural plants have to offer us. They can make tomatoes in a lab today. But are they a food or a fabrication? Most of us have tasted these tomatoes. Even judging by taste alone, the resemblance to an earth and sun grown tomato is pale. We need to keep reminding ourselves that herbs are so much more than a laboratory creation.

• Standardization procedures allow the use of sub-standard materials. Since only one "active constituent" is measured, that constituent may be boosted with a concentration or isolated element to reach the required standard, regardless of the quality of the herb itself. No one constituent, no matter how worthwhile, can do its healing job without the right stuff from the rest of the herb.

• Used in their whole form, herbs, like foods, nourish the body with little danger of toxicity. Potentizing herbal formulas to reach certain standardized constituents makes them more drug-like, without the protection of their natural gentleness and balance. This safety factor means that herbs can be used by everybody, not just herbal experts, without having to worry about harmful interactions. This is a consideration in today's lawsuit-oriented marketplace, where powerful substances carry more risk of abuse and consumer misuse. The slower, long term action of whole herbs is preferable for individual self-treatment.

• Finally, standardization leaves no room for excellence, either in source of supply or in skillful preparation.

Herbs give the body a wealth of subtle healing essences from which to choose. Science can only quantify, isolate and assay to understand. When we say that the standardized constituents are all there is to herbal healing, we lose. An herbal compound is much more than the sum of its parts. Herbs are a natural healing art that can teach your body what to do for its own wellness.

❖

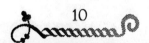

Herbal Preparation & Delivery Methods

Today, hundreds of herbs are available at all quality levels. Worldwide communications and improved storage allow us to simultaneously obtain and use herbs from different countries and different harvests, an advantage ages past did not enjoy. However, because of the natural variety of soils, seeds, and weather, every crop of botanicals is unique. Every batch of a truly natural herbal formula will be slightly different, and offer its own unique benefits and experience.

There must be a firm commitment to excellence from growers and suppliers, because herbal combinations are products for problems. For therapeutic success, herbs must be BIO-ACTIVE and BIO-AVAILABLE.

If you decide to make your own herbal preparations, buy the finest quality you can find. There is a world of disparity between fairly good herbs and the best. Superior stock must go into a medicinal formula so that the herbal product can do its job correctly. Superior plants cost far more than standard stock, but their worth in healing activity is a true value for the health care customer.

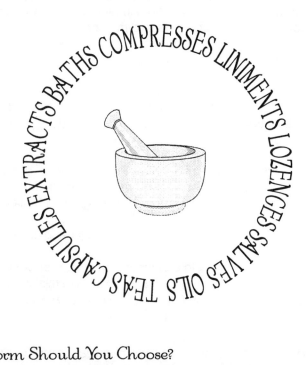

Which Preparation Form Should You Choose?

Whichever herbal preparation form you choose, it is generally more beneficial to take greater amounts at the beginning of your program, in order to build a good internal healing base, and to stimulate the body's vital balancing forces more quickly. As the therapeutic agents establish and build in the body, and you begin to notice good response and balance returning, less and less of the large initial doses should be taken, finally reducing the dosage to long range maintenance or preventive amounts.

"Parts" are a good way to set a common denominator for building an herbal compound. For individual use, one tablespoon is usually adequate as one "part" when using powdered herbs for filling capsules; one handful is common as one part for cut herbs in a tea or bath blend. (See HOW TO MAKE AN HERBAL EXTRACT for quantity information for an extract or tincture).

Herbs can be applied to almost any necessity of life. It is simply a matter of knowing their properties, how they work together and how to use them correctly. But herbs are foods, so your body knows how to use them. Give the herbs time. Give yourself a good diet, some rest and a little less stress for the best results.

Herbal teas are the most basic of all natural healing mediums; they are easily absorbed by the body as hot liquid. They are the least concentrated of all herbal forms, but many herbs are optimally effective when steeped in boiling water. The hot brewing water releases herbal potency and provides a flushing action that is ideal for removing toxic wastes that have been loosened and dissolved by the herbs. Although teas have milder and more subtle effects than capsules or extracts, they are sometimes the only way for a weakened system to accept therapeutic support, and often work synergistically with stronger medicinal forms to boost their value.

NOTE 1: The cutting of herbs for tea bags creates facets on the herb structure causing loss of essential volatile oils. Gently crumble leaves and flowers, and break roots and barks into pieces before steeping.

NOTE 2: Medicinal teas may have bitter tasting properties. Where taste is unpleasant, mint, lemon peel, spices, or stevia (sweet herb), may be added to improve taste without harming therapeutic qualities.

Tips on taking herbal teas:

1. Use 1 packed small teaball to 3 cups of water for medicinal-strength tea. Use distilled water or pure spring water for increased herbal strength and effectiveness.

2. Bring water to a boil, remove from heat, add herbs and steep, covered, off heat; 10 to 15 minutes for a leaf/flower tea; 25 minutes for a root/bark tea. Keep lid closed during steeping so volatile oils won't escape.

3. Use a teapot of glass, ceramic or earthenware, not aluminum. Aluminum can negate the effect of the herbs as the metal dissolves into the hot liquid and gets into the body.

4. Drink medicinal teas in small sips throughout the day rather than all at once. One-half to 1 cup, taken 3 or 4 times over a day allows absorption of the tea, without passing before it has a chance to work.

⚬ **An infusion** is a tea made from dried or powdered herb. Use directions above, or pour 1 cup of boiling water over 1 tablespoon of fresh herb, 1 teaspoon of dried herb, or 4 opened capsules of powdered herb.. Cover and let steep 10 to 15 minutes. Never boil. A cold infusion can be made by simply allowing the herbs, especially powders, to stand in cool water for an hour or more.

⚬ **A decoction** is a tea made from roots and barks. Use directions above, or put 2 tablespoons of cut herb pieces into 1 cup cold water. Bring to a light boil, cover, and simmer gently for 20 to 30 minutes. Strain. For best results, repeat the same process with the same herbs. Strain again and mix both batches.

⚬ **"Sun tea"** is a cold infusion where herbs are put in a covered jar and allowed to stand in the sun.

⚬ For an **herbal broth**, grind dry ingredients in a blender. Mix 2 TBS. of dry mix to 2 cups hot water. Let flavors bloom for 5 minutes before drinking. Herbal broths are rich in minerals and enzymes. Add 1 tsp. BRAGG'S LIQUID AMINOS to each drink for a flavor/nutrient boost if desired. Sip over a $1/_2$ hour period for best assimilation.

❦

Herbal capsules are generally four times stronger than teas, more concentrated in form, convenient to take, and bypass any herbal bitterness. Capsules can make both oil and water soluble herbs available through stomach acid and enzyme alteration. Freeze-dried powdered herbs, with all the moisture removed, are also available in capsules, and are four times more concentrated than regular ground herbs. As noted with herbal teas above, grinding herbs into powders creates facets on the whole herb structure causing potential loss of volatile oils. Effective potency for powdered herbs is six months to a year. (See page 7 for more information on how to take herbal capsules.)

❦

Herbal extracts are 4 to 8 times stronger than capsules. They are effective used as a spray where all the mouth receptors can be brought into play, or as drops held under the tongue, that bypass the digestive system's acid/alkaline breakdown. Their strength and ready availability make extracts reliable emergency measures. Small doses can be used repeatedly over a period of time to help build a strong base for restoring body balance. Holding an extract dose in the mouth as long as possible, 3 or 4 times daily, is effective for the first week of an acute condition.

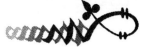

After this first week, the vital force of the body will often have been sufficiently stimulated in its own healing ability, and the dose may be reduced to allow the system to take its own route to balance. As with other forms of herbal mixtures, most extracts should be taken no more than 6 days in a row with a rest on the seventh day, before resuming, to allow the body to do its own work. As the body increases its ability to right itself, the amount, frequency and strength of the dosage should be decreased.

�

Herbal tinctures are also extractions, made using a 25% alcohol and water mixture as the solvent. Tinctures are generally extracted from individual herbs rather than compounds. When they *are* blended into a compound, each separately prepared tincture is added rather than made from the beginning as a compound. Commercial tinctures use ethyl alcohol, and may even be formed from fluid extracts, but diluted alcohol spirits are suitable for home use; vodka is ideal.

Extracts are more concentrated than tinctures, because they distill or filter off some of the alcohol. A tincture is typically a 1:10 or 1:5 concentration (10 or 5 units of extract come from 1 unit of herbs), while a fluid extract is usually 1:1.

Even stronger, *a powdered extract* has the solvent completely removed. Powdered extracts are at least 4 times as potent as an equal amount of fluid extract, and 40 times as potent as a tincture. One gram of a 4:1 powdered extract is equivalent to $\frac{1}{7}$ ounce of a fluid extract, and $1\frac{1}{2}$ oz. of a tincture.

NOTE: *Homeopathic liquid formulas are not the same as herbal tinctures or extracts, and their use is different.*

Here's how to make a simple herbal extraction:

Alcohol, wine, apple cider vinegar, and vegetable glycerine are common mediums for extracting herbal properties for therapeutic use. Alcohol releases the widest variety of essential herbal elements in unchanged form, and allows the fastest sublingual absorption. Alcohol and water mixtures can resolve almost every relevant ingredient of any herb, and also act as a natural preserver for the compound. Eighty to one hundred proof (40-50%) vodka, is an excellent solvent for most plant constituents. It has long term preservative activity and is easily obtainable for individual use. The actual amount of alcohol in a daily dose is approximately $\frac{1}{50}$ oz., but if alcohol is not desired, extract drops may be placed in a little warm water for 5 minutes to allow the alcohol to evaporate before drinking. Most extracts are formulated with 1 gram of herb for each 5ml of alcohol.

Extract directions:

1. Put about 4 ounces dried chopped or ground herb, or 8 ounces of fresh herb, into a quart canning jar.
2. Pour about one pint of 80 to 100 proof vodka over the herbs and close tightly.
3. Keep the jar in a warm place for two to three weeks, and shake well twice a day.
4. Decant the liquid into a bowl, and then pour the slurry residue through several layers of muslin or cheesecloth into the bowl. Strain all the liquid through the layers once again to insure a clearer extract.
5. Squeeze out all liquid from the cloth. (Sprinkle solid residue around your houseplants as herb food. We have done this for years, and they love it.)
6. Pour the extract into a dark glass bottle. Stopper, seal tightly, and store away from light. An extraction made in this way will keep its potency for several years.

�

Herbal wine infusions are a pleasant, effective method of taking herbs, especially as digestive aids with meals, and as warming circulatory tonics by-the-spoonful in winter. The alcohol acts as a transport medium and stimulant to the bloodstream.

Here's how to make a simple wine infusion. Either fresh or dried herbs may be used:

• **Method 1:** For a warming winter circulation and energy tonic, pour off about $\frac{1}{4}$ cup of a fortified wine, such as madeira, cognac or brandy. Place chosen herbs and spices in the wine and recork the bottle. Place in a dark cool place for a week or two. Strain off the solids, and combine the medicinal wine with a fresh bottle. Mix well, and take a small amount as needed for energy against fatigue.

• **Method 2:** For a nerve and brain tonic, steep fresh or dried herbs in a bottle of either white or red wine for about a week. Strain off herbs, and drink a small amount as needed.

🍵

Herbal syrups are well accepted by children, and can greatly improve the taste of bitter herbal compounds. They are also excellent treatment forms for throat coats and gargles, or bronchial, chest/lung infections. Syrups are simple and quick to make.

There are two simple ways to make an herbal syrup:
• **Method 1:** Boil ³/₄ lb. of raw or brown sugar in 2 cups of herb tea until it reaches syrup consistency.
• **Method 2:** Make a simple syrup with ³/₄ lb. of raw sugar in 2 cups of water, boiling until it reaches syrup consistency. Remove from heat, and while the syrup is cooling, add an herbal extract or tincture - one part extract to three parts of syrup.

🍵

Herbal pastes and electuaries are made by grinding or blending herbs in the blender with a little water into a paste. The paste may then be mixed with twice the amount of honey, syrup, butter, or cream cheese for palatability and taste. Other electuaries (mediums that mask the bitter taste of medicinal herbs) include fresh bread rolled around a little of the paste, or peanut butter.

🍵

Herbal lozenges are an ideal way to relieve mouth, throat, and upper respiratory conditions. They are made by combining powdered herbs with sugar and a mucilaginous herb, such as marshmallow or slippery elm, or a gum, such as tragacanth or acacia. Both powdered herbs and essential herbal oils may be used. Proper mucilage preparation is the key to successful lozenges.

Here's how to make an herbal lozenge:
• Soak 1-oz. powdered mucilaginous herb (listed above) in water to cover for 24 hours; stir occasionally.
• Bring 2 cups of water to a boil and add the mucilage herb.
• Beat to obtain a uniform consistency and force through cheesecloth to strain.
• Mix with enough powdered herb to form a paste, and add sugar to taste. Or, mix 12 drops of essential peppermint oil (or other essential oil) with 2-oz. of sugar, and enough mucilage to make a paste.
• Roll on a board covered with arrowroot or sugar to prevent sticking. Cut into shapes and leave exposed to air to dry. Store in an airtight container.

🍵

External Use Preparations:

The skin is the body's largest organ of ingestion. Topical herbal mediums may be used as needed for all over relief and support.

Herbal baths provide a soothing, gentle way to absorb herbal therapy through the skin. In essence, you are soaking in a diluted medicinal tea, allowing the skin to take in the healing properties instead of the mouth and digestive system. The procedure for taking an effective infusion bath is almost as important as the herbs themselves.

There are two good therapeutic bath techniques:
• **Method 1:** Draw very hot bath water. Put bath herbs in an extra large tea ball or small muslin bath bag, (sold in natural food stores). Steep in the bath until the water cools slightly and is aromatic, about 15 minutes.
• **Method 2:** Make a strong tea infusion on the stove as usual with a full pot of water. Strain and add directly to the bath. Soak for at least 30-45 minutes to give the body time to absorb the herbal properties. Rub the body with the solids in the muslin bag while soaking for best herb absorbency.

🍵

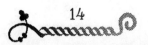

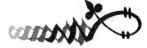

Herbal douches are an effective method of treating simple vaginal infections. The herbs are simply steeped as for a strong tea, strained off, and the liquid poured into a douche bag. Sit on the toilet, insert the applicator, and rinse the vagina with the douche. Use one full douche bag for each application. Most vaginal conditions need douching three times daily for 3 to 7 days. If the infection does not respond in this time, see a qualified health professional.

❦

Herbal suppositories and boluses are an effective way to treat rectal and vaginal problems, acting as carriers for the herbal medicine application. Herbal compounds for suppositories generally serve one of three purposes; to soothe inflamed mucous membranes and aid the healing process, to help reduce swollen membranes and overcome pus-filled discharge, and to work as a laxative, stimulating normal peristalsis to overcome chronic constipation.

For a simple suppository, mix one tablespoon finely powdered herbs with enough cocoa butter to make a firm consistency. Roll into torpedo-shaped tubes an inch long. Place on wax paper, and put in the freezer to firm. Remove one at a time for use, and allow to come to room temperature before using. Insert at night.

❦

Herbal ointments and salves are semi-solid preparations, that allow absorption of herbal benefits through the skin. They may be made with vaseline, *UN-Petroleum Jelly* or cocoa butter for a simple compound; or in a more complex technique with herbal tea, oils and hardening agents such as beeswax, lanolin or lard.

To prepare a simple ointment or salve:
- **Method 1:** Warm about 6 oz. of vaseline, *UN-Petroleum Jelly* or lanolin in a small pan with 2 TBS. of cut herbs; or stir in enough powdered herbs to bring the mixture to a dark color. Simmer gently for 10 minutes, stirring. Then filter through cheesecloth, pressing out all liquid. Pour into small wide-mouth containers when cool but still pliable.

- **Method 2:** This method is best when a carrier base is needed for volatile herbal oils, such as for chest rubs or anti-congestive balms, where the base itself is not to be absorbed by the skin. Steep herbs in water to make a strong tea. Strain off the liquid into a pan. Add your chosen oils and fats, such as almond, sesame, wheat germ, or olive, oils, and cocoa butter or lanolin fats (about 6-oz. total) to the strained tea. Simmer until water evaporates, and the herbal extract is incorporated into the oils. Add enough beeswax to bring mixture to desired consistency; use about 2 oz. beeswax to 5oz. of herbal oil. Let melt and stir until well blended. Add 1 drop of tincture of benzoin (available at most pharmacies), for each ounce of ointment to preserve the mixture against mold.

❦

Herbal compresses and fomentations draw out waste and waste residue, such as cysts or abscesses via the skin, or release them into the body's elimination channels. Compresses are made by soaking a cotton cloth in a strong herbal tea, and applying it as hot as possible to the affected area. The heat enhances the activity of the herbs, and opens the pores of the skin for fast assimilation. Use alternating hot and cold compresses to stimulate nerves and circulation. Apply the herbs to the hot compress, and leave the cold compress plain. Cayenne, ginger and lobelia are good choices for the hot compress.

Make an effective compress by adding 1 teasp. powdered herbs to a bowl of very hot water. Soak a washcloth and apply until the cloth cools. Then apply a cloth dipped in ice water until it reaches body temperature. Repeat several times daily. Green clay compresses, for growths, may be applied to gauze, placed on the area, and left for all day. Simply change as you would any dressing when you bathe.

❦

 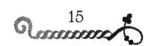

Herbal poultices and plasters are made from either fresh herbs, crushed and blended in a blender with a little olive or wheat germ oil, or dried herbs, mixed with water, cider vinegar or wheat germ oil into a paste. Either blend may be spread on a piece of clean cloth or gauze, and bound directly on the affected area. The whole application is then covered with plastic wrap to keep from soiling clothes or sheets, and left on for 24 hours. There is usually a great deal of throbbing pain while the poultice is drawing out the infection and neutralizing the toxic poisons. This stops when the harmful agents are drawn out, and signals the removal of the poultice. A fresh poultice should be applied every 24 hours.

Make a plaster by spreading a thin coat of honey on a clean cloth, and sprinkling it with an herbal mixture such as cayenne, ginger, and prickly ash, or hot mustard or horseradish. The cloth is then taped directly over the affected area, usually the chest, to relieve lung and mucous congestion.

Herbal liniments are used as warming massage mediums, to stimulate and relieve sore muscles and ligaments. They are for external use only. Choose heat-inducing herbs and spices such as cayenne, ginger, cloves and myrrh, and drops of heating oils such as eucalyptus, wintergreen and cajeput. Steep in rubbing alcohol for two to three weeks. Strain and decant into corked bottles for storage.

Herbal oils are used externally for massage, skin treatments, healing ointments, dressings for wounds and burns, and occasionally for enemas and douches. Simply infuse the herb in oil instead of water. Olive, safflower or almond oil are good bases for an herbal oil.

To make an herbal oil for home use:
- **Method 1:** Cut fresh herbs into a glass container and cover with oil. Place in the sun and leave in a warm place for three to four weeks, shaking daily to mix. Filter into a dark glass container to store.
- **Method 2:** Macerate dried, powdered herbs directly into the oil. Let stand for one or two days. Strain and bottle for use.

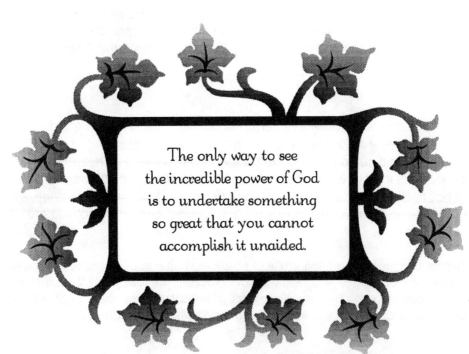

The only way to see
the incredible power of God
is to undertake something
so great that you cannot
accomplish it unaided.

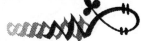

The Herbal Medicine Garden

Growing your own herbal medicines has become increasingly popular as people get "back to the roots" of healing. From our experience in growing herbs for a gourmet kitchen, we see how easy herbs are to grow. Many of our culinary favorites also have healing value. Because most herbs grow wild, an herb garden can be available to almost anyone. Herbs require minimal care, grow in tiny spaces, (virtually every herb will grow in a window box), and are so potent that a little goes a long way. Most herbs are drought resistant, and are evergreen or herbaceous perennials.

Here are a few tips on growing, harvesting and storing your own fresh medicinal herbs:

Herbs can help you get back to the basics, if you take care of their basics first. Good fertile soil structure is extremely important to the potency of herbal medicines, both for mineral and enzyme concentrations. If you don't have good soil, I strongly recommend enriching it before you plant. Add plenty of humus to either clay or sandy soil to improve soil structure and increase its fertility. Most herbs are best planted in the fall before the ground freezes, so they can establish a good root system in loose, well drained soil. If you live in extremely cold climates, where temperatures drop to and stay near zero, you can plant most herbs in early spring as soon as the ground can be worked. (I usually recommend window boxes for cold climates, and for basil anywhere, because you can extend your growing season so much longer.)

Carrot family herbs, like dill, fennel, chervil, coriander (cilantro) and parsley are easy to grow from seeds. Plant these herbs directly into the garden or pot in which they are going to grow because they don't like being transplanted. Annual herbs such as borage, and non-woody perennials like lemon balm, feverfew, chives, elecampane, pennyroyal or sweet violet usually reseed themselves. Woody perennial herbs, such as lavender, rosemary, and the thymes don't self-seed very well and produce far fewer offspring. And some plants, like mint and tarragons don't come up true from seed. They can only be propagated from cuttings or divisions. I recommend purchasing these from a good nursery.

Herbs are wonderful companion plants, not only for each other, but for other plants in your garden. They act as natural pesticides, enhance the growth and flavor of vegetables and help keep soil rich.
- Plant basil with tomatoes to improve flavor and growth, and to repel flies and mosquitoes.
  Don't plant basil near rue.
- Plant hyssop with cabbage and grapes to deter cabbage moths. Don't plant near radishes.
- Put a fresh bay leaf in storage containers of beans or grain to deter weevils and moths.
- Plant borage near tomatoes, squash and strawberries to deter tomato worms.
- Plant caraway to loosen compacted soil.
- Plant catnip to keep away flea beetles.
- Plant chamomile with cabbage and onions to improve flavor.
- Plant chervil with radishes to improve growth and flavor.
- Plant chives with carrots to improve growth and flavor.
- Plant dill with cabbage, but not near carrots.
- Plant gopher purge around your garden to deter burrowing pests.
- Plant horseradish in a potato patch to keep out potato bugs.
- Plant bee balm with tomatoes to improve growth and flavor.
- Plant lovage to improve health of most plants.
- Plant garlic near roses to repel aphids.
- Plant marjoram for more flavor of all vegetables.
- Plant mint for health of cabbage and tomatoes, and to deter white cabbage moths.
- Plant peppermint to deter moths and carrot flies.
- Plant nasturtiums to deter white flies, cabbage moth, squash bugs.

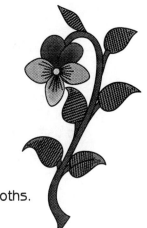

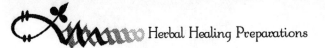

•Plant rue with roses and raspberries to deter Japanese beetles.
•Plant sage to deter cabbage moths, beetles and carrot flies. Dont plant near cucumbers.
•Plant summer savory with beans and onions to improve flavor and deter cabbage moths.
•Plant tansy to deter flying insects, Japanese beetles, cucumber beetles, squash bugs and ants.
•Plant thyme to deter cabbage worms.
•Plant wormwood as a border to keep animals out of your garden.

You can harvest the leaves of medicinal herbs any time during the growing season as long as they look, smell and taste fresh. Avoid harvesting from plants that have begun to discolor, are buggy or diseased. Herbal flowers are best harvested before they are in full bloom.

Harvest roots like burdock, dandelion and comfrey in the spring and fall, when they are full of sap. Wait for a dry spell during rainy seasons because wet roots are difficult to dry and are not as concentrated in medicinal qualities. Look for roots that are fleshy, but not old-looking, woody or fibrous. Roots have to be fully developed, though; immature roots, don't have vital nutritional properties. I don't recommend harvesting roots or corms unless you are something of an expert, because drying and storing techniques are much more difficult, and roots may be contaminated or moldy inside without your being aware of it.

Harvest barks when you harvest roots, in the spring and fall when the sap is moving up and down the plant. Sassafras, birch, willow, oak and witch hazel are common tree barks valued for medicinal qualities.

Harvest seeds late in the day after a few days of dry weather to ensure that all plant parts are dry. Most herb seeds are brown or black when they're ready to harvest. Look for flower stalks that are dry and brown, and seed pods that have turned to brown, gray, or black. Cut off the entire seed head and place it in a large paper bag, cardboard box, or wooden bowl. Place only one kind of seed in each container, and label each container. Set seeds in a dry, warm place with good air circulation. Give them a few weeks of open-air drying before removing the seeds out of the pods or heads; then store them in airtight containers. Check seeds periodically for mold.

Drying herbs is the time-honored way of preserving their medicinal qualities. Harvesting herbs in the traditional way means cutting the stems with leaf, flower and all, tying the stalks in bundles and hanging them upside down in an attic or drying shed I think a food dehydrator is by far the best way to dry herbs today. It provides you with a clean, thoroughly dried product, and it doesnt take up much space.

Once dry, put the herbs in airtight, glass containers away from light and heat. I dont recommend either metal canisters or paper bags for medicinal herbs, because the qualities are either changed or lost.

Freezing fresh dried herbs retains their medicinal qualities very well. Here's how to do it.

Rinse the herbs and let them drain until dry. I usually strip the leaves off the stems, and snip them with kitchen shears for better storage and later use in teas. Lay the herb pieces in a single layer on baking sheets and freeze until rigid, about an hour. Pour the rigid herbs into small freezer plastic bags, press out air, seal, and return to the freezer.

To use, simply take out what you need, reseal, and return the rest to the freezer. Its so easy.

An Herbal First Aid Kit For Your Medicine Chest

As we rediscover the value of herbs for healthy healing, one of the best health invest ments is a basic herbal medicine chest kit, so that useful remedies will be on hand when you need them. An herbal first aid kit is a safe way to cope with everyday healing problems, and temporary or non-serious health conditions. It can handle many problems immediately and simply, save you hundreds of dollars in doctor bills, and keep you from a traumatic, time consuming visit to a medical clinic. The choices in the following kit are easy to use, inexpensive, gentle enough for children and effective for adults.

❧ **For colds, flu and chest congestion:** elder/yarrow/peppermint tea for sniffles; mullein oil for earaches, lavender or eucalyptus steams or hot ginger compresses for chest congestion, a echinacea/golden seal/myrrh combination as a natural antibiotic.

❧ **For coughs, and sore throat:** loquat syrup or licorice/wild cherry/slippery elm tea for coughs, zinc source herbal extract for sore throat, herbal throat drops, aloe vera juice or tea tree oil gargle.

❧ **For burns:** aloe vera gel, calendula gel, pau d'arco gel, tea tree oil, comfrey root/wheat germ oil/honey compress, St. John's wort oil, dip cotton balls in strong fresh ginger juice or strong black tea and apply.

❧ **For allergies:** bee pollen granules (begin with small doses and gradually increase to about 1 teaspoon), ginkgo biloba (helps inactivate allergens). Antioxidants are a key: consider grape seed extract, quercetin with bromelain, CoQ10, Ester C powder with bioflavonoids).

❧ **For cold/canker sores:** L-lysine; *dumontiaceae*, a red marine algae, an immunomodulatory and antiviral agent works topically as well as internally in controlling and reducing *herpes simplex* virus populations; aloe vera, an antiviral soothes and dries out sores, and promotes healing; peppermint oil and lemon balm are antiviral against herpes.

❧ **For immune support and to rebuild the system from illness:** panax ginseng, echinacea, ashwagandha, siberian ginseng, licorice root, astragalus, ligustrum, goldenseal, ginger, codonopsis, suma, yellow dock, dandelion, cayenne, aloe vera, propolis and immune-enhancing mushrooms (reishi, maitake and shiitake).

❧ **For cuts, wounds, scrapes and scars:** ginseng skin repair gel, pau d' arco/calendula gel, witch hazel compresses, comfrey/aloe salve, aloe vera gel, Deva Flowers First Aid Remedy extract, tea tree oil.

❧ **For fungal infections like athlete's foot, ringworm and nail fungus:** tea tree oil, grapefruit seed extract, black walnut extract, golden seal/myrrh solution, pau d'arco/dandelion/gentian gel.

❧ **For parasite infections (intestinal worms, amoebic dysentery, giardia):** black walnut hulls or pau d'arco/echinacea extract, and cayenne/garlic caps after every meal for 2 weeks. Effective vermifuge herbs include myrrh, valerian, una da gato extracts, barberry tea . Goldenseal caps work especially for giardia.

❧ **For minor bacterial and viral infections:** echinacea/golden seal/myrrh combination, white pine/bayberry capsules for first aid; osha root tea, usnea extract, St. John's wort/lomatium extract.

❧ **For rashes, itching, swelling from insect bites or other histamine reactions:** antihistamine marshmallow/bee pollen/white pine capsules, calendula/pau d'arco gel, comfrey/plantain ointment, tea tree oil, aloe vera gel, echinacea/St. John's wort/white willow capsules.

❧ **For pain, cramping and headache relief:** lavender compresses, black cohosh/scullcap extract, peppermint oil rubs, comfrey compresses, rosemary tea or steam, ginkgo biloba or feverfew extract.

∼ **For strains, sprains and muscle pulls:** White willow/St John's wort capsules or salve, Tiger Balm analgesic gel, CHINESE white flower oil, tea tree or wintergreen/cajeput oil, and Fo-Ti (ho-shu-wu).

∼ **For periodic constipation and diarrhea:** fiber and herbs butternut/cascara capsules, senna/fennel laxative tea, milk thistle seed extract to soften stool, Ayurvedic Triphala formula, aloe vera juice.

∼ **For sleep aids for insomnia:** rosemary/chamomile/catnip, or passion flower/spearmint tea, hops/rosemary sleep pillow, wild lettuce/valerian extract, ashwagandha/black cohosh/scullcap capsules.

∼ **For calming stress and tension:** ginseng/licorice extract, rosemary/chamomile tea; Bach Flower Rescue Remedy drops, lemon balm/lemongrass tea, valerian/wild lettuce extract; chamomile aromatherapy.

∼ **For depression:** St. John's wort, one of the most widely used antidepressant herbs, can be taken with Kava Kava (relaxes & calms the body and mind quickly); ginkgo biloba, Bach Flower Rescue Remedy.

∼ **For indigestion, gas and upset stomach relief:** ginger tea or capsules; catnip/fennel tea; mint mix tea or extract, comfrey/pepsin capsules; aloe vera juice with herbs, spice mix tea or extract.

∼ **For eye infections and inflammations:** aloe vera juice wash, eyebright/parsley/bilberry capsules or wash, echinacea/golden seal wash, chamomile/elder compress; witch hazel/rosemary solution.

∼ **For earaches:** mullein oil ear drops, warm garlic oil ear drops, warm lobelia extract in the ear, castor oil drops, calendula oil ear drops.

∼ **For toothaches and gum problems:** tea tree oil, apply clove oil directly onto tooth or gums.

∼ **For concentration and memory enhancement:** ginkgo biloba, gotu kola, rosemary, evening primrose oil.

∼ **For overcoming fatigue, nerve exhaustion and mental burn out:** panax ginseng, siberian ginseng, suma, gotu kola, ginkgo biloba, bee pollen, royal jelly, green grasses (barley, wheat grass, alfalfa) and micro-algae (chlorella, spirulina, & blue green algae) are some of the most nutrient-rich and restorative foods.

∼ **For shock** *(beneficial emergency measures until medical help arrives)*: Cayenne - dilute cayenne powder or extract in water - 2-4 capsules or 1 to 3 teasp.- give with an eyedropper on the back of the tongue if necessary every 10 minutes to restore normal heart rate. Bach Flowers Rescue Remedy or Deva Flowers First Aid remedy (2 to 4 drops on the tongue every 5 minutes until breathing normalizes) Consciousness-reviving herbs include; camphor, bay oil or musk, used under the victim's nose as aromatherapy for revival; gingko biloba extract (a few drops in water, given on the tongue helps with stroke and allergic reactions.

∼ **Antiviral herbs:** St. John's wort, bee propolis, echinacea, yarrow, lomatium, osha root, una de gato, licorice, goldenseal, garlic, myrrh, dumontiaceae - a red marine algae (selectively supports the immune system to fight viruses such as Herpes & Epstein Barr), cinchona (natural source for quinine until the drug was synthetically produced), peppermint (more than 30 pathogenic micro-organisms have yielded to the influence of peppermint - including herpes simplex, staphlococcus aureus and candida albicans)

∼ **Antibacterial herbs** (antibiotic, antiseptic, antimicrobial): usnea, licorice, chaparral, echinacea, bee propolis, goldenseal, tea tree oil, garlic, myrrh, cyani flowers, marshmallow, St John's wort, lomatium, yarrow, marigold cream (calendula), kelp, bayberry root bark, oregon grape root, yellow dock, chickweed (effective against certain respiratory pathogens), mullein, red clover (possesses activity against several bacteria, the most significant of which is the pathogen that causes tuberculosis), peppermint, pau d'arco

∼ **Antifungal herbs:** tea tree oil, garlic extract, black walnut extract, turmeric extract, lomatium extract, echinacea cream, thuja (thrush and ringworm), bee propolis, licorice root, marigold cream, and pau d'arco .

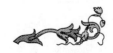

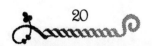

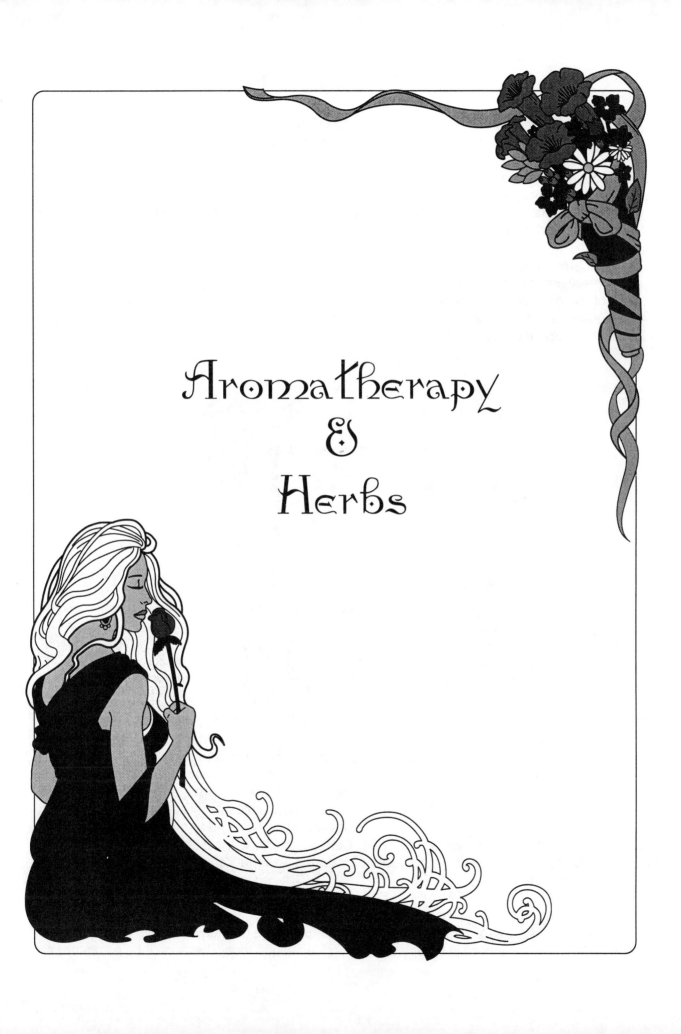

Aromatherapy & Herbs

Aromatherapy & Herbs

Aromatherapy, a branch of herbal medicine that uses essential plant oils to produce physical and emotional effects in the body, is both an ancient art and science. Aromatherapy works on different levels to accelerate healing, especially restoring energy and body balance through the nervous system. Aromatherapy oils have deep subconscious effects on emotions, triggering memory, and altering attitudes. Depending on the oils chosen, they may either calm and relax, or stimulate and energize. On the spiritual plane, aromatherapy elevates and soothes the spirit to restore harmony between mind and body.

The term "aromatherapy" was coined in 1937, by the French chemist René-Maurice Gattefossé, who accidentally burned his hand while he was working in his lab. The nearest cold liquid happened to be a bowl of lavender oil and Gattefossé plunged his hand into it. He immediately noticed pain relief and that afterwards, his burn healed remarkably fast. He became inspired to devote his life to studying the influence of essential oils on healing.

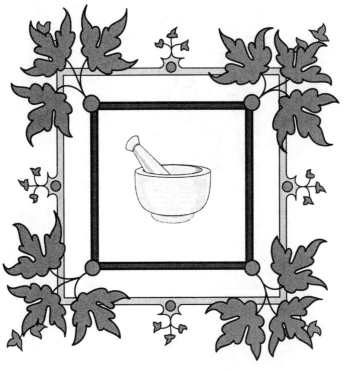

Records of aromatherapy date back thousands of years. Every ancient civilization used some form of aromatherapy to improve health and daily life. Egyptians burned scented oils 5,000 years ago, and also embalmed their corpses with resin and essence compounds. Hippocrates, the father of modern Western medicine, successfully fought a plague in Athens 2,000 years ago using aromatic fumigations throughout the city. In the middle ages, people burned pine oil in the streets during disease epidemics, and rubbed their bodies with oil of garlic, a powerful antibacterial agent. Aromatic frankincense was as precious as gold in the ancient world. Its vapor was believed to elevate the spirit, linking the human psyche with higher energies. In 1981, German scientists investigated the "mind-altering" effects of frankincense, and found that its vapor produced a powerful consciousness-expanding, psychoactive reaction in the brain.

As modern lifestyles become more chaotic and medical costs keep rising, many people are rediscovering aromatherapy as a natural, self-help means to restore harmony between mind and body. Aromatherapy is widely practiced in Europe as a healing technique today, because it helps restore the

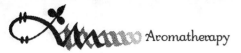
natural balance of the body instead of merely suppressing the symptoms of an ailment. In England, for instance, it is used in hospitals with diffusers, which pump the relaxing aroma of lavender through the wards to help boost patient morale. Lavender relaxes stress, so it is felt that patients are able to heal faster. At night, patients are given a choice of a tranquilizer drug or an aromatherapy oil massage.

Essential oils, 75 to 100 times more concentrated than dried herbs and flowers, are the heart of aromatherapy. During the life of the plant, essential oils deliver messages through the plant structure to regulate its functions, trigger immune response to environmental stress, protect it from harm and attract insects for pollination and propagation. In essence, aromatherapy oils act in plants much like hormones do in humans. They are some of the most potent of all herbal medicines.

Essential oils affect people first through the sense of smell. Smell is the most rapid of all the senses because its information is directly relayed to the hypothalamus. Motivation, moods and creativity all begin in the hypothalamus, so odors affect all of these processes. Scents are intimately intertwined with our emotions, feelings, and memories. A familiar scent can instantly flood your head with a field of flowers, or paint pictures of your past on the movie screen of your mind.

Scents also influence the endocrine system responsible for hormone levels, metabolism, insulin production, stress levels, sex drive, body temperature and appetite. The volatile molecules of essential oils work through hormone-like chemicals to produce their sensations. Certain oils can enhance your emotional equilibrium merely by inhaling them. (The smelling salts of Victorian days were used for more than just reviving a fainting lady.)

When scents enter through the nose, the molecules of the essential oil stimulate a sensory cell in the back of the nose that sends a message to the olfactory nerve which then sends a message to the limbic brain, the section of the brain that controls emotion and sexual response. Limbic brain neurochemicals also trigger memory and create subtle mood changes. In fact, the fastest way to alter mood state is with smell, and according to neurologists, the healing response from this process can last for hours or days (even though the oils usually do not remain in the body for more than three or four hours.) Studies done on brain-waves show that scents (like lavender) increase alpha brain waves associated with relaxation; scents (like jasmine) boost beta waves linked with alertness.

Essential oil fluids are volatile, non-oily essences. They are highly active, and may be taken in by inhalation, steams and infusers, or applied topically in massages, compresses or baths. The therapeutic effects of essential oils are due both to their pharmacological properties and their small molecular size, which allows penetration through the skin, the walls of the blood vessels, the lymph system and body tissues. Essential oils are also effective when rubbed on the skin. These pathways allow essential oils to strengthen and tone the body's organ, hormonal, nervous and immune systems.

Essential oils combine healing, psychological and beautifying benefits. They are often synergistic, working well together in a blend. Combining two to six oils is the norm in aromatherapy (using more than six is, in some instances, counter-productive, decreasing instead of increasing potency). Blends do not always achieve synergism, but when they do, the effect of the oils can be considerably greater than the sum of its parts.

Essential oils are best known for counteracting stress, and the many conditions in which stress plays a part. Indications of stress usually include mental tension, poor sleep and unexplained physical fatigue. Other warning signs may include back, neck and shoulder pain, lack of appetite and chronic irritability. I have found that the best natural solutions for relieving stress are eating healthfully, regular exercise, relaxation techniques like imaging, and herbal aromatherapy. Aromatherapy relieves stress by promoting mental relaxation and alertness, good-quality sleep, physical relaxation, and by increasing overall energy. Aromatherapy also makes us feel good in part by releasing certain mood-inducing neurochemicals in the brain.

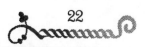

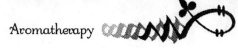

Here is just a partial list of the specific benefits aromatherapy has to offer:

Stimulates tissue regeneration by nourishing the growth of new healthy skin, resulting in rapid healing from burns, wounds, sores and ulcers.

Stimulates the immune system (partly by invigorating the production of white blood cells). A recent study found that all essential oils stimulate phagocytosis, the ability of white blood cells to eat up invading microbes.

Stimulates the electromagnetic charge of the aromatic molecules of the essential oils for a sharp influence on cellular magnetic fields, which new studies have found very effective in healing.

Increases effectiveness against bacteria, viruses, fungi and parasites. All essential oils have antibacterial properties, but each oil is effective against different pathogens. While most essential oils are toxic to bacteria, they are non-toxic to the human organism. (For example: tea tree oil is one of the most effective and least harmful anti-microbial essential oils.) One way to test the effectiveness of essential oils against a particular bacteria is the aromatogram. A bacteria is cultured in clear dishes and one measured drop of each essential oil to be tested is placed on the culture (each in its own dish). After a few hours a visible circle around each oil drop appears. The size of the diameter of the circle around the drop represents the zone of inhibition - the larger the zone area, the more effective that essential oil is against the bacteria.

Viruses, because they invade and take control of our body cells, are more difficult than bacteria for the immune system to identify and attack. While there are few substances (natural or synthetic) which are effective aginst viruses, certain essential oils have shown effectiveness against them. Thyme, cinnamon, black pepper, eucalyptus, tea-tree, lavender (against herpes simplex virus or cold sores) and geranium are good examples.

Essential oils have proven effective against parasite infections, like lice, crabs, scabies, intestinal worms, trichomonas, and more; and against fungi like ringworm, athlete's foot and thrush. The same type of anti-toxic action also may be seen against the poison from insect bites and stings. Tea tree and lavender are two oils that are effective against mosquito bites and bee and wasp stings, for instance. (Lavender is also reputed to have a neutralizing effect on the bite of the black widow spider and the funnel-web spider, two very poisonous spiders.)

Helps lower blood pressure, and stimulates sluggish circulation to help promote detoxification.

Acts as a blood cleanser and purifies. Rose oil helps counteract the toxic blood effects of alcohol.

Acts as an expectorant which stimulates the removal of heavy mucous in the lungs and bronchial tubes.

Stimulates the drainage ducts (the cutaneous glands, the lungs, kidneys and intestines), for the elimination of metabolic residues and toxins. For example, juniper an effective diuretic acts by enhancing the filtration action of the kidneys, and by increasing the amount of potassium, sodium and chlorine excreted.

Relieves pain by helping to relieve muscular aches, period pains, headaches and more. Essential oils also act indirectly, by stimulating the release of the body's own natural analgesics.

Encourages body chemistry normalization. Essential oils of garlic and hyssop have a normalizing effect on blood pressure. If the blood pressure is too high, the oils help reduce blood pressure; if the blood pressure is too low the oils help increase it. The normalizing effect on the nervous system are common with essential oils. For example, Bergamot or geranium oil will either stimulate or sedate according to the needs of the individual. Rose oil and yarrow also can help normalize a system invaded by allergens, such as pollens and spores.

Aromatherapy oils aren't really oils, but distilled condensations, formed by rushing steam through plant material. Although steam distillation is the most common method, a process using carbon dioxide, a cold process, can capture all the notes lost in steam distillation. Another process, called "expression," is a mechanical pressing used to produce citrus oils; solvents like hexane may be used to produce an "absolute." It takes over 200 pounds of jasmine flowers to produce a single pound of jasmine absolute.

Essential oils can be diluted or extended by adding them to vegetable or carrier oils, like jojoba oil, sweet almond oil, olive oil, carrot seed, avocado and wheat germ oils, borage seed, evening primrose and rose hip seed oils, apricot kernel, grapeseed, hazelnut, sunflower, sesame and canola oils.

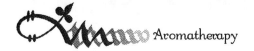

Using Aromatherapy Oils

REMEMBER: ESSENTIAL OILS ARE VERY CONCENTRATED, AND SHOULD ONLY BE USED IN 1 TO 5 DROP DOSES.

Skin Care

Skin is the body's largest organ, both for ingestion and elimination. It is a major part of the immune system, too, protecting against the elements, and preventing harmful chemicals or too much water from entering the body. Stress, poor nutrition and pollution all take a heavy toll on skin.

Essential oils are especially effective for the skin. They act as transporters to carry therapeutic benefits to the skin layers; and they penetrate the skin, weaving their way through the intercellular fluids. Aromatherapy helps improve the skin's condition by stimulating circulation. It encourages cell growth through phytohormone activity and cell regeneration, creating a fresher, more vibrant complexion. Stress-reducing benefits also keep skin looking clear and calm.

Floral waters are the easiest way to use essential oils on the skin. Waters have the healing properties of the oil itself, and are well-suited to sensitive skin. Make floral waters in a spray bottle if possible, for convenience. Simply blend 5 to 10 drops of the essential oil into 4 oz. distilled water, and use as needed. Essential oils may also be added to your lotions and moisturizers. However, because the oils are volatile, you cannot make up the preparation in advance. Pour some lotion into your hand; add 3 drops of oil and apply to skin.

Oils for general skin care - chamomile, geranium, lavender, lemon, ylang-ylang.
Oils for dry, or aging skin - rose, carrot seed, rosemary, jasmine, red sage, sandlewood.
Oils for oily skin - lavender, eucalyptus, geranium, ylang ylang, basil, camphor, lemon.
Oils for sensitive skin - chamomile, neroli, rose.
Oils for wrinkled skin - lemon, fennel, palmarosa, carrot seed, myrrh.
Oils to promote the growth of healthy skin cells - lavender, rose

Facial Oil for Dry to Normal Skin: in a base of $\frac{1}{4}$ ounce Jojoba or vitamin E oil, add 2 drops geranium oil, 1 drop frankincense oil, and 1 drop myrrh oil. Massage several drops into your skin twice daily.

Facial Oil for Normal to Oily Skin: in a base of $\frac{1}{4}$ ounce Jojoba or vitamin E oil, add 3 drops lavender oil and 1 drop ylang-ylang oil.

Aromatherapy Facial Steam Cleanse: add 3 drops lemongrass oil and 1 drop eucalyptus oil to a bowl of steaming water. Put your face 6 to 10 inches above the water, and tent a towel over your head.

Aromatherapy Skin Wash: in a base of 4 ounces of liquid soap, add 5 drops peppermint oil, 1 drop eucalyptus oil, 1 drop chamomile oil, and 2 drops sage oil to revitalize troubled skin.

NOTE: A DROP OF ANY OF THE FOLLOWING IS PARTICULARLY EFFECTIVE FOR TREATING A BLEMISH THAT IS JUST ERUPTING. PUT ON A COTTON SWAB AND APPLIED DIRECTLY.

Oils for inflamed skin - chamomile, lavender, neroli, rosewood, geranium, cedarwood.
Oils for acne - eucalyptus, juniper, lavender, cajeput, palmarosa, tea tree.
Oils for eczema or psoriasis - cedarwood, patchouli, lavender, chamomile.

Hair Care

The easiest way to use the aromatherapy oils for your hair is to mix 12 to 15 drops of oils into an 8 oz. bottle of your favorite shampoo or conditioner.

NOTE: SOME ESSENTIAL OILS MAY STRIP PEROXIDE-BASED HAIR COLORING. DO A SAMPLE TEST AREA IF YOU ARE CONCERNED.

Oils for dry hair - cedarwood, lavender
Oils for oily hair - lemongrass, rosemary

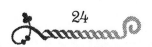

Oils for dandruff - rosemary, cedarwood
Oils to reduce hair loss - cedarwood, lavender, rosemary, sage, juniper.

Essential Brushing Oil: to balance, shine, and scent hair and scalp; add equal amounts rosemary and lavender oil to a small perfume bottle; shake out 2 drops on a brush and run several times through hair.

Aromatherapy Scalp Rub For Scalp Diseases: to 2-oz. sweet almond oil, add 2 drops rosemary oil, 2 drops sage oil and 2 drops cedarwood oil to relieve scalp distress.

Oral Hygiene

Follow directions exactly when using aromatherapy oils in the mouth.

For fresh breath and better digestion - use 1 drop peppermint oil on the tongue; or blend five drops peppermint oil with 1 oz. of cider vinegar and 3 oz. water, and use as a regular mouthwash.
For toothache - blend 20 drops clove oil with 1-oz. brandy and apply with a cotton swab.
For gum problems - Put 3 or 4 drops of sage or tea tree oil on a cotton swab and apply to gums.

Mental, Emotional & Spiritual Health

Use in a massage oil, in a diffuser, in an aromatic bath, or inhale aromas from the bottle.

Oils for refreshment and invigoration - sage, lemon, lime, pine, eucalyptus, vervain.
Oils to calm nervous tension and emotional stress - sage, pine, geranium, rosemary, pennyroyal.
Oils for pleasant dreams and insomnia - anise, chamomile, ylang ylang.
Oils for libido - ylang ylang, patchouli, sandalwood, cinnamon.
Oils for stimulating intellect and memory - rosemary, petitgrain.
Oils for serenity and calmness - lavender, pine, chamomile, orange.
Oils for positive motivation - peppermint, lemon, eucalyptus.

Stress Reduction & Relaxation

Reducing stress is an aromatherapy specialty. Essential oils appear to influence hormones that regulate body metabolism and insulin production. Chronic stress lowers immunity, elevates blood pressure, and raises cholesterol levels. Stress depletes all your body's energies, and nutrient supplies. Signs of stress are anger, anxiety, depression, paranoia, hostility, lethargy, and mental fatigue.

Stress-Soothing Massage Oil - to 2 ounces sweet almond oil, add 4 drops bergamot oil, 4 drops chamomile oil, 4 drops lavender oil, 4 drops sandalwood oil, 3 drops marjoram oil and 2 drops elemi oil.

Stress-Buster Diffuser Oil - in a small glass bottle, combine 15 drops lavender oil, 10 drops sage oil, 10 drops elemi oil, 10 drops geranium oil, 8 drops bergamot oil, 8 drops orange oil, 8 drops rosewood oil, 6 drops ylang ylang oil and 5 drops coriander oil. Add a few drops to your diffuser or lamp bowl to reduce tension.

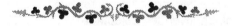

One of the best ways to use aromatherapy is in a relaxing, therapeutic bath. Regular aromatherapy baths can help control stress, alleviate tension, and minimize muscular aches and pains. Simply swish oils in warm bath water and soak.

Winter Bath: help ward off colds and stimulate circulation, use 3 drops juniper oil, 2 drops pepper oil and 5 drops lavender oil.

Summer Bath: cool your skin, refresh and invigorate - use 3 drops peppermint oil, 4 drops bergamot oil and 2 drops basil oil.

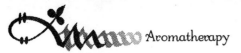

Morning Bath: start the day with an invigorating tonic - use 5 drops rosemary oil, 5 drops juniper oil and 2 drops peppermint oil.

Evening Bath: get sweeter, better quality sleep - use 2 drops chamomile oil, 5 drops lavender oil, 2 drops orange blossom oil.

Aphrodisiac Bath: put yourself in the mood for love - use 2 drops ylang-ylang oil, 8 drops sandalwood oil and 2 drops jasmine oil.

Lemon Detox Bath: freshen and cleanse the body - use the juice from 1 lemon, 5 drops lemon oil and 2 drops geranium oil.

Relaxing Mineral Bath Salts: soak away stress - add 1 cup Dead Sea salts, 1 cup Epsom salts, $\frac{1}{2}$ cup regular sea salt and $\frac{1}{4}$ baking soda to a tub; swish in 3 drops lavender oil, 2 drops chamomile oil, 2 drops marjoram oil and 1 drop ylang-ylang oil.

Aromatherapy For Energy & Stimulation. Some essential oils have a direct effect on the central nervous system. Peppermint energizes while easing headaches. Ginger and fennel stimulate circulation. Rose influences hormonal activity. Lavender and geranium can either stimulate or sedate, according to the individual's physiological needs.

Rosemary Fatigue-Fighting Bath: Use 4 drops rosemary oil, 2 drops orange oil, 1 drop thyme oil.

Energizing Body Oil: mix, then massage into skin in the morning, 2 ounces sweet almond oil, 6 drops lavender oil, 4 drops rosemary oil, 3 drops geranium oil, 3 drops lemon oil, 2 drops coriander oil, 2 drops patchouli oil

Energy Inhalant Oil: in a small glass bottle, combine 8 drops rosemary oil, 6 drops elemi oil, 4 drops peppermint oil, 3 drops basil oil, 1 drop ginger oil. Inhale directly from the bottle for an energy boost.

Energy Boosting Diffuser Blend: in a small glass bottle, combine 15 drops rosemary oil, 12 drops pine oil, 10 drops lavender oil, 10 drops lemon oil, 2 drops peppermint oil. Add a few drops to your diffuser or lamp bowl.

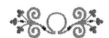

Aromatherapy Oils For Healing. Hunreds of laboratory tests have demonstrated the effectiveness of essential oils against infections. Studies at France's Pasteur Institute found that oils of clove, thyme, mint, marjoram, pine and oregano strongly inhibit microbes that cause tuberculosis, cholera and many staphylococcal infections. Amazingly enough, oil of lavender has more than four times, rosemary has more than five times, clove has more than nine times, and thyme has more than twelve times the germ-killing power of phenol, a common disinfectant. Blend just before using for most effectiveness.

Body cleansing and rejuvenation - massage skin with a blend of 15 drops geranium, 35 drops neroli and 1-oz. vegetable oil, to promote cell regeneration, rid the body of toxins and relieve tension.

Antiseptic activity - lemon, clove, eucalyptus, pine, cinnamon, rosemary, thyme, tea tree. Note: These are excellent in a diffuser to keep harmful bacteria count down. Effective for upper respiratory infections, colds and flu. Use approximately 30 to 50 drops oils, and let diffuser run for 30 minutes twice a day.

Skin abrasions - apply one drop of sage or lavender oil to speed healing. If used for first aid to cuts or bruises, put a few drops on a cotton swab and apply to area.

Sore throat and cough - oils such as eucalyptus and tea tree may be applied topically to the throat. Cypress may be taken as a "tea", at a dose of 1 drop to a cup of hot water every hour.

Chest congestion - make a vapor rub, using 50 drops eucalyptus, 15 drops peppermint, and 10 drops wintergreen to 1 oz. vegetable oil. Rub into chest for relief.

Allergy and asthma relief - add a few drops of eucalyptus, lavender, sage, peppermint or wintergreen oil to a pot of boiling water or a vaporizer.

Bladder problems - use 2 drops each of lavender, juniper, thyme oil in a cup of hot water.

Indigestion - take 1 to 2 drops with meals of either rosemary, peppermint or lemon oil.

Intestinal or bowel irritation - use a "tea" with 1 drop geranium oil to a cup of hot water.

Sunburn - use 1 part tea tree oil to 1 part aloe vera gel and apply.

Headache - apply 1 drop of lavender, peppermint or rosemary oil to back of the neck and temples.

Analgesic rub for sore joints and muscles - use 20 drops each of clove, eucalyptus, tea tree, and wintergreen oils in 1 oz. vegetable oil. Rub into affected area, or add $\frac{1}{4}$ oz. to a bath.

Anxiety - blend ylang-ylang (which soothes nervous tension) with rose or lavender oils and a sweet almond oil for a full-body massage or a few drops of the essential oils can be added to bathwater.

Depression - add a few drops of jasmine or bergamot into sunflower, olive or another carrier oil for a full-body massage or a few drops of the essential oils can be added to the bathwater to help uplift and rejuvenate.

Fatigue - add a few drops of rosemary oil for an invigorating boost. Rosemary enlivens the brain, clears the head, aids memory, is good for weakness, exhaustion and lethargy.

Insomnia/stress - a few drops of lavender on your shoulders, neck or near your face can help ease stress and induce sleep. It can also be added to a carrier oil for massage or added to a hot bath.

Menopause - add a drop each of geranium, fennel, sage, basil, roman chamomile and cypress to a carrier oil and rub daily on pulse points.

THERE'S A WIDE RANGE OF THERAPEUTIC OILS FOR YOU TO CHOOSE FROM. HERE ARE SOME OF THE EASIEST TO USE:

Basil: Ocimum basilicum - useful for headaches and allergies. A brain stimulant and tonic for the nerves that helps concentration, circulation and heart problems. Contains plant estrogens. Contra-Indications: avoid during pregnancy. May irritate the skin.

Bergamot: Citrus bergamia - eases digestion; relaxes the nervous system; helps with eczema, psoriasis, acne and wounds; antiseptic for urinary tract; uplifting anti-depressant, and good for anxiety. Contra-Indications: can cause photosensitivity. Avoid hot sun right after use on skin.

Cedarwood: Juniperus virginiana - strong antiseptic and expectorant for coughs. Useful as an astringent for urinary infections, cystitis. A tonic for the nervous system. Gives deep relaxation and is a sedative for anxiety and stress. Has been found to be good for meditation; spiritually uplifting.

Chamomile: Matricaria recutita - stimulates the mind, memory and respiratory system; helps overcome exhaustion; used for a wide range of complaints including eczema and asthma. True chamomile oil is a deep blue because of the azulenes it contains.

Clary sage: Salvia sclarea - a hormone balancer. Helpful for painful cramps, PMS, and muscle spasms. Brings feelings of well-being; lifts the mind and reduces stress. Useful for all types of skin inflammation and for aging skin and wrinkles.

Clove: Eugenia caryophyllata - rejuvenates, soothes irritability and allays temper; relieves pain of toothache and arthritis; anti-bacterial; may be used to alleviate infectious wounds. Contra-Indications: Can be irritating to the skin. Use in low doses and dilute in a carrier oil.

Cypress: Cupressus sempervirens - harmonizes the fluids of the body, good for excess fluids. Helps nose bleeds, heavy periods, incontinence, sweating. Soothes sore throats. Helps reduce cellulitic skin; an astringent for oily skin, hemorrhoids and varicose veins. Calms irritability and helps with transitions. Contra-Indications: Avoid in pregnancy.

Eucalyptus: Eucalytus globulus - anti-viral action works on the respiratory tract and loosens mucous, treats asthma, bronchitis and sinusitis. Good for flu, throat infections and coughs. Steam can be inhaled, or can be massaged onto chest. Also good for herpes, burns, pus eruptions in wounds. Contra-Indications: Do not use when there is high blood pressure or epilepsy. May antidote homeopathic medication.

Geranium: Pelargonium graveolens - stimulates the psyche, acts as an anti-depressant, averts tension and stress; tonic to the nervous system. Helps the pituitary gland to regulate the endocrine system. Regulates the hormonal system during menopause, PMS and heavy periods. Diuretic, and astringent - helps stem bleeding. A helpful tonic in overcoming addictions. Helpful for diabetes and urinary infections; and for circulation to the skin, eczema, burns and shingles. A good skin cleanser. Contra-Indications: Avoid during pregnancy. Test for skin sensitivity.

Ginger: Zingiber officinalis - helps settle the digestive system, and stimulates the appetite. Helps colds, flu and reduces fever. Helps motion sickness, nausea, gas and pain. May be added to massage rubs for rheumatic pains and bone injuries. It sharpens senses and aids memory. Dilute with carrier oil for sores and bruises. Contra-Indications: Can irritate skin.

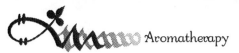 *Aromatherapy*

Jasmine: Jasminum grandiflorum - uplifting and soothing, very good for depression; known for its erogenous quality. Harmone balancer. Helpful for menstrual pain, uterine disorders and childbirth. Helpful for respiratory problems such as: breathing difficulties, bronchial spasm, catarrh, cough and hoarseness. Good for all types of skin, especially dry and sensitive skin.

Juniper: Juniperus communis - a diuretic thta relieves pain in back, legs and feet. Helps arthritis and gout. Aids kidneys and liver. Helps clear the nervous system. A tonic for oily skin, acne, eczema and seborrhea of the scalp. Contra-Indications: Avoid during pregnancy. Prolonged use may overstimulate the kidneys.

Lavender: Lavendula angustifolia - induces sleep, alleviates stress, reduces depression, nervous tension and hyperactiviy. May also be used to calm animals. Balances the central nervous system and the emotions; pain relief for headaches. Has a sedative action on the heart; lowers high blood pressure. Rub on stomach for painful menstrual periods. Promotes new cell growth; a tonic for the hair.

Lemongrass: Cymbopogon citratus - helps sedate the nervous system, soothes headaches, stimulates thyroid and energizing for states of exhaustion. Lifts the spirits; has tonic effects, especially when recovering from illness. Helpful for aching muscles as it reduces lactic acid and stimulates circulation. Tones the skin, is helpful for tightening loose skin after dieting.

Marjoram: Origanum majorana - a warming analgesic for pain, stiff joints, colds, asthma, and painful periods. A tonic for heart that lowers high blood pressure and calms anxiety. Promotes blood flow in the skin. Note: Take a break after one month of usage.

Neroli: Citrus aurantium - relieves stress, depression, anxiety, nervous tension and insomnia. Helps headaches. A heart tonic, that improves circulation and helps nerve pain. Useful for dry and sensitive skin.

Orange: Citrus sinensis - helps clear depression; has a cheering, uplifting quality. Calming action on stomach; encourages appetite. Helps diarrhea and constipation. Lowers cholesterol.

Patchouli: Pogostemon patchouli - a nerve sedative and antidepressant. Balances the central nervous system. A mild aphrodisiac. Helps reduce appetite. Has a cell regenerative action, good for aging, wrinkled and cracked skin and for athlete's foot. Note: A low dose has a sedative action - a high dose has a stimulant action.

Peppermint: Mentha piperita - cools fevers; the steam decongests sinuses, and helps asthma and colds. Soothes headaches and calms the mind. Helps concentration. Useful as a digestive for nausea, motion sickness and food poisoning, Good for bad breath. An antibacterial that helps combat infections. Capillary constriction on the skin relieves itching, inflammation and sunburn. Stimulant action is useful for numb limbs, shock, anemia, dizziness and fainting. The oil contains large amounts of menthol. Contra-Indications: Avoid during pregnancy. Avoid eye contact. Undiluted it may irritate skin. Can antidote homeopathic remedies.

Pine: Pinus sylvestris - antiseptic for respiratory tract, the steam is a good expectorant that helps bronchitis, flu, laryngitis and sinusitis. Soothes mental stress and relieves anxiety. Regenerates a tired mind; stimulates the adrenal glands. Contra-Indications: Undiluted may irritate sensitve skin.

Rosemary: Rosmarinus officinalis - encourages intuition, enlivens the brain, clears the head and enhances memory. Useful for exhaustion, weakness and lethargy, especially when there are headaches. A good decongestant. Pain relieving properties are useful for arthritis, gout, and sore muscles. A heart tonic that normalizes low blood pressure and helps anemia. Often used in hair products for hair growth and to relieve dandruff. Contra-Indications: Avoid during pregnancy, with high blood pressure or epilepsy.

Sage: Salvia officinalis - a cleansing and detox oil; good for mental strain and exhaustion.

Sandalwood: Santalum album - enhances the immune system. A sedative that relaxes for meditation and sleep quality. Massage the oil over the bladder area for cystitis and kidney problems. Healing to the skin, moisturizing for cracked and dry skin, relieving for itching and inflammation. Sometimes used as an aphrodisiac.

Tangerine: Citrus reticulata - soothes psyche, calms, eases nervous tension.

Tea Tree: Melaleuca alternifolia - one of the most useful anti-bacterial, anti-viral, anti-fungal and anti-parasitic essential oils available. Strongly antiseptic for colds, flu, fever and cold sores. Steam can be inhaled for sinusitis and lung congestion. Strenthens the immune system. Is also anti-inflammatory, a venous decongestant, neurotonic and analgesic. Very effective for cuts, minor burns, and insect bites and stings. Useful as a rub for arthritis and muscle aches. Tea tree has so many uses it is been refered to as "a medicine chest in a bottle".

Thyme: Thymus vulgaris - a strong immune stimulant; fortifies on all levels - physical, emotional and mental. Good for colds and arthritis. Raises low blood pressure. A tonic for anemia, fatigue. Enlivens the mind. Heals wounds, sores and boils. Contra-Indications: Can irritate skin, dilute with a carrier oil.

Vanilla: Vanilla planifolia - calming and soothing with aphrodisiac qualities.

Ylang Ylang: Cananga odorata - a depression diminisher that brings an uplifting mood; eases anxiety and feelings of anger, shock, panic and fear. Balances the hormones. Helps high blood pressure and insomnia. Balances sebum flow, and stimulates scalp for hair growth.

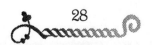

Here's How To Use Aromatherapy Oils For The Best Results. Aromatherapy oils are customarily used by adding a few drops to a massage oil or facial care product, or using a diffuser or lamp, or in a steam inhaler to ease respiratory distress. When inhaled into the lungs, molecules of essential oils attach to oxygen molecules, enter the blood stream and journey throughout the body with therapeutic activity.

Oils evaporate easily and completely. They don't leave marks on your clothing or towels.

Use only pure essential oils. Never substitute synthetics.

Buy your essential oils from reliable sources that guarantee the purity of their oils.

Always dilute essential oils in a carrier oil, such as almond, apricot, canola, jojoba, or sunflower oil, before applying them. Essential oils are highly concentrated - sometimes as much as 100 times stronger than the fresh or dried plant. Even one drop of pure essential oil applied directly to your skin may cause irritation.

Uncap the bottle for a few seconds only. Drop oils into the palm of your hand or a clean container for blending. Keep bottles tightly capped and away from sunlight and heat when not in use.

Follow the directions for the aromatherapy blends carefully. Never add more than the recommended number of drops. When using essential oils on infants or children, dilute them.

Use glass containers for all blends of essential oils. Oils can damage plastic containers.

Do not shake essential oils. Just gently roll the bottle between your hands for a few minutes.

Trust your nose. If you dislike the smell of a certain oil, don't use it. Inhale essential oils for short periods only; run a diffuser for only five to ten minutes at a time.

If you experience any irritation, sensitivity, or reaction, discontinue use of the suspect oil.

Never take essential oils internally, except as directed by a professional of medical aromatherapy.

The essential oils and aromatherapy blends discussed in this book are safe for most people to use.

As always, people with certain medical conditions should be cautious. Some essential oils can trigger asthma attacks or epileptic seizures in susceptible people. Some can elevate or depress blood pressure. Consult a health care professional before using aromatherapy if you have any of these conditions. Essential oils can also counteract or diminish the effectiveness of homeopathic remedies. If you are using any homeopathic preparations, check with a homeopathic physician.

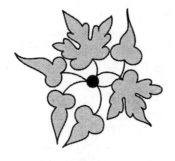

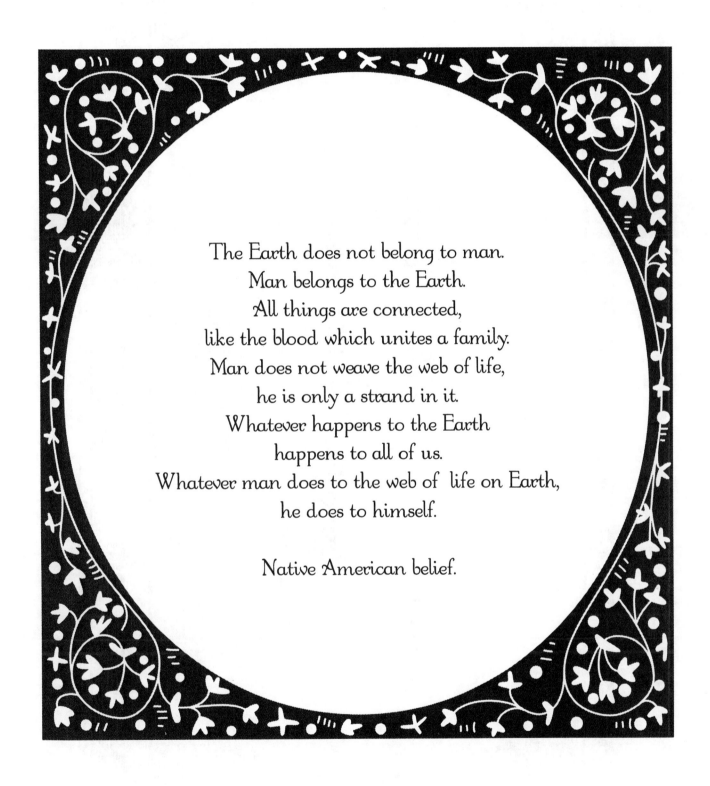

The Earth does not belong to man.
Man belongs to the Earth.
All things are connected,
like the blood which unites a family.
Man does not weave the web of life,
he is only a strand in it.
Whatever happens to the Earth
happens to all of us.
Whatever man does to the web of life on Earth,
he does to himself.

Native American belief.

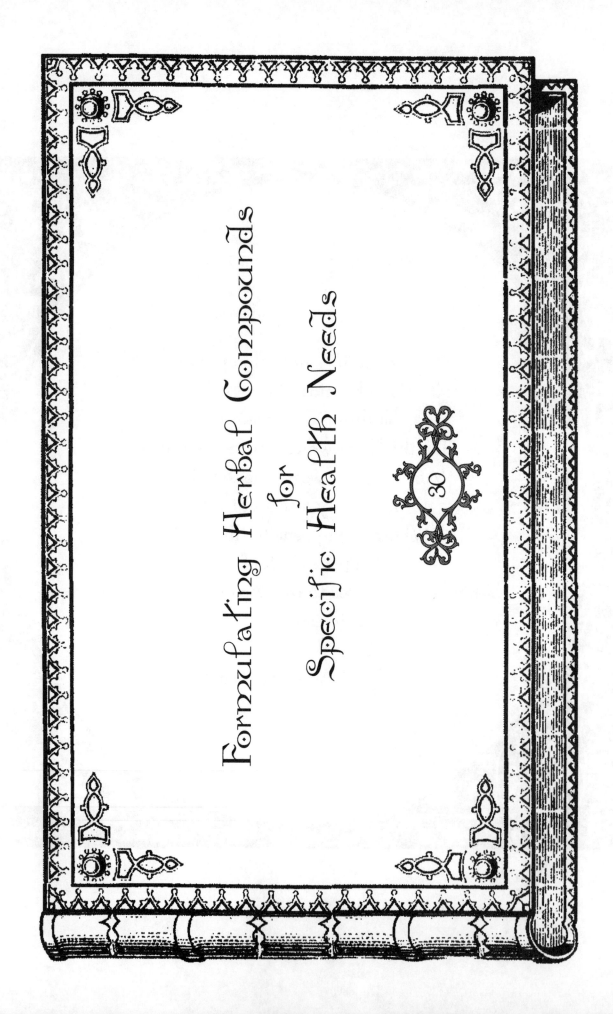

Formulating Herbal Compounds

for

Specific Health Needs

30

An Important Message About Your Health Care Responsibility

The material on the following pages is intended as an educational tool to offer information about alternative healing and health maintenance options available to the health care consumer today.

I believe we must be respectful of all ways of healing. The crisis intervention measures of drug therapy are sometimes needed to stabilize an emergency or life-threatening situation, but for long term well-being, disease prevention, and many common, self-limiting problems, diet improvement, exercise, and natural medicine choices make good sense. They are gentle, non-invasive, and in almost every case, free of any side effects.

The herbal recommendations in this section are not intended as a substitute for the advice and treatment of a physician or other licensed health care professionals. In many cases, they may be used as complementary medicines to professional care, to help shorten the time you may have to use drug treatment, and to help overcome any side effects.

Are there interactions between drugs and herbs? It is important to remember that herbs are foods, remarkably safe in their naturally-occurring state, and especially in combinations. They do not normally interact with drugs any more than a food would interact. However, be fair to your doctor and yourself. Discuss your alternative choices with your physician, and always inform your doctor or pharmacist of any other medication you are taking. Pregnant women are especially urged to consult with their health care provider before using any therapy.

I feel that education is the key to making wise health decisions. Part of the job of taking more command of your own health care is using your common sense, intelligence, and adult judgement based on the knowledge of your own body experiences. Ultimately, you must take the full responsibility for your choices and how you use the information presented here.

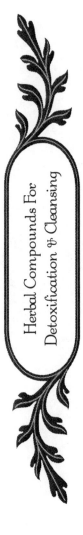

Herbal Compounds For Detoxification & Cleansing

Today, Americans are exposed to synthetic, often toxic substances on an unprecedented scale. Industrial chemicals and their pollutant by-products, pesticides, additives in our foods, heavy metals, anesthetics, residues from drugs, and environmental hormones are trapped within the human body in greater concentrations than at any other point in history. Every system of the body is affected, from tissue damage to sensory deterioration.

Many chemicals are so widely spread that we are unaware of them. But they have worked their way into our bodies faster than they can be eliminated, and are causing allergies and addictions in record numbers. More than 2 million synthetic substances are known, 25,000 are added each year, and over 30,000 are produced on a commercial scale. Only a tiny fraction are ever tested for toxicity. A lot of them come to us on the winds from developing countries that have few safeguards in place. And these things don't even count the second-hand smoke, caffeine and alcohol overload, or daily stress that is an increasing part of our lives.

The molecular structure of many chemical carcinogens interacts with human DNA, so long term exposure can result in metabolic and genetic alteration that affects cell growth, behavior and immune response. New research by the World Health Organization implicates toxic environmental chemicals in 60 to 80% of all cancers. Studies also link pesticides and pollutants to hormone dysfunctions, psychological disorders, birth defects, still births and now breast cancer. The wide variety of toxic substances means that every system of the body is affected - from deep level tissue damage to sensory deterioration.

As toxic matter saturates our tissues, anti-oxidants and minerals in vital body fluids are reduced, so immune defenses are thrown out of balance, and eventually disease begins. Circumstances like this are the prime factor in today's immune compromised diseases like candidiasis, lupus, fibromyalgia, chronic fatigue syndrome, and cancer.

Chemical oxidation is the other process that affects body degeneration and allows disease. The oxygen that "rusts" and ages us also triggers free radical activity, a destructive cascade of incomplete molecules that damages DNA and other cell components. And if you didn't have a reason to reduce your fat intake before, here is a critical one: oxygen combines with fats in body storage cells to speed up the free radical deterioration process.

How do you know if you need to detoxify? Almost everybody does. It's one of the best ways to remain healthy in a destructive environment. Not one of us is immune to environmental toxins, and most of us can't escape to a remote, unpolluted habitat. In the last few decades we have become dangerously able to harm the health of our planet, even to the point of making it uninhabitable for life. We must develop further and take even larger steps... those of cooperation and support. The well-being of the world depends on the cooperation of mankind and the Earth together, to save it all for us all. It starts with ourselves. We can take positive steps to keep our own body systems in good working order, so that toxins are eliminated quickly. (We can also take a closer look at our own air, water and food, and keep an ever watchful eye on the politics that control our environment. Legislation on health and the environment follows two pathways in America today…the influence of business and profits, and the demands of the people for a healthy environment and responsible stewardship of the Earth.)

Our bodies are clearly created as self-cleaning, self-healing mechanisms. Internal detoxification is an ongoing process performed on a daily basis. Just as our hearts beat nonstop and our lungs breathe automatically, so our metabolic processes continually dispose of wastes and poisons. Detoxification is the body's natural process of eliminating and neutralizing toxins, by the liver, the kidneys, urine, feces, exhalation, and perspiration. If you keep immune response high, elimination regular, circulation sound, and stress under control, your body can handle a great deal of toxicity and regularly prevent disease.

Unfortunately, body systems and organs that were once completely capable of detoxification are now so overloaded that they are largely unable to rid us of the daily poisons that assault us. So toxicity builds and builds in our systems, and eventually disease results.

In the past, detoxification was used either clinically for recovering alcoholics and drug addicts, or individually as a once-a-year mild "spring cleaning" for general health maintenance. Today, a regular detoxification program two or three times a year can make a big difference in the way your body performs. In fact, it might be the missing link for preventing chronic opportunistic diseases like cancer, arthritis, diabetes and fatigue syndromes like candida albicans.

Most people eat too much animal protein, fat, caffeine, alcohol, and chemicalized foods that inhibit optimum cell function. But even if your diet is good, a cleanse can restore body vitality against environmental toxins. Detoxification is becoming necessary not only for health, but for the quality of our lives.

Here are some signs that you may need to detoxify:

•If you get frequent, unexplained headaches or back pain; •If you have chronic respiratory problems, sinus problems or asthma; •If you have abnormal body odor, bad breath or coated tongue; •If you have food allergies, poor digestion, or constipation with chronic intestinal bloating, or gas; •If you have brittle nails and hair, psoriasis, adult acne, or unexplained weight gain over 10 pounds; •If you have joint pain, or arthritis; •If you are depressed and irritable, and always out of energy; •If you have unusually poor memory and chronic insomnia.

Here are some of the benefits you can expect from a body cleanse:

•Your digestive tract is cleansed of accumulated waste and fermenting bacteria; •liver, kidney and blood purification take place, impossible under ordinary eating patterns; •mental clarity is enhanced, impossible under chemical overload; •dependency on habit-forming substances, such as sugar, caffeine, nicotine, alcohol and drugs is reduced as the blood is purified; •bad eating habits are often turned around, and the stomach has a chance to reduce to normal size for weight control.

Cleansing also releases hormone secretions that stimulate immune response, and encourages a disease-preventing environment. After a cleanse, the body starts rebalancing, energy levels rise physically, psychologically and sexually, and creativity begins to expand. You start feeling like a "different person" - and of course, you are. See HEALTHY HEALING, 10TH EDITION, by Linda Rector Page for detailed programs on a broad range of cleansing regimens. See COOKING FOR HEALTHY HEALING, by Linda Rector Page for complete diets and recipes to help you get the most from your cleansing program

A good detox program should be in 3 stages ... cleansing, rebuilding and maintaining. Herbs in their abundance of diversity, along with the specific nature of their activity, are optimally suited to these tasks. Herbs are effective for a broad spectrum of body cleansing goals. Herbs are rich in food-source minerals, vitamins, amino acids, and enzyme precursors. In the dried state, herbs provide concentrated, whole food nutrition that becomes part of the body to stimulate cleansing, fuel regrowth, and build resistance to disease. Herbs are unique among therapeutic mediaums in these abilities, in a way that drugs, or even partitioned substances like vitamins are not. They work with the body's own action as a source of life and growth. This is the key to their success as natural medicines. Use unsprayed or wildcrafted herbs for the most benefits.

✦FORMULAS FOR DETOXIFICATION ARE EFFECTIVE FOR THE FOLLOWING CONDITIONS:

•Alcohol & Drug Abuse •Nicotine Addiction •Liver & Spleen Disease •Bacterial, Staph & Strep Infections •Hypoglycemia •Environmental Pollution & Heavy Metal Poisoning •Kidney Stones & Infection •Eczema & Psoriasis •Herpes •Meningitis & Rheumatic Fever •Acne & Dermatitis •Mononucleosis & Hepatitis •Malignant Tumors •Warts, Abscesses & Cysts •HIV Virus/AIDS •Epilepsy •Internal Parasites & Worms.

✦COMPOUNDS FOR FORMULATION SHOULD INCLUDE:

•Herbal compounds for (a) blood purification, (b) mucous and (c) bowel cleansing. During a cleanse, the body decomposes and burns only the substances and tissues that are damaged, diseased or unneeded, such as abscesses, tumors, excess fat deposits, and congestive wastes. Even a relatively short fast accelerates elimination, often causing dramatic changes as masses of accumulated waste are expelled. Living medicinal foods like therapeutic plants literally pick up dead matter from the body and carry it away.

You will be very aware of this if you experience the short period of headaches, fatigue, body odor, bad breath, diarrhea or mouth sores that commonly accompany accelerated elimination. However, digestion usually improves right away as do many gland and nerve functions.

•Herbal compounds for rebuilding liver, organ and glandular health. The second part of a good cleansing program is rebuilding healthy tissue and restoring body energy. This phase allows the body's regulating powers to become active with obstacles removed, so it can rebuild at optimum levels.

•Herbal compounds for long term rebuilding and maintenance. The final part of a good cleansing program is keeping your body clean and toxin-free - very important after all the hard work of detoxification. Modifying lifestyle habits to include high quality nutrition from both food and supplement sources is the key to a strong resistant body.

Note: A full spectrum combination might encompass herbs for each of these objectives, and may be used as a long term detoxification requiring several months. A more recommended program would include two or more different combinations, to be used consecutively for better focus and strength.

33

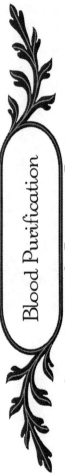

Blood Purification

Detoxification & Cleansing Compounds

Your blood is your river of life. The health of your blood is critical. It is the chief neutralizing agent for bacteria and toxic wastes. Many diseases are the result of blood toxins, because toxins ingested in sub-lethal amounts can eventually add up to disease-causing amounts. This is especially true in the three blood cleansing systems: the liver, the kidneys and the lymph glands. While the body has its own self-purifying complex for maintaining healthy blood, the best way to protect yourself from disease is to keep those cleansing systems in good working order. Herbs provide strengthening support for a successful blood cleanse. Detoxifying herbs can maintain energy levels and nerve stability during heavy metabolic waste elimination. They can supply concentrated chlorophyll benefits and alkalize body acidity. The molecular composition of chlorophyll is so close to that of human hemoglobin that a series of "green supplements" is almost like giving yourself a purifying transfusion.

❧ ESSENTIAL CATEGORIES FOR AN EFFECTIVE BLOOD PURIFYING COMPOUND:

Lymph Stimulation	Detoxification Herbs	Body Chemistry Balancers	Antihistamine & Liver Stimulation	Anti-Viral Herbs	Anti-Bacterial Herbs
Echinacea root	Pau d'arco bark	Dandelion root	Oregon grape root	St. John's wort	Goldenseal root
Goldenseal root	Burdock root	Alfalfa	Milk thistle seed	Reishi mushroom	Usnea
Myrrh	White Sage	Kelp/other sea plants	Red sage	Bee pollen & propolis	Aloe vera
Ginger root	Red Clover Blossom	Marshmallow root	Bupleurum	Osha root	Myrrh
Licorice root	Licorice root	Yellow dock root	Wild Yam root	Garlic	Black walnut hulls
Capsicum	Sarsaparilla root	Chlorella	Bee pollen	Echinacea root	Garlic
Prickly ash	Japanese green tea	Barley grass	Bayberry	Lomatium dissectum	Chaparral
Burdock root	Butternut bark	Chamomile	Rose hips	Astragalus bark	Echinacea root
Hawthorn lf. flr. & bry.	Nettles	Barberry bark	Yellow dock root	Maitake mushroom	Propolis

❧ ESSENTIAL HERBS FOR AN EFFECTIVE BLOOD PURIFYING COMPOUND:

Primary Herbs		Assisting & Complementary Herbs	Catalyst & Transporting Herbs	
Echinacea root	Chlorella	Alfalfa	Capsicum	Bayberry
Licorice root	Barley Grass	Marshmallow root	Kelp	Rosemary
Goldenseal root	Sarsaparilla root	Oregon grape root	Ginger root	Parsley root & leaf
Dandelion	Hawthorn lf. flr. & bry.	Yellow dock root	Fennel seed	Chamomile
Red clover blossom	Nettles	Prickly ash bark	Cinnamon	Chaparral
Burdock root	White sage	Aloe vera juice	Poria mushroom	Propolis/Bee pollen
Pau d'arco bark	Kelp & ocean plants	St. John's wort	Gotu kola	Black walnut hulls
Milk thistle seed	Panax ginseng	Garlic	Ginkgo biloba	Osha root
Reishi mushroom	Japanese green tea	Barberry bark	Usnea	Rose hips

❧ EXAMPLE FORMULAS OF BLOOD PURIFYING COMPOUNDS:

A TEA COMPOUND			(CD - 5120)	A CAPSULE COMPOUND		(CD - 2000)
Red clover blossom	White sage	Pau d'arco bark	Yerba santa	Red clover blossom	Butternut bark	Yellow dock root
Hawthorn lf. flr. bry.	Horsetail	Gotu kola		Licorice root	Garlic	Buckthorn bark
Alfalfa	Echinacea root	Lemongrass		Burdock root	Goldenseal root	Prickly ash bark
Nettles	Milk Thistle seed	Blue malva		Pau d'arco bark	Astragalus	Panax ginseng

SEE PAGE 1 FOR FORMULATING INSTRUCTIONS.

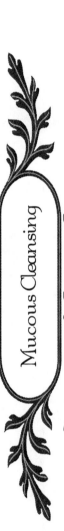

Mucous Cleansing

Detoxification & Cleansing Compounds

A lung and mucous congestion cleanse can help if you have chronic colds, allergies or asthma. Excess mucous may be a sign that the body is trying to bring itself to health. Human beings take about 22,000 breaths a day, and along with the oxygen, we take in dirt, pollen, disease germs, smoke and other pollutants. Mucous gathers up these irritants as they enter the nose and throat, protecting the mucous membranes that line the upper respiratory system. The lungs are on the front line of toxic intake from viruses, pollutants, and mucous-forming congestives. Herbal supplements are a good choice during a mucous and congestion cleanse. They act as premier broncho-dilators and anti-spasmodics to open congested airspaces. They can soothe bronchial inflammation and cough. They have the ability to break up mucous. They are expectorants to remove mucous from the lungs and throat.

ESSENTIAL CATEGORIES FOR AN EFFECTIVE MUCOUS CLEANSING COMPOUND:

Loosen & Flush Mucous	Increase Oxygen Uptake	Expectorant Herbs	Soothing, Demulcent Herbs	Dissolve Congestion & Obstruction	Stimulate Lymph & Circulation
Elecampane	**Rosemary**	**Horehound**	**Marshmallow root**	**Elder Flower & Berry**	**Echinacea root**
Boneset	**Mullein**	**Eucalyptus**	White willow bark	**Myrrh**	**Goldenseal root**
Garlic	**Ginkgo biloba**	**Licorice root**	Passionflower	**Fenugreek seed**	**Capsicum**
Fenugreek seed	**Ma huang**	Horseradish	**Slippery elm**	**Usnea barbata**	**Ginger root**
Marshmallow root	**White pine bark**	**Pleurisy root**	Parsley root	Elecampane	Peppermint
Eyebright	Wild cherry bark	**Coltsfoot**	**Wild cherry bark**	Peppermint	Garlic
Lobelia	Bee pollen	Anise seed	**Comfrey root**	**Lobelia**	Cloves
Yarrow	Red sage	Hyssop	Irish moss	Sage	Nettles
Pleurisy root	Chaparral	Fennel seed	Flax seed	Ginger root	Peppermint

ESSENTIAL HERBS FOR AN EFFECTIVE MUCOUS CLEANSING COMPOUND:

Primary Herbs		Assisting & Complementary Herbs		Catalyst & Transporting Herbs	
Echinacea root	Slippery elm	Garlic	Licorice root	Capsicum	Aloe vera juice
Boneset	Eyebright	Horehound	Rose hips	Gotu kola	Rosemary
Marshmallow root	Wild cherry bark	Fenugreek seed	Peppermint	Elecampane	Lobelia
Mullein	Coltsfoot	Pleurisy root	Myrrh	Ginkgo biloba	Garlic
Ma huang	Nettles	Eucalyptus	Passionflower	Ginger root	Cloves
Elder flower & berry	Chaparral	Sage	Angelica root	Cinnamon	Calendula
Elecampane	Mullein	Goldenseal root	Usnea barbata	Lemon peel	Fennel
Comfrey root	Yarrow	Anise seed	Hyssop	Green tea	Hyssop
Parsley root	White willow bark	Yarrow	White pine bark	Bee pollen	Horseradish

EXAMPLE FORMULAS FOR MUCOUS CLEANSING COMPOUNDS:

A BRONCHO-DILATING TEA TO OPEN BREATHING PASSAGES (B - 5010)			AN EXPECTORANT TEA TO RELEASE MUCOUS (B - 5930)		
Marshmallow root	Ma Huang	Rosemary	Ma Huang	Mullein	Peppermint	Ginger root
Fenugreek seed	Wild Cherry	Angelica root	Licorice root	Rose Hips	Fennel	Calendula
Mullein	Ginkgo Biloba	Lobelia	Pleurisy root	Marshmallow	Boneset	
	Cinnamon bark	Passionflower				

SEE PAGE 1 FOR FORMULATING INSTRUCTIONS.

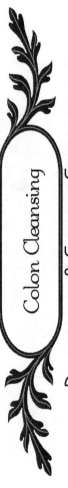

Colon Cleansing

DETOXIFICATION & CLEANSING COMPOUNDS

A colon elimination cleanse is something most of us need. The bowel and colon are essential to body detoxification. When colon health is compromised, there is greater release of toxins from the bowel into the bloodstream, causing diseases, organ dysfunction and accelerated aging. Constipation is usually a chronic problem, and while body cleansing progress can be felt fairly quickly with a diet change, it takes from three to six months to rebuild bowel and colon elasticity with good systole/diastole action. The rewards of a regular, energetic life are worth it. Look for reduced immunity, tiredness, coated tongue, bad breath, body odor, mental dullness and sallow skin. **You can easily combine a colon cleanse with a cholesterol cleanse.** If your cholesterol numbers are too high, a colon cleanse is a good choice because it increases absorption of cholesterol-lowering foods and also helps you lose colon congestive weight.

ESSENTIAL CATEGORIES FOR AN EFFECTIVE COLON CLEANSING COMPOUND:

LOOSEN & FLUSH WASTES	DETOXIFY THE COLON	IMPROVE BODY CHEMISTRY	SOOTHING DEMULCENT HERBS	REGULATE WASTE FILTERING FUNCTIONS	NORMALIZE PERISTALSIS
Cascara sagrada	**Sarsaparilla root**	**Aloe vera**	**Marshmallow root**	**Yellow dock root**	**Capsicum**
Senna leaf & pods	**Licorice root**	**Pau d' arco**	**Slippery Elm**	**Dandelion root**	Butcher's broom
Butternut bark	**Pau d' arco bark**	**Miso**	Flax seed	**Oregon grape root**	**Ginger root**
Psyllium husks	Echinacea root	Marshmallow root	**Irish moss**	Ginger root	Buckthorn bark
Flax seed	**Barberry bark**	**Peppermint**	Fenugreek seed	Buckthorn bark	**Peppermint**
Rhubarb root	Burdock root	**Green tea**	Comfrey root	Red sage	**Boneset**
Barberry bark	Horsetail	Fennel seed	Papaya	Burdock root	**Butternut bark**
Buckthorn bark	Chaparral	Calendula flowers	Calendula	Gotu kola	Miso
Aloe vera juice	Irish moss	Wild yam root	Lobelia	Nettles	Black walnut hulls

ESSENTIAL HERBS FOR AN EFFECTIVE COLON CLEANSING COMPOUND:

PRIMARY HERBS	ASSISTING & COMPLEMENTARY HERBS	CATALYST & TRANSPORTING HERBS
Butternut bark	Marshmallow root	Capsicum
Turkey rhubarb root	Gotu kola	Calendula
Cascara sagrada	Slippery elm	Miso
Psyllium husks	Calendula flowers	Peppermint
Barberry bark	Irish moss	Ginger root
Flax seed	Papaya	Lobelia
Buckthorn bark	Burdock root	Lemon balm
Aloe vera juice	Fenugreek seed	Hibiscus
Pau d' arco	Green tea	Butcher's broom

				Aloe vera juice		
				Black walnut hulls		
				Parsley root		
				Kelp		
				Lemon peel		
				Chaparral		

EXAMPLE FORMULAS FOR COLON CLEANSING COMPOUNDS:

AN EVACUATING FORMULA THAT RESTORES PERISTALSIS (CD - 2350)				A GENTLE CAPSULE FORMULA FOR AN IRRITABLE BOWEL (CD - 1560)		
Butternut bark	Psyllium husks	Licorice root	Capsicum	Peppermint	Slippery Elm	Lobelia	Ginger root
Cascara sagrada	Barberry bark	Ginger root		Peppermint oil	Marshmallow	Wild yam root	
Turkey rhubarb	Fennel seed	Irish moss		Aloe vera	Pau d' arco bark		

SEE PAGE 1 FOR FORMULATING INSTRUCTIONS.

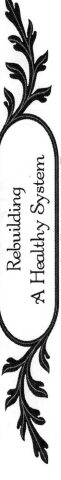

Rebuilding A Healthy System

Detoxification & Cleansing Compounds

The second part of a good cleansing program is rebuilding healthy tissue and restoring body energy. This stage usually begins after two to three weeks of waste and toxin elimination. Effective herbal compounds make a big difference in the success and rapidity with which the body rebuilds its strength. Targets for rebuilding a healthy system should include stimulating deep body areas like the glands, (especially the adrenals), organs, muscles and immune response. A broad spectrum herbal gland-balancing formula can nourish, regulate and extend gland and cell life. Mineral rich herbs are specifics for strong body building blocks. They provide a regular, daily way to get absorbable minerals, silica and iodine. As the herbal minerals accumulate in the body, a noticeable improvement may be seen in outwardly in hair and skin health and inwardly in overall immune response.

❧ ESSENTIAL CATEGORIES FOR SYSTEM REBUILDING COMPOUNDS:

BUILD RED BLOOD CELLS	BALANCE BODY CHEMISTRY	STRENGTHEN & REGENERATE	ENHANCE LIVER & ORGAN HEALTH	ENHANCE GLAND & HORMONE HEALTH	IMPROVE MUSCLE & SKIN TONE
Chlorella	Alfalfa	Bee pollen	**Milk thistle seed**	**Panax ginseng**	Sarsaparilla root
Spirulina	**Spirulina**	**Panax/Siber.ginseng**	**Dandelion root**	**Dong quai**	**Siberian ginseng**
Barley grass	**Kelp & sea vegetables**	**Miso & rice protein**	Barley grass	**Wild yam root**	Bee pollen
Dandelion leaf & root	**Bee pollen**	Marshmallow root	Yellow dock root	**Saw palmetto berry**	**Royal Jelly**
Hawthorn bry. & lf.	Ginkgo biloba	**Barley grass**	Alfalfa	**Burdock root**	Bilberry
Yellow dock root	Burdock root	Ginkgo biloba	**Sarsaparilla root**	**Licorice root**	Licorice root
Red clover	Prickly ash	Horsetail	**Red sage**	Kelp & sea vegetables	Alfalfa
Parsley leaf	Rose hips	Gotu kola	Black cohosh	**Red raspberry**	**Gotu kola**
Suma root	Reishi mushroom	Ashwagandha	Echinacea root	St. John's wort	Prince ginseng root

❧ ESSENTIAL HERBS FOR SYSTEM REBUILDING COMPOUND:

PRIMARY HERBS		ASSISTING & COMPLEMENTARY HERBS		CATALYST & TRANSPORTING HERBS	
Siberian ginseng	Ginkgo biloba	Gotu kola	Wild yam root	Sea plants - kelp, irish	Aloe vera juice
Hawthorn lf. & bry.	Dandelion root & lf.	Bee pollen	Horsetail	moss, dulse, etc.	Nettles
Spirulina	Licorice root	Chinese ginseng	Prince ginseng root	Ginger root	Bee pollen
Chlorella	Kelp & sea plants	Milk thistle seed	Black cohosh	Capsicum	Bilberry berries
Sarsaparilla root	Reishi mushroom	Burdock root	Saw palmetto berry	Ma huang	Fennel seed
Yellow dock root	Astragalus	Ashwagandha	Pau d' arco bark	Rose hips	Watercress
Barley grass	Panax ginseng root	Prickly ash bark	St. John's wort	Red raspberry	Uva ursi
Alfalfa	Suma root	Dong quai	Echinacea root	Miso	Parsley leaf
Royal Jelly	Red clover	Marshmallow root	Red sage	Rice protein	

❧ EXAMPLE FORMULAS FOR SYSTEM REBUILDING COMPOUNDS:

A REBUILDING ADRENAL SUPPORT FORMULA			(E - 1000)
Licorice root	Uva ursi	Astragalus root	Bee pollen
Sarsaparilla root	Irish moss	Capsicum	
Bladderwrack	Ginger root	Rose hips	

A RESTORATIVE GINSENG SUPER TEA FORMULA			(PD - 6380)
Prince ginseng root	Pau d' arco	St. John's wort	Reishi Mushroom
Kirin ginseng root	Echinacea Ang.	Ephedra	Fennel seed
Suma root	Echinacea Purp.	Chinese ginseng	Tienchi root
Aralia root	Astragalus root	Siberian ginseng	Ginger root

SEE PAGE 1 FOR FORMULATING INSTRUCTIONS.

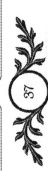

37

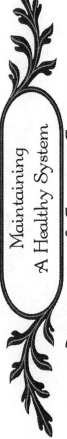

Maintaining A Healthy System

Detoxification & Cleansing Compounds

The final part of a cleansing program is keeping the body clean and toxin-free - very important after all the hard work of detoxification. High quality nutrition from both food and supplement sources is the key to a strong, resistant body. Remember that cleansing helps release hormone secretions that stimulate the immune system, and encourage a disease-preventing environment. The foods for a good immune defense diet should rely heavily on fresh fruits and vegetables for regulating fiber and body chemistry health. It should include cooked vegetables, whole grains and seeds for strength; sea foods, eggs, and low-fat cheeses as sources of quality protein; and lightly cooked sea foods and vegetables with a little dinner wine for circulatory health. A good, long range herbal formula can be a whole body tonic supplement to help rebuild tissue, strengthen muscle, maintain stamina and body tone, and enhance immunity.

❧ ESSENTIAL CATEGORIES FOR LONG TERM MAINTENANCE COMPOUNDS:

BODY BALANCE & ALKALINITY	LIVER & ORGAN HEALTH	GLAND & HORMONE HEALTH	MINERAL-RICH HERBS	CHLOROPHYLL-RICH ENZYME-RICH HERBS	TONIC ADAPTOGEN HERBS
Lemongrass	Watercress	Licorice root	Kelp/sea vegetables	Kelp/sea vegetables	All ginseng types
Bee pollen	Licorice root	Saw palmetto berry	Nettles	Spirulina	Rosemary
Garlic	Gotu kola	Black cohosh	Garlic	Chlorella	Astragalus
All ginseng types	Milk thistle seed	Red raspberry	Dandelion root & lf.	Barley grass	Gingko biloba
Hawthorn bry. & lf.	Hyssop	Sarsaparilla	Yellow dock root	Alfalfa	Siberian ginseng
Ginger root	Burdock root	Wild yam root	Oatstraw	Watercress	Suma root
Bilberry	Capsicum	Burdock root	Irish moss	Parsley	Gotu kola
Chlorophyll-rich herbs	Horsetail	Ashwagandha	Horsetail	Nettles	Ashwagandha
Kelp/sea vegetables	Wild yam root	Panax ginseng	Miso powder	Papaya	Panax ginseng

❧ ESSENTIAL HERBS FOR LONG TERM MAINTENANCE COMPOUNDS:

PRIMARY HERBS		ASSISTING & COMPLEMENTARY HERBS		CATALYST & TRANSPORTING HERBS	
Siberian Ginseng	Ginkgo biloba	Wild yam root	Aloe vera	Capsicum	Rosemary
Panax ginseng	Alfalfa	Ashwagandha	Schizandra berry	Ginger root	Nettles
Bee pollen	Pau d' arco	Yellow Dock root	Prince ginseng root	Kelp	Borage seed
Dandelion root & leaf	Hawthorn Bry. & Lf.	Garlic	Black cohosh	Miso powder	Parsley rt. & lf.
Spirulina	Reishi mushroom	Burdock root	Saw palmetto berry	Acidophilus	Red raspberry
Licorice root	Astragalus	Milk thistle seed	Oatstraw	Bilberry berries	Spearmint
Kelp & sea plants	Chlorella	Gotu kola	Lemongrass	Fennel seed	Stevia Herb
Barley grass	Suma root	Horsetail	Sage	Watercress	Nutritional yeast
Kelp/sea vegetables	Panax ginseng	Nettles	Hyssop	Fennel seed	Cranberry

❧ EXAMPLE FORMULAS FOR LONG TERM MAINTENANCE COMPOUNDS:

A SYSTEM STRENGTHING CAPSULE FORMULA		(SA - 4080)	A "FEEL GREAT" TEA FORMULA		(E - 5330)
Bee pollen	Barley grass	Siberian ginseng	Red clover blossom	Prince ginseng	Licorice root
Nutritional yeast	Dandelion root	Nettles	Alfalfa	Spearmint	Stevia herb
Alfalfa	Licorice root	Bilberry berry	Hawthorn bry. & lf.	Dandelion root	Dulse
Oatstraw	Pau d' arco	Rosemary			
	Spirulina	Sea plants			
	Chlorella	Red raspberry			

SEE PAGE 1 FOR FORMULATING INSTRUCTIONS.

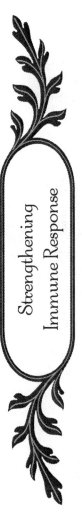

Strengthening Immune Response

We hear so much about immune system breakdown today. Yet, most of us don't know very much about it, or how it works. It's really an amazing part of our bodies. The immune system is the body's most complex and delicately balanced infrastructure. While the workings of other body systems have been well known for some time, the complex nature and dynamics of the immune system have been largely a mystery. One of the problems in comprehending immune response is its highly individual nature. It's a personal defense system that comes charging to the rescue at the first sign of an alien force, such as a harmful virus or pathogenic bacteria. Personal immune response shows us that there is so much more to our healing than the latest wonder drug. It shows us that we are the ultimate healer of ourselves.

The immune system is not responsive to drugs for healing. Even doctors admit that most drugs really just stabilize the body, or arrest a harmful organism, to allow the immune system to gather its forces and take over. The character of immune response varies widely between people, making it almost impossible to form a drug that will stimulate immunity for everyone. But natural nutritive forces, like healing foods and herbal medicines **can and do** support the immune system. They enhance its activity, strengthen it, and provide an environment through cleansing and detoxification for it to work at its best.

Immune defense is autonomic and subconscious. It's a system that works on its own to fend off or neutralize disease toxins, and set up a healing environment for the body. It is this quality of being a part of us, yet not under our conscious control, that is the great power of immune response. It is also the dilemma of medical scientists as they struggle to get control of a system that is all pervasive and yet, in the end, impossible to completely understand. It is as if God shows us his face in this incredibly complex part of us, where we are allowed to glimpse the ultimate mind-body connection.

Maintaining strong immune defenses in today's world is not easy. Daily exposure to environmental pollutants, the emotional and excessive stresses of modern lifestyles, chemicalized foods, and new virus mutations are all a challenge to our immune systems. Devastating, immune-deficient diseases are rising all over the world. Reduced immunity is the main factor in opportunistic diseases, like candida albicans, chronic fatigue syndrome, lupus, HIV, hepatitis, mononucleosis, herpes II, sexually transmitted diseases and cancer. These diseases have become the epidemic of our time, and most of us don't have very much to fight with. An overload of antibiotics, antacids, immunizations, cortico-steroid drugs, and environmental pollutants eventually affect immune system balance to the point where it cannot distinguish harmful cells from healthy cells.

I see traditional, drug-based medicine as "heroic" medicine. Largely developed in wartime, its greatest strengths are emergency measures - the ability to arrest a crisis, destroy or incapacitate pathogenic organisms, reset and re-attach broken body parts, and stabilize the body so it can gather its healing forces. Because drugs work in an attempt to directly kill harmful organisms, it is easy to see that their value would be for emergency measures, and for short term use.

But, three unwanted things often happen with **prolonged** drug use: 1) Our bodies can build up a tolerance to the drug so that it requires more of it to get the same effect. 2) The drug slowly overwhelms immune response so the body becomes dependent upon it, using it as a crutch instead of doing its own work. 3) The drug misleads the body's defense system to the point that it doesn't know what to assault, and attacks everything in confusion. This type of over-reaction often happens during an allergy attack, where the immune system may respond to substances that are not really harmful. Most of the time, if we use drugs wisely to stimulate rather than over kill, if we "get out of the way" by keeping our bodies clean and well nourished, the immune system will spend its energies rebuilding instead of fighting, and strengthen us instead of constantly gathering resources to conduct a "rear guard" defense.

The very nature of immune strength means that it must be built from the inside out. The immune system is the body system most sensitive to nutritional deficiencies. Giving your body generous, high quality, natural remedies at the first sign of infection improves your chances of overcoming disease before it takes serious hold. Powerful, immune-enhancing superfoods and herbs can be directed at "early warning" problems to build strength for immune response. Building good immune defenses takes time and commitment, but it's worth it. The inherited immunity and health of you, your children and your grandchildren is laid down by you.

FORMULAS FOR IMMUNE STRENGTH ARE EFFECTIVE FOR THE FOLLOWING CONDITIONS:

•Viral & Bacterial Infections •Staph & Strep Infections •Measles •Chronic Fatigue Syndromes •Fibromyalgia •Environmental Pollution & Heavy Metal Poisoning •Candida Albicans •Chronic Colds •Pneumonia •Lupus •Normalizing After Overuse of Prescription or Recreational Drugs •Cervical Dysplasia & HPV •Mononucleosis & Hepatitis •Tumors •Warts, Abscesses & Cysts •Herpes •Meningitis & Rheumatic Fever •Toxic Shock •Internal Parasites & Worms.

COMPOUNDS FOR FORMULATION SHOULD INCLUDE:

•Herbal compounds to improve body chemistry and composition.
•Herbal compounds to detoxify and cleanse the liver, organs and lymph system.
•Herbal compounds to rebuild immunity after surgery or illness.
•Herbal enzymes for maintaining immune vitality.

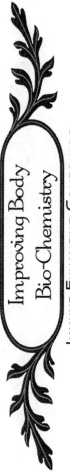

Improving Body Bio-Chemistry

IMMUNE ENHANCING COMPOUNDS

The challenges to our body's defense system are great. Can plants really boost human immunity? Herbs are excellent choices for immune enhancement. The highly complex nature of therapeutic herbs is a good match for that of the immune system. Their value in renewing immune response is unequalled because they are able to support and nourish the body while it rebuilds and normalizes, something drugs are not able to do. We know that the body is basically a self-healing organism. Modern herbal therapy uses herbs to normalize body systems, to give the body a clean slate to better heal itself. Herbal "power plants," are really nutriceuticals. They offer concentrated nutrients with superior absorbability for the human body. They may be used over a long period of time without side effects. As inexpensive, nutrient-rich food supplements, they are becoming more and more relevant in a world that is becoming almost hostile to our health.

❧ ESSENTIAL CATEGORIES FOR IMPROVING BODY BIO-CHEMISTRY:

LYMPH STIMULATION	DETOXIFICATION HERBS	BODY CHEMISTRY BALANCERS	ANTIHISTAMINE & LIVER STIMULATION	ANTI-VIRAL HERBS	ANTI-BACTERIAL HERBS
Echinacea root	Pau d'arco bark	**Dandelion root**	**Oregon grape root**	**St. John's wort**	**Goldenseal root**
Goldenseal root	**Barley grass**	Alfalfa/Barley grass	**Milk thistle seed**	**Reishi mushroom**	**Usnea**
Myrrh	**White sage**	**Kelp/other sea plants**	Red sage	Bee pollen/ Royal jelly	Reishi mushroom
Ginger root	Red clover blossom	Hawthorn lf. flr. & bry.	**Bupleurum**	**Propolis**	Myrrh
Licorice root	Licorice root	Spirulina/**Chlorella**	Wild yam root	**Garlic**	**Black walnut hulls**
Capsicum	Sarsaparilla root	Astragalus	**Bee pollen**	**Echinacea root**	**Garlic**
Prickly ash bark	Japanese green tea	Ginkgo biloba	Gotu kola	Lomatium dissectum	Kelp & sea plants
Nettles	**Aloe vera**	Ginseng - all types	Rose hips	**Aloe vera**	**Echinacea root**
Reishi mushroom	**Burdock root**	White pine bark	**Yellow dock root**	**Maitake mushroom**	**Propolis**

❧ ESSENTIAL HERBS FOR IMPROVING BODY BIOCHEMISTRY:

PRIMARY HERBS		ASSISTING & COMPLEMENTARY HERBS		CATALYST & TRANSPORTING HERBS	
Echinacea root	Chlorella	Red clover blossom	Astragalus	Capsicum	Aloe vera juice
Licorice root	Barley Grass	Pau d'arco bark	Goldenseal root	Kelp	Rosemary
Spirulina	Sarsaparilla root	Dandellon	Horsetall	Ginger root	Parsley root
Reishi mushroom	Hawthorn lf. flr. & bry.	Yellow dock root	Myrrh	Fennel seed	Parsley leaf
Bee pollen	Nettles	Prickly ash bark	Ginkgo biloba	Japanese green tea	Lemon peel
Siberian ginseng	Gotu kola	Wild yam	Bilberry	Propolis	Apple pectin
Alfalfa	Kelp & ocean plants	St. John's wort	Lemon balm	Rose hips	Acerola cherry
White pine bark	Panax ginseng	Garlic	Royal jelly	Lemongrass	Black walnut hulls
Maitake mushroom	Burdock root	White sage	Bupleurum	Oregon grape root	Usnea

❧ EXAMPLE FORMULAS OF BODY BIO-CHEMISTRY ENHANCING COMPOUNDS:

AN ENERGY GREEN DRINK COMPOUND		(SA - 8150)	AN ANTI-OXIDANT CAPSULE COMPOUND		(PD - 3840)
Barley grass/sprouts	Acerola cherry	Dandelion lf./rt.	Lemon peel	White pine bark	Rosehips Vit. C	Licorice root	Hawthorn
Alfalfa grass/sprouts	Sarsaparilla root	Gotu kola	Spirulina	Rosemary	Echinacea Ang..	Astragalus	Bilberry
Bee pollen	Chlorella	Licorice root	Rice protein	Siberian ginseng	Pau d'arco bark	Lemon balm	Spirulina
Siberian ginseng	Dulse	Hawthorn	Apple pectin	Ginkgo biloba	Red clover	Garlic	

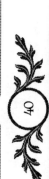

SEE PAGE 1 FOR FORMULATING INSTRUCTIONS.

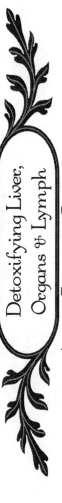

Detoxifying Liver, Organs & Lymph

IMMUNE ENHANCING COMPOUNDS

The health and vitality of the body depend to a large extent on the health and vitality of the liver. A liver and organ cleanse can get to the bottom of a lot of health problems. A healthy liver produces natural antihistamines to keep immunity high. A healthy liver, organs and lymph system can deal with a wide range of toxic chemicals and pollutants that continually assail us in our food, water and air. The liver has amazing rejuvenative powers, and continues to function when as many as 80% of its cells are damaged. Even more remarkable, the liver regenerates its own damaged tissue. **Do you need a liver and organ cleanse?** Body signals that your liver and organs need some TLC include great fatigue, unexplained weight gain, depression or melancholy, mental confusion, sluggish elimination system, food and chemical sensitivity, PMS, jaundiced skin or liver spots on the skin, repeated nausea, dizziness and dry mouth.

❧ ESSENTIAL CATEGORIES FOR LIVER AND ORGAN CLEANSING COMPOUNDS:

LIVER & ORGAN TONIC HERBS	ACID/ALKALINE BALANCE	ANTI-INFECTIVE HERBS	THYMUS & LYMPH STIMULATION	GLAND & ADRENAL STIMULANTS	ANTIOXIDANT HERBS
Nettles	**Alfalfa/Watercress**	**Garlic**	**Echinacea root**	**Licorice root**	Kelp/ocean plants
Milk thistle seed	Fennel seed	**Myrrh**	**Goldenseal root**	**Sarsaparilla root**	**Rosemary**
Oregon grape root	Barley grass	Capsicum	**Kelp/sea plants**	Bladderwrack/Kelp	Siberian ginseng
Yellow dock root	**Dandelion root**	St. John's wort	Hawthorn lf., bry., flr.	**Bee pollen**	**Barley grass**
Barberry bark	**Burdock root**	**Turmeric**	Chlorella/Spirulina	**Royal jelly**	**Spirulina**
Red sage	**Japanese green tea**	Alfalfa	Garlic	Wild yam root	**Garlic**
Hyssop	Chamomile	Bilberry	**Reishi mushroom**	Yarrow	**Chlorella**
Beet root	Ginger root	White willow bark	Royal jelly	Ginger root	Parsley leaf
Gotu kola	Lemongrass	Pau d'arco bark	Red clover	Astragalus	Ginsengs - all types

❧ ESSENTIAL HERBS FOR LIVER AND ORGAN CLEANSING COMPOUNDS:

PRIMARY HERBS	ASSISTING & COMPLEMENTARY HERBS	CATALYST & TRANSPORTING HERBS
Echinacea root	Goldenseal root	Reishi mushroom	Astragalus	Aloe vera juice
Licorice root	Gotu kola	Wild cherry bark	Rosemary	Turmeric
Milk thistle seed	St. John's wort	White sage	Kelp	White willow bark
Kelp/ocean plants	Barberry bark	Myrrh	Capsicum	Cloves
Pau d'arco bark	Hyssop	Lemongrass	Parsley lf.	Calendula
Watercress	Red sage	Alfalfa	Yerba santa	Fennel
Yellow dock root	Sarsaparilla root	Ginkgo biloba	Ginger root	Bilberry
Oregon grape root	Wild yam root	Burdock root	Lecithin	Chamomile
Chlorella/Spirulina	Garlic	Japanese green tea	Brewer's yeast	Lobelia

(Note: Primary Herbs table has additional entries: Siberian ginseng, Bee pollen/Royal jelly, Beet root, Hawthorn lf., bry., flr., Nettles, Dandelion rt. & lf., Red clover, Yarrow, Barley grass)

❧ EXAMPLE FORMULAS OF LIVER AND ORGAN CLEANSING COMPOUNDS:

A CLEANSING & PURIFYING TEA FOR LIVER & ORGANS			(CD - 5120)
Red clover blsm.	White sage	Pau d'arco bk.	Blue malva
Hawthorn	Horsetail	Gotu kola	Yerba santa
Alfalfa	Echinacea root	Lemongrass	
Nettles	Milk thistle seed		

A LIVER DETOX CAPSULE			(CD - 3000)
Beet root	Milk thistle seed	Licorice root	Barberry bark
Oregon grape root	Yellow dock root	Gotu kola	Lecithin granules
Dandelion rt.	Ginkgo biloba	Ginger root	
Wild yam root	Wild cherry bark		

SEE PAGE 1 FOR FORMULATING INSTRUCTIONS.

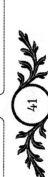

41

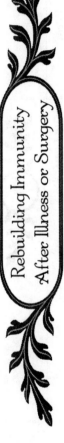

Rebuilding Immunity After Illness or Surgery

IMMUNE ENHANCING COMPOUNDS

Herbal remedies can do a great deal toward minimizing the damage and rebuilding the body after surgery, chemotherapy and radiation. Herbal support is a good choice for faster and better healing, cleansing the body of drug residues, overcoming drug side effects, and rebuilding immune strength. Your body has wonderful self-healing powers, but after injury or illness, it often needs extra help to do it. Herbs pave the way for the body to do its own work, by breaking up toxins, cleansing, lubricating, toning and nourishing. Healing/mending herbs supply minerals for building blocks and nutrient assimilation, carotenes as anti-infectives, B and C vitamins for tissue regrowth, and amino acids as protein precursors for body strength. Many healing herbs have antibiotic properties to help overcome harmful bacteria and infections. Many are effective anti-oxidants to discourage illness relapse, and to create a high tissue oxygen environment where disease cannot flourish.

✦ ESSENTIAL CATEGORIES FOR REBUILDING AFTER SURGERY OR ILLNESS:

BLOOD & LYMPH CLEANSING HERBS	LIVER & ORGAN TONIC HERBS	GLAND & ADRENAL STIMULANTS	CHLOROPHYLL SOURCE HERBS	IMMUNE-ENHANCING PROTECTORS	ANTIOXIDANT HERBS
Echinacea root	**Milk thistle seed**	**Licorice root**	**Chlorella**	**Astragalus**	**White pine bark**
Goldenseal root	**Red sage**	**Kelp/sea vegetables**	**Spirulina**	**Suma**	**Gotu kola**
Kelp/sea plants	**Dandelion root & lf.**	**Ginger root**	**Kelp/Bladderwrack**	**Ginseng - all types**	**Chlorella**
Hawthorn lf., bry., flr.	**Chlorophyll-rich herbs**	**Gotu kola**	**Nettles**	**Pau d'arco bark**	**Spirulina**
Chlorella/Spirulina	Wild yam root	**Barley grass**	**Barley grass**	**Reishi mushroom**	Alfalfa
Red clover	Yellow dock root	**Bee pollen/royal jelly**	**Alfalfa**	**Schizandra berry**	Siberian ginseng
Garlic	**Oregon grape root**	Sarsaparilla root	**Watercress**	Garlic	Garlic
Reishi mushroom	Flax seed	Bayberry bark	Parsley leaf	Capsicum	Rosemary
Royal jelly	Lobelia	Hawthorn lf., bry., fl.	Comfrey leaf	Burdock root	**Ginkgo biloba**

✦ ESSENTIAL HERBS FOR REBUILDING AFTER SURGERY OR ILLNESS:

PRIMARY HERBS		ASSISTING & COMPLEMENTARY HERBS		CATALYST & TRANSPORTING HERBS	
Garlic	Schizandra	Spirulina	Black cohosh	Aloe vera	Garlic
Siberian ginseng root	Bee pollen & royal jelly	Yellow dock root	Wild yam root	Peppermint	Lobelia
Chlorella	Licorice root	Reishi mushroom	Peppermint	Capsicum	Calendula
Astragalus	Suma	Goldenseal root	Myrrh	Rosemary	Fennel
Echinacea root	Nettles	White pine bark	Dandelion rt. & lf.	Ginger root	Wild cherry bk.
Gotu kola	Alfalfa	Dandelion root & lf.	Milk thistle seed	Bayberry bark	Comfrey leaf
Pau d'arco bark	Ginseng - all types	Burdock root	Yarrow	Acidophilus powder	Guggul
Kelp/sea vegetables	Barley grass	Red sage	Horsetail	Nutritional yeast pwr.	Elecampane
Hawthorn lf., bry., fl.	Ginkgo biloba	Red clover	Sarsaparilla root	Parsley leaf	Miso powder

✦ EXAMPLE FORMULAS FOR REBUILDING AFTER SURGERY OR ILLNESS:

A REBUILDING, FEEL GREAT, CAPSULE COMPOUND			(E - 2250)	AN HERBAL DEFENSE EXTRACT COMPOUND			(PD - 4780)
Bee pollen	Licorice	Wild cherry bk.	Hawthorn	Garlic	Hawthorn lf./bry.	Pau d'arco bk.	Peppermint
Siberian ginseng	Suma	Black cohosh	Panax ginseng	Echinacea Rt.	Goldenseal rt.	Astragalus rt	
Gotu kola	Schizandra	Kelp	Spirulina	Siberian ginseng	Guggul	Elecampane	
Sarsaparilla	Alfalfa	Goldenseal root	Barley grass	Rose Hips			

SEE PAGE 1 FOR FORMULATING INSTRUCTIONS.

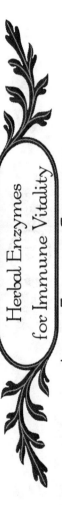

Herbal Enzymes for Immune Vitality

IMMUNE ENHANCING COMPOUNDS

The very nature of immune strength means that it must be built from the inside out. Nowhere is enzyme activity more important. No substances in our bodies are more important than enzymes. They make life possible. Without them we cannot breathe, digest food, or move a muscle. No vitamin, mineral, or hormone can do its job without enzymes. They are involved in every biochemical process. One of the most important functions of enzymes is to neutralize toxins in the body through their anti-oxidant activity. Giving your body generous, high quality plant nutrients at the first sign of infection or ill health improves your chances of destroying pathogenic bacteria. Immune-enhancing plants can be directed at "early warning" problems to build strength for immune response. Herbs and superfoods are excellent choices for enzyme therapy because they carry their own plant enzymes along with their medicinal properties.

ESSENTIAL CATEGORIES FOR AN IMMUNE SYSTEM VITALITY COMPOUND:

STRENGTHEN & REBUILD BLOOD	ACID/ALKALINE BALANCERS	ENZYME-RICH HERBS	CHLOROPHYLL-RICH HERBS	TONIC ADAPTOGEN HERBS	PROTECTIVE ANTIOXIDANT HERBS
Chlorella	Pau d'arco	Echinacea root	**Chlorella**	**Ginsengs - all kinds**	**Garlic**
Dandelion root	**Ginger root**	**Goldenseal root**	**Spirulina**	Astragalus	**Ginkgo biloba**
Barley grass	**Kelp & sea vegetables**	St. John's wort	**Barley grass**	**Ashwagandha**	**Rosemary**
Nettles	**Bee pollen/Royal Jelly**	Ginkgo biloba	**Parsley leaf**	**Hawthorn lf. & bry.**	Bilberry
Yellow dock root	**Aloe vera**	Horsetail	**Alfalfa**	**Siberian ginseng**	Yarrow
Licorice root	Nutritional yeast	Sages - red and white	**Comfrey leaf**	Sarsaparilla root	**Alfalfa**
Hawthorn lf., bry., flr.	Lemongrass	**Chlorophyll-rich plants**	**Nettles**	Schizandra berry	**Gotu kola**
Wild yam root	Marshmallow root	**Kelp & sea vegetables**	**Kelp & sea vegetables**	Reishi mushroom	Rose hips
Alfalfa	Miso	Garlic	**Dandelion leaf**	Gotu kola	Red clover blsm.

ESSENTIAL HERBS FOR AN IMMUNE SYSTEM VITALITY COMPOUND:

PRIMARY HERBS		ASSISTING & COMPLEMENTARY HERBS		CATALYST & TRANSPORTING HERBS	
Echinacea root	Ginsengs - all kinds	Suma root	Nettles	Sea plants - kelp, irish	Aloe vera juice
Hawthorn lf. & bry.	Astragalus	Licorice root	Yellow dock root	moss, dulse, etc.	Garlic
Chlorella	Ginkgo biloba	Burdock root	Boneset	Ginger root	Bilberry berry
Bee pollen/royal jelly	Oatstraw	Schizandra bry.	White sage	Capsicum	Parsley root
Spirulina	Wild yam root	Alfalfa	Myrrh	Rose hips	Lemongrass
Pau d'arco bark	Nettles	Red raspberry	Marshmallow root	Anise seed	Lemon peel
Barley grass	Sarsaparilla root	St. John's wort	Red sage	Rosemary	Acidophilus pwdr.
Kelp & sea vegetables	Dandelion root & lf.	Red clover blsm.	Horsetail	Borage seed	Comfrey leaf
Gotu kola	Goldenseal root	Ashwagandha	Reishi mushroom	Nutritional yeast	Yarrow

EXAMPLE FORMULAS FOR IMMUNE SYSTEM VITALITY COMPOUNDS:

A SYSTEM STRENGTHENING ENZYME DRINK COMPOUND (SA - 8230)			AN HERBAL DEFENSE TEAM ENZYME TEA FORMULA (PD - 5540)		
Miso	Barley grass	Siberian ginseng	Spirulina	Red clover blsm.	Suma rt.	Aralia rt.	St. John's wort
Nutritional yeast	Dandelion root	Nettles	Sea plants	Hawthorn lf. & bry.	Schizandra bry.	Lemongrass	Anise seed
Alfalfa	Licorice root	Bilberry berry	Chlorella	Burdock rt.	Astragalus	Marshmallow	
Oatstraw	Pau d'arco	Rosemary	Red raspberry	Licorice rt.	White sage	Boneset	

SEE PAGE 1 FOR FORMULATING INSTRUCTIONS.

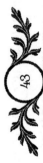

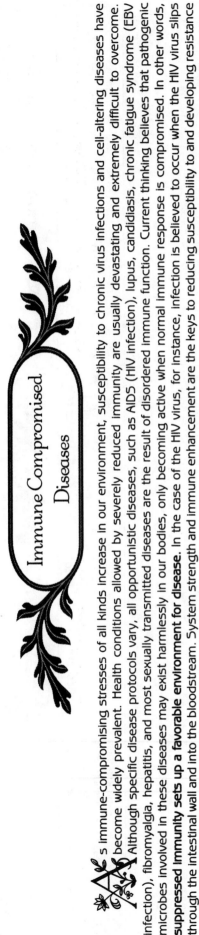

Immune Compromised Diseases

s immune-compromising stresses of all kinds increase in our environment, susceptibility to chronic virus infections and cell-altering diseases have become widely prevalent. Health conditions allowed by severely reduced immunity are usually devastating and extremely difficult to overcome. Although specific disease protocols vary, all opportunistic diseases, such as AIDS (HIV infection), lupus, candidiasis, chronic fatigue syndrome (EBV infection), fibromyalgia, hepatitis, and most sexually transmitted diseases are the result of disordered immune function. Current thinking believes that pathogenic microbes involved in these diseases may exist harmlessly in our bodies, only becoming active when normal immune response is compromised. In other words, **suppressed immunity sets up a favorable environment for disease.** In the case of the HIV virus, for instance, infection is believed to occur when the HIV virus slips through the intestinal wall and into the bloodstream. System strength and immune enhancement are the keys to reducing susceptibility to and developing resistance against opportunistic pathogens. Natural therapies and especially herbal remedies are clearly more therapeutic than prescription drugs in rebuilding immune response. Healing emphasis should be on system detoxification, enhancing liver function and immune support.

✤ COMMON LIFESTYLE CAUSES AND RISKS THAT COMPROMISE IMMUNITY:

• Prolonged use of antibiotics, prescription or pleasure drugs, infected needles, cortico-steroids, birth control pills, unnecessary childhood vaccinations or travel immunizations. These things may alter thymus gland activity, and its immune-controlling ability.

• Once immunity is severely compromised, you can continually re-infect yourself if you don't change destructive lifestyle practices. Repeating exposure to opportunistic pathogens through sexual excess, multiple sex partners, and excessive use of chemicals, drugs and alcohol, reduces your ability to overcome them dramatically.

• Immune compromised diseases often cascade from one to another. Hepatitis, for instance, predisposes a person to AIDS, because the liver is so weakened it cannot play its part in resisting infection. Syphilis is also usually present in AIDS victims, as are parasites and other herpes viruses.

• Parasites are becoming an epidemic in the U.S. and are many times a co-factor in immune compromised disease development. If you are frequently diagnosed with a bacterial infection and treated with antibiotics that don't help, have your stool tested for parasites. If your lifestyle is immuno-suppressing, parasites can easily take hold.

• Sexual contact with infected, contagious persons who pass on immune-compromising organisms. Symptoms can appear anywhere from 6 months to 3 years after infection.

• A high stress lifestyle that depletes basic body reserves.

• Poor diet with too many refined and junk foods, causing poor cell health and nutritional deficiencies on a wide scale.

• Auto-toxemia through poor waste elimination and constipation.

• Exhausted liver and adrenal glands; general gland/hormone depletion and imbalance.

• Our water, air and soil are now full of chemicals that affect delicate immune balance. You must consciously make healthy choices for yourself.

✤ FORMULAS FOR IMMUNE COMPROMISED DISEASES HELP IN THE FOLLOWING CONDITIONS:

•Viral & Bacterial Infections •Normalizing After Overuse of Drugs •HIV Virus •Chronic Fatigue Syndromes •Fibromyalgia •Tumors •Candidiasis (Candida Albicans) •Rheumatic Fever •Lupus •Eczema & Psoriasis •Cervical Dysplaysia & HPV •Mononucleosis •Toxic Shock Syndrome •Hepatitis •Herpes •Lyme Disease •Internal Parasites & Worms •Sexually Transmitted Diseases.

✤ COMPOUNDS FOR FORMULATION SHOULD INCLUDE:

•Purifying herbal compounds to accelerate toxin release.
•Enzyme therapy compounds to strengthen cells, organs and deep body tissue.
•Herbal compounds to rebuild healthy new blood and immune defenses.

44

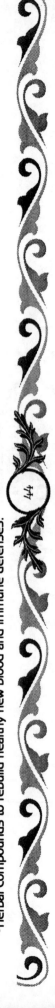

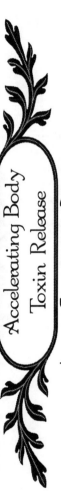

Accelerating Body Toxin Release

IMMUNE-COMPROMISED DISEASES

In immune-compromised syndromes the body is unable to defend itself against retro-viruses that affect DNA and T-cells. Infection often occurs in stages: an asymptomatic state (when the disease is often passed), an acute mononucleosis-like stage, a state with one or more immune-related diseases, and then the full blown infection. The herbal suggestions here are most beneficial for people in the asymptomatic stages, or for people who have tried orthodox medical treatment, but have showed no improvement and decided to take charge of their own health with alternative remedies. If you decide to use a combination of orthodox and alternative treatments, be quite careful.... ask a knowledgeable naturopath. Mixing natural products with powerful drugs can be dangerous. It is absolutely necessary to detoxify the liver for holistic healing to be effective. Compromised nutrition is bound to immune dysfunction. Diet improvement is the primary step in preventing the asymptomatic stage from becoming full-blown.

✒ ESSENTIAL CATEGORIES FOR ACCELERATING BODY TOXIN RELEASE:

BLOOD CLEANSING & PURIFICATION	THYMUS & LYMPH STIMULATION	CHLOROPHYLL SOURCES	BODY BIOCHEMISTRY BALANCERS	ANTI-VIRAL HERBS	ANTIOXIDANT HERBS
Red clover	Myrrh	**Alfalfa**	**Ginseng-all types**	St. John's wort	**Kelp/sea vegetables**
Reishi mushroom	**Echinacea root**	**Barley grass**	**Spirulina & Chlorella**	Reishi mushroom	Goldenseal root
Chlorophyll-rich herbs	**Goldenseal root**	Aloe vera	Alfalfa	**Lomatium dissectum**	Black walnut hulls
Kelp/sea vegetables	**Garlic**	**Kelp/sea vegetables**	Gotu kola	**Myrrh**	Myrrh
Aloe vera	Mullein	**Parsley leaf**	**Hawthorn lf., bry., fl.**	**Una da gato**	Garlic
Dandelion root	Licorice root	**Spirulina**	Chamomile	**Bee pollen & propolis**	Burdock root
Milk thistle seed	Capsicum	**Chlorella**	Kelp/sea vegetables	Pau d' arco bark	Ginger root
Burdock root	Oregon grape root	**Dandelion leaf**	**Sarsaparilla root**	Echinacea root	**Chlorophyll-rich herbs**
Licorice root	**Sarsaparilla root**	Nettles	**Miso**	Goldenseal root	Aloe vera

✒ ESSENTIAL HERBS FOR ACCELERATING BODY TOXIN RELEASE:

PRIMARY HERBS		ASSISTING & COMPLEMENTARY HERBS		CATALYST & TRANSPORTING HERBS	
Echinacea root	Pau d'arco bark	Alfalfa	Butternut bark	Capsicum	Aloe vera juice
Garlic	Sarsaparilla root	Yellow dock root	Goldenseal root	Chamomile	Rosemary
Una da gato	Myrrh	Oregon grape root	St. John's wort	Kelp/sea vegetables	Parsley root
Siberian ginseng	Kelp/sea vegetables	Nettles	Prickly ash bark	Ginkgo biloba	Parsley leaf
Chlorella	Hawthorn lf. flr. & bry.	Dandelion root	Ginkgo biloba	Ginger root	Miso powder
Spirulina	Astragalus	Gotu kola	Bilberry	Acerola cherry	
Burdock root	Kelp & ocean plants	Nettles	Bee pollen	Rosehips	
Licorice root	Ginseng - all types	Milk thistle seed	Royal jelly/Propolis	Rosemary	
Reishi mushroom	Barley grass	Red clover	Mullein	Black walnut hulls	

✒ EXAMPLE FORMULAS OF BODY TOXIN RELEASE ACCELERATION:

AN ENERGY GREEN CAPSULE COMPOUND			(SA - 2135)	AN ALL-OVER DETOX CXAPSULE COMPOUND			(CD - 2000)
Barley grass/sprouts	Siberian ginseng	Chlorella	Dulse	Red clover	Rosehips Vit. C	Echinacea root	Astragalus
Alfalfa grass/sprouts	Sarsaparilla root	Licorice root	Kelp & sea plants	Licorice root	Sarsaparilla root.	Butternut bark	Yellow dock rt.
Bee pollen	Acerola cherry	Hawthorn	Oat/Alfalfa sprouts	Burdock root	Kelp	Garlic	Buckthorn
Spirulina	Dandelion lf./rt	Gotu kola		Pau d' arco bark	Alfalfa	Golden seal root	Prickly ash

SEE PAGE 1 FOR FORMULATING INSTRUCTIONS.

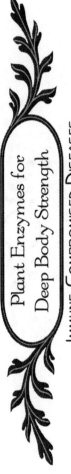

Plant Enzymes for Deep Body Strength

IMMUNE-COMPROMISED DISEASES

Enzymes in the saliva and intestinal tract produce a hostile environment that destroys the virulence of many harmful organisms. Because there is no such protection in the colon, it is relatively easy to transfer the HIV virus through anal intercourse. Immune suppression is believed to occur when a virus slips through the intestinal wall and into the bloodstream. Normal immune response is for macrophages to attack and kill pathogenic organisms which are then removed through the lymphatic system. As toxic wastes, the microphages are dumped into the colon on its last leg of clearance from the body. But in an unprotected colon without a good defensive environment, new organisms hatch from the dead macrophages and repeat the cycle all over again. The immune system does not detect the virus in the colon nor marshal its forces until the infection is in the bloodstream; often too late if body defenses are exhausted. Plant enzymes, anti-virals and antioxidants have been among the most effective treatments against opportunistic organisms.

ESSENTIAL CATEGORIES FOR DEEP BODY STRENGTHENING COMPOUNDS:

Blood Composition Tonics	Essential Fatty Acid Sources	Gland & Organ Stimulation	Immune Stimulating Herbs	Mineral-Rich Herbs	Antioxidant Herbs
Pau d' arco	Flax seed	Dandelion root & lf.	Astragalus	Chlorophyll-rich herbs	Ginkgo biloba
Licorice root	Aloe vera	Goldenseal root	Echinacea root	Barberry bark	Rosemary
Chlorophyll-rich herbs	Evening primrose oil	Yellow dock root	Reishi mushroom	Yellow dock root	Sage
Burdock root	Borage seed oil	Kelp/sea vegetables	Myrrh	Kelp/sea vegetables	Barley grass
Nettles	Black currant oil	Hawthorn lf., bry., flr.	Siberian ginseng	Pau d' arco	Spirulina
Aloe vera	Fenugreek seed	Bee pollen/royal jelly	Barberry bark	Alfalfa	Garlic
Capsicum	Schizandra	Milk thistle seed	Garlic	Nettles	Chlorella
Ginseng - all types	Ginger root	Sarsaparilla root	Bupleurum	Horsetail	Kelp/sea vegetables
Kelp/sea vegetables	Lemongrass	Dong qual	Ashwagandha	Watercress	Aloe vera juice

ESSENTIAL HERBS FOR DEEP BODY STRENGTHENING COMPOUNDS:

Primary Herbs		Assisting & Complementary Herbs		Catalyst & Transporting Herbs	
Chlorella	Oregon grape rt.	Sarsaparilla root	Suma root	Aloe vera juice	Thyme
Burdock root	Nettles	Gotu kola	White sage	Fenugreek seed	Rosemary
Ginseng - all types	Pau d' arco bark	Dong qual	Bupleurum	Turmeric	Lobelia
Red sage	Hawthorn lf. & bry.	Barberry bark	Myrrh	Capsicum	Damiana
Echinacea root	Milk thistle seed	Watercress	Red clover	Peppermint	Calendula
Alfalfa	Dandelion rt. & lf.	Spirulina	Garlic	Cranberry powder	Fennel
Kelp & sea vegetables	Licorice root	Astragalus	Ginkgo biloba	Ginger root	Flax seed
Goldenseal root	Yellow dock rt.	Wild yam root	Ashwagandha	Schizandra berry	Yellow dock root
Barley grass	Reishi mushroom	Bee pollen/royal jelly	Evening primrose oil	Lemongrass	Borage seed oil

EXAMPLE FORMULAS FOR DEEP BODY STRENGTHENING COMPOUNDS:

A LIVER-NORMALIZING EXTRACT COMPOUND		(CD - 4880)	A DEEP BODY NORMALIZING CAPSULE COMPOUND		(CD - 1650)
Oregon grape rt.	Ginkgo biloba	Fennel seed	Pau d' arco bark	Barberry bark	Rosemary
Milk thistle seed	Wild yam root		Vegetable acidophilus	Spirulina	Dong qual
Yellow dock rt.			Black walnut hulls	Cranberry pdr.	Damiana
Dandelion rt.			Garlic	Licorice root	Rosehips
Licorice root					
Red sage					

SEE PAGE 1 FOR FORMULATING INSTRUCTIONS.

46

Rebuilding Healthy New Blood

IMMUNE-COMPROMISED DISEASES

Rebuilding immune response is critical to success in overcoming opportunistic diseases. These conditions are so virulent and invade at such deep tissue levels, that the self-healing activity of the body and the immune system are the only answer to permanent remission. Normalizing the bioactive environment is an effective protocol no matter what the etiology of the specific disease is. Two powerful herbal qualities are keys to building new body biochemistry. **Antioxidant activity from herbs** scavenges damaging free radicals. **Herbal enzyme activity** works biochemically to speed up the rate of metabolic activity, and raise the body's defense mechanisms to fight disease. The herbs recommended in this section may be used for 6 months to a year, in order to change and then stabilize the internal environment. They can help 1) strengthen and improve immune response, 2) enzymatically balance body chemistry, and 3) increase tissue oxygen.

❧ ESSENTIAL CATEGORIES FOR REBUILDING HEALTHY NEW BLOOD COMPOUNDS:

STRENGTHEN/REBUILD NEW BLOOD	STRENGTHEN & REBUILD IMMUNE RESPONSE	CHLOROPHYLL-RICH DIGESTIVE TONIC HERBS	IODINE/POTASSIUM HERB SOURCES	ADRENAL SUPPORT HERBS	PROTECTIVE ANTIOXIDANT HERBS
Alfalfa	**Ginseng - all kinds**	**Chlorella**	**Kelp**	**Licorice root**	White pine bark
Chlorella/spirulina	**St. John's wort**	**Spirulina**	**Dulse**	**Sarsaparilla root**	Bilberry
Barley grass	**Reishi mushroom**	**Barley grass**	Horsetail	**Kelp/Bladderwrack**	Siberian ginseng
Siberian ginseng	Echinacea root	**Parsley leaf**	Watercress	**Astragalus**	**Garlic**
Sarsaparilla root	Dandelion root	**Alfalfa**	**Chlorophyll-rich herbs**	Hawthorn bry., lf., flr.	**Rosemary**
Yellow dock root	Alfalfa	Acidophilus pwdr.	**Black walnut hulls**	Borage seed	Pau d' arco bark
Beet root	Red clover blsm.	**Nettles**	Scullcap	Bee pollen/Royal jelly	**Chlorophyll-rich herbs**
Barberry bark	**Astragalus**	**Kelp & sea vegetables**	Burdock root	Gotu kola	**Kelp/sea vegetables**
Kelp/sea vegetables	Bupleurum	**Dandelion leaf**	Nettles	Marshmallow root	Chaparral

❧ ESSENTIAL HERBS FOR REBUILDING HEALTHY NEW BLOOD COMPOUNDS:

PRIMARY HERBS		ASSISTING & COMPLEMENTARY HERBS		CATALYST & TRANSPORTING HERBS	
Ginseng - all kinds	Kelp & sea vegetables	Watercress	Nettles	Capsicum	Aloe vera juice
Barley grass/Chlorella	Astragalus	Schizandra Bry.	Lemongrass	Miso	Bilberry berry
Echinacea root	Ginkgo biloba	Astragalus	Bilberry	Lobelia	Lecithin
Hawthorn bry., lf., flr.	Burdock rt.	Gotu kola	White sage	Rosemary	Lemon peel
Siberian ginseng	Yellow dock root	Boneset	Myrrh	Garlic	Acidophilus pwdr.
Licorice root	Spirulina	White pine bark	Marshmallow root	Ginger root	Heartsease
Pau d' arco	Sarsaparilla root	St. John's wort	Barberry bark	Scullcap	Calendula
Alfalfa	Dandelion root & lf.	Bupleurum	Horsetail	Anise seed	Chaparral
Ashwagandha	Red clover blsm.	Beet root	Black walnut hulls	Bee pollen/royal jelly	Borage seed

❧ EXAMPLE FORMULAS FOR REBUILDING NEW BLOOD COMPOUNDS:

A BLOOD STRENGTHENING ENZYME-RICH CAPSULE COMPOUND (PD - 1700)		
Hawthorn lf. & Bry	Bilberry	Lecithin	Heartsease
Siberian ginseng	Capsicum	Kelp/sea plants
Motherwort	Astragalus bark	Ginkgo biloba

AN HERBAL DEFENSE ENZYME-RICH TEA COMPOUND (PD - 5540)		
Red clover blsm.	Suma rt.	Aralia rt.	St. John's wort
Hawthorn lf. & Bry.	Schizandra Bry.	Lemongrass	Anise seed
Burdock rt.	Astragalus	Marshmallow
Licorice rt.	White sage	Boneset

SEE PAGE 1 FOR FORMULATING INSTRUCTIONS.

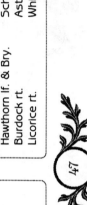

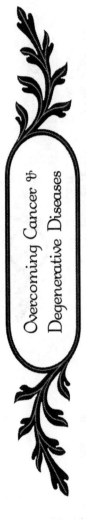
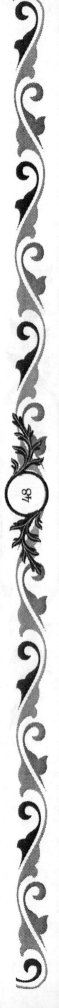

Overcoming Cancer & Degenerative Diseases

By the turn of the century, cancer is expected to be the number one cause of death in America. **One in every three Americans will get some kind of cancer; one in four will die from it.** Cancer used to be extremely rare. The dramatic increase is only minimally due to new diagnostic tests, or to calling old diseases, like consumption, cancers. The devastating disease we know as cancer today emerged gradually and then started rising at extraordinary rates as industrial societies became more dependent on technology instead of nature. At least 20,000 of the 70,000 chemicals people come in contact with regularly, are toxic.

Cancer in not a single entity with a single cause, but a complex, multi-dimensional disease. Over 200 different diseases are now classified as cancer. Chasing every cancer classification with a drug for the different characteristics of each one is futile. I feel the only chance for success is to use every part of our lifestyle to normalize tissue that is out of control. Herbal remedies in particular acknowledge the intelligence of the human body as a self-healing entity against degenerative, life-style related diseases.

The link between cancer and lifestyle is undeniable and scientifically proven. New evidence is indicates that 90% of all cancer is environmentally caused and therefore preventable. Diet and nutrition are by far the most important preventive factors, and many cancers respond well to diet improvement. America's enormous incidence of breast and colon cancer, 500% more compared to the rest of the world, is overwhelmingly felt to be due to poor nutrition and food choices. Lifestyle causes mean that we can positively affect many cancer source factors ourselves - both to prevent cancer from occurring and helping ourselves when it has.

LIFESTYLE CHOICES YOU CAN MAKE TO IMPROVE YOUR CHANCES AGAINST CANCER AND DEGENERATIVE DISEASE:

• Most cancers are caused or aggravated by poor diet and nutrition. Nutritional deficiencies accumulate over a long period of time, eventually changing normal body chemistry. You can improve your nutrition: **1)** Reduce your intake of fat. Environmental toxins become lodged in the fatty tissue of the animals in our food chain, and in tissue of humans who are exposed to them. Fat from cancer tissue regularly tests almost double the safe amount of chlorinated pesticides. **2)** Reduce your intake of red meats. Cancer onset is closely related to the protein and fat in red meats, fast foods and fried foods. **3)** Eat vegetables every day. The more fruits and vegetables you eat, the less your cancer risk, regardless of the type of cancer. People who eat plenty of fruits and vegetables have half the risk of people who eat few fruits and vegetables. Even small to moderate amounts of fruits and vegetables make a big difference. Two fruits and three vegetable servings a day have shown amazing anti-cancer results. Eating fruit twice a day, instead of twice a week, can cut the risk of lung cancer by 75%, even in smokers. **4)** Use plant enzyme therapy against cancer: Have a fresh green salad every day as a source of hydrolytic enzymes to stimulate immune response.

• Detoxify at least twice a year. Certain superfoods and juices accelerate natural body detox activity and prevent the genetic ruin of cells, a prelude to cancer.

• Keep your liver in top condition. It is a powerful chemical plant that keeps immune defense strong and healthy red blood cells forming.

• Regular exercise is almost a "cancer defense" in itself. It enhances oxygen use and accelerates passage of material in the colon. Exercise at least 3 times a week. While one out of three Americans falls victim to cancer, only one out of seven **active** Americans does.

• Stress reduction is significant. Relaxation techniques such as guided imagery give you a measure of control over your body's ability to fight off disease.

• Keep your immune system strong. U.S. industries alone generate **88 billion pounds of toxic waste per year.** The EPA estimates 90% of them are improperly disposed of. Environmental toxins can damage cell DNA, which leads to cell mutation and tumor development. Avoid tobacco in any and all forms.

FORMULAS FOR OVERCOMING CANCER HELPS IN THE FOLLOWING CONDITIONS:

•Systemic Cancers - Colon, Bowel, Stomach, Organ and Lungs •Malignant Tumors •Lupus •Melanoma •Parkinson's Disease •Leukemia •Lyme Disease Syndrome •Skin Cancers •Multiple Sclerosis •Muscular Dystrophy.

COMPOUNDS FOR FORMULATION SHOULD INCLUDE:

•Purifying herbal compounds to accelerate toxin release in the liver, organs and endocrine system.
•Normalizing herbal compounds to deter cancer cell proliferation.
•Herbal compounds to rebuild the body after chemotherapy and radiation treatments.

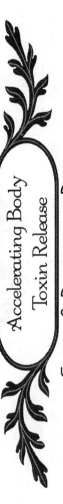

Accelerating Body Toxin Release

Cancer & Degenerative Diseases

Cancer and degenerative disease are usually created or allowed by the accumulation and saturation of toxic matter in the body, throwing defense mechanisms and vital body operations out of balance. Cancer cells seem to live and grow in unreleased waste and mucous deposits in the body. Indications that you might benefit from a toxin-releasing cleanse include chronic constipation or diarrhea, the sudden appearance or enlargement of growths, internal bleeding (especially blood passing in the stool), non-healing wounds and unexplained chronic pain in a specific area. Herbal detoxifiers along with a cleansing diet are documented methods for reversing disease symptoms of this kind. It is a type of therapy that allows the body to decompose substances and tissue that are damaged, diseased or unneeded, such as abscesses, tumors, and congestive wastes, and allow the body to clean out enough waste to maintain health.

✦ ESSENTIAL CATEGORIES FOR ACCELERATING BODY TOXIN RELEASE:

Blood Cleansing & Purification	Thymus & Lymph Stimulation	Chlorophyll Sources	Body Biochemistry Balancers	Anti-Pathogen Herbs	Antioxidant Herbs
Red clover	**Siberian ginseng**	**Alfalfa**	Calendula	**St. John's wort**	**White pine bark**
Green tea leaf	**Echinacea root**	**Barley grass**	Ginger root	**Reishi Mushroom**	**Rosemary**
Licorice root	**Goldenseal root**	**Aloe vera**	**Alfalfa**	Lomatium dissectum	**Bilberry**
Kelp/sea vegetables	**Kukicha Twig/Bancha**	**Kelp/sea vegetables**	Miso	Astragalus bark	**Barley grass**
Burdock root	Mullein	**Parsley leaf**	**Dandelion root**	Una de gato	**Spirulina/Chlorella**
Sarsaparilla root	Yarrow	Spirulina	**Lemongrass**	Propolis	**Garlic**
Yellow dock root	Capsicum	Chlorella	Bladderwrack/sea plants	**Osha root**	**Ginkgo biloba**
Hawthorn lf., bry., fl.	Sage	**Dandelion leaf**	Peppermint	**Echinacea root**	**Kelp/sea vegetables**
Nettles	Green tea	Nettles	Ginseng - all types	Usnea	Chaparral

✦ ESSENTIAL HERBS FOR IMPROVING BODY TOXIN RELEASE:

Primary Herbs		Assisting & Complementary Herbs		Catalyst & Transporting Herbs	
Echinacea root	Siberian ginseng	Sheep sorrel	Red sage/white sage	Capsicum	Aloe vera juice
Goldenseal root	Green tea	Una de gato	Yellow dock root	Lobelia	Orange peel & blsm.
Licorice root	Kelp/sea vegetables	Spirulina	Buckthorn bark	St. John's wort	Calendula
Ginseng - all types	Hawthorn lf. flr. & bry.	Barley grass	Prickly ash bark	Peppermint	Rosemary
Burdock root	Astragalus	Mullein	Reishi Mushroom	Ginger root	Parsley root & lf.
Pau d'arco bark	Dandelion root/leaf	Ginger root	Bilberry	Spearmint	Cinnamon
Chlorella	Green tea leaf	Yarrow	Slippery elm	Fennel seed	White pine bark
Sarsaparilla root	Garlic	Gotu kola	Spirulina	Rosemary	Osha root
Red clover	Alfalfa	Chaparral	Nettles	Miso	Lemongrass

✦ EXAMPLE FORMULAS OF BODY TOXIN RELEASE:

A BLOOD & CIRCULATORY CLEANSING TEA COMPOUND		(PD - 5100)
Hawthorn lf. & bry.	Heartsease	Licorice root	Peppermint
Bilberry	Ginkgo biloba	White sage	Astragalus
Kukicha twig	Pau d'arco bark	Calendula	
Ginger root	Red sage	Yellow dock root	

A TRADITIONAL STRONG PATHOGEN HERBAL CLEANSER		(PD - 1675)
Sheep sorrel	Panax ginseng	Slippery elm	Turkey rhubarb
Burdock root	Pau d' arco bk.		
Red clover blossom			

SEE PAGE 1 FOR FORMULATING INSTRUCTIONS.

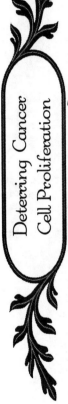

Deterring Cancer Cell Proliferation

Cancer & Degenerative Diseases

The natural healing world regards cancer as an unhealthy body whose defenses can no longer destroy abnormal cells - a view that has engendered remarkable healing success. We know that the body possesses natural cancer-fighting substances because most cancer patients do not die. We know that the body can use certain herbs to help it stimulate a cancer-fighting response. Enzyme therapy from herbs is a key to building healthy new blood, and normalizing body biochemistry so the immune system can defend the body properly. Encouraging the body's natural ability to fight cancer through biological therapies offers the best chance of dealing with the environmental and lifestyle conditions that helped caused the cancer in the first place. **Herbal enzymes** 1) improve immune response, 2) chemically alter by-products of a tumor to lessen cancer's side effects, and 3) change the surface of a tumor to make it more recognizable to the immune system.

Essential Categories for Deterring Cancer Cell Proliferation:

Blood Composition Tonics	Essential Fatty Acid Sources	Gland & Organ Stimulation	Immune Stimulating Herbs	Tumor Growth Inhibitors	Antioxidant Herbs
Pau d' arco	**Flax seed**	Dandelion root & lf.	**Astragalus**	**Panax ginseng**	**Ginkgo biloba**
Milk thistle seed	**Aloe vera**	Goldenseal root	**Reishi mushroom**	Echinacea root	**Rosemary**
Chlorophyll-rich herbs	**Evening primrose oil**	Parsley lf. & rt.	**Myrrh**	Bladderwrack/Kelp	**Rosehips vitamin C**
Burdock root	**Borage seed**	**Kelp/sea vegetables**	**Ginseng - all types**	**Pau d' arco**	**Barley grass**
Nettles	**Black currant oil**	**Hawthorn lf., bry., flr.**	Turmeric	Alfalfa	**Spirulina**
Aloe vera	Fenugreek seed	**Bee pollen & royal jelly**	Garlic	**Bilberry**	**Garlic**
Capsicum	Schizandra bry.	**Licorice root**	Bupleurum	**Ashwagandha**	**Chlorella**
Ginseng - all types	Ginger root	**Sarsaparilla root**	Ashwagandha	Watercress	Kelp/sea vegetables
Red sage	Lemongrass	Red raspberry leaf	Chlorella	Calendula	Chaparral

Essential Herbs for Deterring Cancer Cell Proliferation:

Primary Herbs

Spirulina/Chlorella	Oregon grape rt.
Burdock root	Nettles
Ginseng root	Pau d' arco bark
Astragalus	Hawthorn lf. & bry.
Bee pollen/Propolis	Milk thistle seed
Alfalfa	Dandelion rt. & lf.
Kelp & sea vegetables	Siberian ginseng
Goldenseal root	Licorice root
Aloe vera	Barley grass

Assisting & Complementary Herbs

Sarsaparilla root	Parsley lf. & rt.
Gotu kola	Bilberry
Wild cherry bk.	Rose hips vitamin C
Barberry bark	Myrrh
Watercress	Schizandra bry.
Hyssop	Bupleurum
Reishi mushroom	Ginkgo biloba
Yellow dock root	White sage
Red sage	Mullein

Catalyst & Transporting Herbs

Garlic	Ashwagandha
Fenugreek seed	Hibiscus
Turmeric	Rosemary
Capsicum	Lobelia
Parsley root & lf.	Calendula
Ginger root	Fennel
Carrot powder	Flax seed
Red raspberry lf.	Borage seed
Evening primrose oil	Lemongrass

Example Formulas for Deterring Cancer Cell Proliferation:

A Normalizing Compound to Rebuild the Body (SA - 1450)

Spirulina	Hawthorn lf. & flr.	Siberian ginseng	Chlorella
Bee pollen	Kelp/sea plants	Sarsaparilla root	Goldenseal root
Alfalfa	Barley grass	Red raspberry lf.	Mullein
Rose hips vitamin C	Carrot powder	Wild cherry bk.	Spirulina

A Liver Detoxifying Tea Compound (CD - 5780)

Dandelion root	Pau d' arco bark	Red sage	Hibiscus
Dandelion lf.	Hyssop	Licorice root	White sage
Watercress	Parsley lf. & rt.	Milk thistle seed	
Yellow dock root	Oregon grape rt.		

See page 1 for formulating instructions.

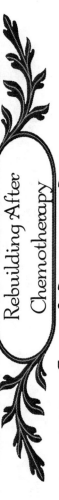

Rebuilding After Chemotherapy

CANCER & DEGENERATIVE DISEASES

Chemotherapy and radiation are both the oldest recorded medicines and the newest scientific trend for cancer treatment. In studies for breast, ovarian and prostate cancer, herbs rich in phyto-hormones (plant hormones) are showing enormous promise in their ability to bind to estrogen receptor sites and inhibit tumor growth, while allowing cell structure to remain normal. Chemotherapy, radiation and even tamoxifen regularly kill surrounding healthy cells as they kill off cancer cells, making it extremely difficult for the body to generate new, healthy tissue. Cancers are opportunistic, attacking when immune defenses and bloodstream health are low. Every new test and research study points to rallying the immune system as the best protection against cancer.

Are herbal medicines effective for cancer? Herbal or phyto-pharmaceuticals are both widely used by the medical community for treating cancerous growth.

✤ ESSENTIAL CATEGORIES FOR REBUILDING AFTER CHEMOTHERAPY COMPOUNDS:

LIVER & BLOOD BUILDING HERBS	ANTI-INFLAMMATORY HERBS	CHLOROPHYLL-RICH DIGESTIVE TONIC HERBS	VITAMIN C/BIOFLAVONOID SOURCES	ADRENAL SUPPORT HERBS	PROTECTIVE ANTIOXIDANT HERBS
Alfalfa	**White willow bark**	**Chlorella**	**Hawthorn bry., lf., flr.**	**Licorice root**	**White pine bark**
Chlorella & spirulina	**St. John's wort**	**Spirulina**	**Rose hips**	**Sarsaparilla root**	**Gotu kola**
Barley grass	**Reishi mushroom**	**Barley grass**	**Acerola cherry**	**Kelp/Bladderwrack**	**Chlorella**
Nettles	Echinacea root	Acidophilus pwdr.	Ginkgo biloba	**Astragalus**	**Spirulina**
Milk thistle seed	Dandelion root	**Alfalfa**	**Bilberry**	Hawthorn bry., lf., flr.	Siberian ginseng
Yellow dock root	Alfalfa	Fennel seed	**Cranberry concentrate**	Borage seed	**Garlic**
Beet root	Burdock root	Aloe vera juice	Lemon peel	**Bee pollen**	**Rosemary**
Barberry bark	Prickly ash bark	**Kelp & sea vegetables**	**Hibiscus flower**	**Royal jelly**	**Pau d' arco bark**
Panax ginseng	**Turmeric**	**Dandelion leaf**	Aloe vera juice	**Gotu kola**	Alfalfa

✤ ESSENTIAL HERBS FOR REBUILDING AFTER CHEMOTHERAPY COMPOUNDS:

PRIMARY HERBS		ASSISTING & COMPLEMENTARY HERBS		CATALYST & TRANSPORTING HERBS	
Panax Ginseng	Kelp & sea vegetables	Yellow dock root	Nettles	Capsicum	Aloe vera juice
Barley grass	Astragalus	Alfalfa	St. John's wort	Turmeric	Bilberry
Echinacea root	Ginkgo biloba	Rose hips	Bilberry	Rosemary	Acerola cherry
Hawthorn bry., lf., flr.	Burdock rt.	Gotu kola	Chamomile	Garlic	Acidophilus pwdr.
Siberian ginseng	Yellow dock root	Garlic	Licorice root	Ginger root	Cranberry powder
Licorice root	Spirulina	White pine bark	Beet root	Parsley root & lf.	Calendula
Pau d' arco	Sarsaparilla root	Prickly ash bark	Bugleweed	Vitamin C powder	Lemongrass
Chlorella	Dandelion root & lf.	Parsley root & lf.	Barberry bark	White willow bark	Lemon peel
Milk thistle seed	Reishi mushroom	Borage seed	Bee pollen/Royal Jelly	Fennel seed	Hibiscus

✤ EXAMPLE FORMULAS FOR REBUILDING AFTER CHEMOTHERAPY COMPOUNDS:

FOUR DETOXIFYING DOUBLE-HERB EXTRACT COMPOUNDS			
#1 Panax ginseng	#2 Chlorella	#3 Panax ginseng	#4 Pau d' arco
Licorice root	Panax ginseng	Reishi mushroom	Echinacea root

A HEAVY METAL RELEASE COMPOUND FOR RADIATION		(PD - 2450)
Ascorb. vit. C pwdr.	Bugleweed	Parsley root
Bladderwrack	Astragalus	Parsley lf.
Kelp	Barley grass	
Prickly ash bark		
Licorice root		

SEE PAGE 1 FOR FORMULATING INSTRUCTIONS.

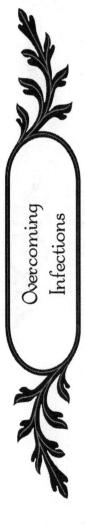

Overcoming Infections

Most infections are signs of a depressed immune system or a chronic system imbalance. Infective organisms enter the body through the gastro-intestinal tract, the respiratory tract, or through a wound, sore, or insect bite. If identified early, many infection types respond to a mild, short term blood and body cleanse. However, early and/or correct identification is not always clear cut.

It is difficult to correctly identify an infection. In truth, there is no comprehensive rule of thumb for diagnosis. •Many illnesses with the same symptomology, such as a cold, the flu, and bronchitis, can actually stem from different infectious causes, and need different treatments. •Some illnesses may also begin as one form of infection and extend into another. This is true of diseases that begin as a bacterial infection, and become overwhelmed by a viral infection because of today's virulent, mutating strains. Upper respiratory infections, pneumonia and immune deficiency diseases are good examples of this type. •Still other diseases have a root cause, like an over-acid condition, or yeast overgrowth, but the symptoms show up as infections, like mouth sores or vaginal infections. •Infections related to immuno-suppression may revolve around cortico-steroid or antibiotic drug therapy. Healthy immune response is often compromised by prolonged courses of these drugs, because normal system checks and balances become upset, allowing relatively harmless microbes to multiply out of control and cause infections.

However, there are well-known symptoms that can indicate treatment action. Inflammation and swelling of the infected area are usually the first signs of every infection type. In most cases, the severity and duration of the infection may be gauged by the severity and duration of the inflammation and swelling. Other signs include area pain and/or pressure, body heat and fever, redness and body malfunction. Chronic, recurring infections indicate low thyroid function.

Herbs can come to the rescue against many kinds of infections. As anti-bacterial agents, herbs contain powerful natural substances to flush and cleanse the lymph glands, allowing the body to process out harmful pathogenic wastes. Herbs are effective internally in overcoming both acute and chronic infections, and externally as poultices or compresses, to draw out infection through the skin.

Herbal antibiotic combinations are also beneficial when used in conjunction with other therapeutic herbal formulas to increase their efficacy, especially at the beginning or acute stages of an illness. Antibiotic combinations are especially effective in cases of oncoming colds and fever, swollen glands, bronchitis, inflamed lung and chest ailments, heavy post-nasal drip, low grade throat and sinus infections, and "hanging on" conditions where the body can't seem to "get over" a problem on its own. All infections regularly cause painful inflammation as the body reacts to isolate and overcome the infection.

Herbs are at their best as products for problems. As an herbalist, I look carefully at a wide range of symptoms, side effects and stages of a health condition before constructing a formula to address it. Even though many herbs have antibiotic properties, they do not work with a shotgun approach like antibiotic drugs. Instead, the herbs in a well-crafted compound work together as a whole, synergistically, to concentrate on the different aspects of a problem. Assistant and catalyst herbs have great effect in the way the primary herbs act against a specific infection.

❋FORMULAS FOR IMMUNE STRENGTH AGAINST OPPORTUNISTIC DISEASES HELP IN THE FOLLOWING CONDITIONS:

•Colds •Flu •Bronchitis •Bacterial Infections •Viral Infections •Staph Infections •Strep Infections •Pneumonia & Pleurisy •Sore Throat •Chronic Cough •Sinusitis •Candida Albicans Infections •Fungal Infections •Adrenal Exhaustion •Chronic Low Grade Throat & Sinus Infections.

❋COMPOUNDS FOR FORMULATION SHOULD INCLUDE:

•Herbal compounds to overcome bacterial,strep and staph infections.
•Herbal compounds to fight viral infections.
•Herbal compounds to get rid of fungal infections.
•Uerstanding chronic respiratory infections.
•Herbal compounds to overcome cold infections and flu infections.
•Herbal compounds to overcome pneumonias and bronchitis.

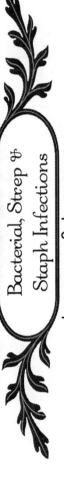

Bacterial, Strep & Staph Infections

INFECTIONS & INFLAMMATION

Bacterial infections are usually caused by a pathogenic organism, but may also be an opportunistic infection, in which a normally innocuous microbe grows out of control because of body imbalances. Examples of a bacterial infection include upper respiratory infections, bacterial cystitis, abscesses, acne, rheumatic fever, sore throat and most chronic low-grade infections. Staphylococcus, streptococcus organisms and gardnerella fall under this category. **A staph infection** involves a staphylococcus organism, usually virulent, often food-borne. Herbs with antibiotic properties are very effective for both short term and chronic needs. Medical anti-biotics are effective in the short term. Herbal antibiotic compounds are also effective in conjunction with other herbal medicines to increase their efficacy, especially at the beginning or acute stages of an illness.

❧ ESSENTIAL CATEGORIES FOR BACTERIAL, STAPH & STREP INFECTIONS:

BLOOD & LYMPH CLEANSING HERBS	VITAMIN C & BIOFLAVONOID SOURCES	ANTIBACTERIAL HERBS	ANTI-INFLAMMATORY HERBS	ENZYME THERAPY & DIGESTIVE HERBS	ANTIOXIDANT HERBS
Echinacea root	Parsley root & leaf	**Echinacea root**	**St. John's wort**	**Aloe vera**	**White pine bark**
Maitake mushroom	**Rose hips**	**Pau d' arco bark**	**White willow bark**	Acidophilus powder	**Rosemary**
Panax ginseng	**Barley grass**	**Goldenseal root**	Una da gato	Garlic	**Bilberry**
Elecampane	Hawthorne lf., bry., fl.	Una da gato	**Calendula**	**Barley grass**	**Barley grass**
Prickly ash bark	**Lemon peel**	Myrrh	Marshmallow root	**Spirulina**	**Spirulina**
Spirulina	Alfalfa	Turmeric	Chamomile	**Ginger root**	**Garlic**
Reishi mushroom	Bilberry	Propolis	Alfalfa	**Chlorella**	Astragalus
Capsicum	**Watercress**	Elecampane	Comfrey root	Milk thistle seed	**Kelp/sea vegetables**
Licorice root	Pau d' arco	Garlic	**Turmeric**	Barberry bark	Chaparral

❧ ESSENTIAL HERBS FOR BACTERIAL, STAPH & STREP INFECTIONS:

PRIMARY HERBS	ASSISTING & COMPLEMENTARY HERBS	CATALYST & TRANSPORTING HERBS
Echinacea root	Reishi mushroom	Capsicum
Chlorella	Marshmallow root	Acidophilus powder
Goldenseal root	Prickly ash bark	White pine bark
Licorice root	Alfalfa	Aloe vera
Burdock root	Barberry bark	Ginger root
Pau d'arco bark	Una da gato	Osha root
Elecampane	Propolis	Black walnut hulls
Myrrh	Astragalus	Rosemary
Turmeric	Yarrow	Rose hips
		Calendula
		Turmeric
		Chamomile
		Parsley root & lf.
		Lemon peel
		Chaparral
		Comfrey root
		Milk thistle seed
		Lemongrass
	Red sage	
	Yellow dock root	
	Buckthorn bark	
	Maitake mushroom	
	Ginkgo biloba	
	Bilberry	
	Spirulina	
	Barley grass	
	White willow bark	

❧ EXAMPLE FORMULAS OF BACTERIAL, STAPH & STREP INFECTION COMPOUNDS:

AN HERBAL ANTIBIOTIC CAPSULE COMPOUND		(PD - 1150)
Echinacea A. root	Black walnut hulls	Turmeric
Goldenseal root	Elecampane	Kelp
Capsicum	Echinacea Pur. rt.	
Myrrh		
Yarrow		
Marshmallow root		

AN HERBAL ANTIBIOTIC EXTRACT COMPOUND		(PD - 4678)
Echinacea Ang. root	Goldenseal root	Myrrh
Echinacea Pur. rt.	Pau d'arco bark	Wiintergreen

SEE PAGE 1 FOR FORMULATING INSTRUCTIONS.

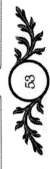

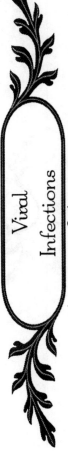

Viral Infections

Infections & Inflammation

Viral Infections are caused by simple, but virulent, tenacious living organisms that have a rapid replication mechanism, with the ability to move and mutate their structure in order to escape being overcome. Severe viral infections are becoming increasingly prevalent and insidious in America, as environmental pollutants, chemically-laced foods, over-use of drugs and generally poor nutrition lower our immune defenses. A viral infection can infiltrate the deepest regions of the body, living off the cell enzymes of the host. Examples of a viral infection include human papilloma virus (HPV), causing sexually transmitted genital warts, Epstein Barr virus (EBV), causing chronic fatigue syndrome and mononucleosis, Human Immunodeficiency Virus (HIV), causing AIDS, Herpes Simplex Type 2, causing genital herpes, hepatitis virus, causing acute liver disease, viral flu and pneumonia. Medical antibiotics are not effective. Herbs with anti-viral properties are very effective.

✦ ESSENTIAL CATEGORIES FOR VIRAL INFECTION COMPOUNDS:

ANTI-VIRAL HERBS	ESSENTIAL FATTY ACID SOURCES	IMMUNE RESPONSE STIMULANTS	BODY CHEMISTRY BALANCERS	VITAMIN C/BIOFLAV. SOURCES	ENZYME THERAPY & DIGESTIVE HERBS
St. John's wort	**Flax seed**	**Siberian ginseng**	**Panax ginseng**	Hawthorn fl., bry., lf.	**Aloe vera**
Lomatium	**Chlorella**	**Pau d' arco bark**	**Kelp/sea vegetables**	**Rosehips**	Acidophilus powder
Myrrh	**Barley grass**	Una da gato	Ginkgo biloba	**Barley grass**	Garlic
Echinacea root	Bee pollen	**Ashwagandha**	Lemongrass	**Pau d' arco**	**Barley grass**
Astragalus	Capsicum	**Reishi mushroom**	Garlic	Alfalfa	**Spirulina**
Aloe vera	Alfalfa	**Bee pollen & royal jelly**	**Burdock root**	Parsley leaf	**Ginger root**
Garlic	Garlic	Propolis	**Bee pollen**	**Lemon peel**	Chlorella
Osha root	**Evening primrose oil**	Schizandra berry	Turmeric	Watercress	Milk thistle seed
Usnea	**Borage seed**	**Maitake mushroom**	Chlorella	**Bilberry**	**Peppermint**

✦ ESSENTIAL HERBS FOR VIRAL INFECTION COMPOUNDS:

PRIMARY HERBS		ASSISTING & COMPLEMENTARY HERBS		CATALYST & TRANSPORTING HERBS	
St. John's wort	Reishi mushroom	Una da gato	Ashwagandha	Kelp/sea vegetables	Hibiscus
Echinacea root	Propolis	Suma root	Panax ginseng	Acidophilus powder	Rosemary
Astragalus	Bupleurum	Burdock root	Maitake mushroom	Peppermint	Calendula
Bee pollen	Usnea	Barberry bark	Turmeric	Lemon grass	Fennel
Pau d' arco bark	Kelp/sea vegetables	Alfalfa	Ginkgo biloba	Capsicum	Flax seed
Lomatium dissectum	Garlic	Aloe vera	White sage	Parsley root & lf.	Evening primrose oil
Barley grass	Siberian ginseng	Osha root	Schizandra Bry.	Ginger root	Borage seed
Chlorella	Licorice root	Goldenseal root	Bilberry	Lobella	Royal jelly
Myrrh	Barley grass	Dandelion root	Chaparral	Dandelion lf.	Lemon peel

✦ EXAMPLE FORMULAS OF VIRAL INFECTION COMPOUNDS:

AN ANTI-VIRAL TEA COMPOUND			(PD - 6350)
Osha root	Echinacea root	Peppermint	
ST. John's wort			

AN ANTI-VIRAL EXTRACT COMPOUND		(PD - 4688)
Lomatium dissectum	St. John's wort	Propolis

Prince ginseng rt.
Astragalus

SEE PAGE 1 FOR FORMULATING INSTRUCTIONS.

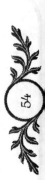

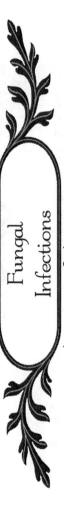

Fungal Infections

INFECTIONS & INFLAMMATION

Fungal Infections are caused by a fungus microbe, sometimes appearing as a growth that resembles fungi. They are very difficult for drugs to overcome because fungus cell structure is so similar to normal human cells. Fungal infections are characterized by moist, weepy, red patches on the body with bacterial odor. They don't dry out, and may look like non-healing cuts. A fungal infection may only be a symptomatic reaction to an overall body imbalance. Stimulating and rebuilding immune response is the key to controlling them. Examples of localized fungal infections include athlete's foot, nail and skin fungus, vaginitis and ringworm. Examples of systemic fungal infections where the organisms are found throughout the body include thrush and candidiasis. Many are caused by broad spectrum antibiotics or prescription drugs use that kill friendly digestive flora and lower immune defenses.

❧ ESSENTIAL CATEGORIES FOR FUNGAL INFECTIONS COMPOUNDS:

ANTI-FUNGAL HERBS	ENZYME THERPY & DIGESTIVE HERBS	CHLOROPHYLL SOURCES	IMMUNE STIMULATING HERBS	ANTI-INFLAMMATORY HERBS	ANTIOXIDANT HERBS
Black walnut hulls	**Peppermint**	**Chlorella**	**Siberian ginseng**	**St. John's wort**	**White pine bark**
Barberry bark	Garlic	Alfalfa	**St. John's wort**	**White willow bark**	**Gotu kola**
Maithake mushroom	**Ginger root**	**Barley grass**	**Pau d' arco bark**	**Una da gato**	**Chlorella**
Tea tree oil	**Fennel seed**	**Kelp & sea weeds**	Astragalus	**Calendula**	**Spirulina**
Garlic	Goldenseal root	Spirulina	Suma	Marshmallow root	**Bilberry**
Myrrh	Alfalfa	**Parsley leaf**	**Garlic**	Chamomile	**Siberian ginseng**
Thyme	**Catnip**	Nettles	**Echinacea root**	Alfalfa	**Garlic**
Una da gato	**Papaya**	**Watercress**	Capsicum	Aloe vera	**Rosemary**
Wormwood	**Lemongrass**	**Comfrey leaf**	Chaparral	**Turmeric**	**Pau d' arco bark**

❧ ESSENTIAL HERBS FOR FUNGAL INFECTIONS COMPOUNDS:

PRIMARY HERBS	ASSISTING & COMPLEMENTARY HERBS	CATALYST & TRANSPORTING HERBS
Garlic	St John's wort	Aloe vera
Burdock root	Wormwood	Peppermint
Chlorella	Marshmallow root	Capsicum
Spirulina	Calendula	Fennel seed
Black walnut hulls	Barley grass	Ginger root
Alfalfa	White willow bark	Acidophilus powder
Pau d' arco	Parsley leaf	Bilberry
Tea tree oil	Nettles	Red raspberry lf.
Myrrh	Suma	Wild cherry bk.
		Cranberry ext
		Rosemary
		Lobelia
		Kelp & sea weeds
		Lemongrass
		Chamomile
		Dong Qual
		Nettles
		Spearmint

❧ EXAMPLE FORMULAS OF FUNGAL INFECTIONS COMPOUNDS:

AN ANTI-FUNGAL TOPICAL SKIN COMPOUND (BB - 7880)			AN ANTI-FUNGAL COMPOUND FOR SYSTEMIC FUNGUS (CD - 1650)		
Pau d'arco bk.	Myrrh	Lomatium Diss.	Pau d'arco bark	Barberry bark	Dong Qual
Dandelion rt.	Goldenseal rt.	Grapefruit seed	Acidophilus powder	Spirulina	Damiana
Gentian root	Witch hazel		Black walnut hulls	Cranberry ext.	Rose hips vit. C
	Aloe vera gel		Garlic	Licorice root	
	Lecithin				
	Veget. glycerine		SEE PAGE 1 FOR FORMULATING INSTRUCTIONS.		

Understanding Chronic Respiratory Infections

Chronic respiratory infections are more than common in our society today. It is estimated that at any one time, over a third of our population has had a cold or flu within the last two weeks. The national average is 2.5 colds per person per year -- more than 600 million colds in all!

A "cold" is often a cleansing attempt by the body to rid itself of waste overload. Toxins and bacteria build up to a point where natural immune response cannot cope. So the wonderful, complex immune system opens up, and drains the body of excess mucous accumulation and bacterial colonies, through coughing, runny nose, sneezing or diarrhea. Then it begins to rebuild a stronger, cleaner system. The glands are barometers of infection; since the endocrine system is on a six day cycle, a normal cold runs for about a week as the body works through its detoxification process.

Many of today's respiratory infections come from lifestyle habits that depress the immune system. Smoking, environmental pollutants, and poor diet are the most influential causes. The person who suffers frequently from sinus headaches, bronchitis, constant colds and sore throat, flu, or chronic congestion, is almost invariably one who eats a lot red meats and fatty dairy products, who likes plenty of salty, sugary, fatty foods, and is a heavy coffee drinker. Fresh fruits and vegetables are almost off this person's diet chart. A diet like this causes too much mucous to be formed in the body, and although some mucous is beneficial for membrane and tissue health, most Americans carry around 12 to 15 pounds of it. Mucous deposits become filled with toxic impurities and unreleased wastes from preservatives, chemical additives, pesticide residues, etc. They are a perfect breeding ground for harmful bacteria and virus growth.

Drugs and over-the-counter medicines only relieve the symptoms of respiratory infections. They do not cure them, and often make the situation worse by depressing immune response, drying up necessary mucous elimination, and keeping harmful bacteria, virus, or allergens, inside the body. (Yet another case of "fooling Mother Nature" that doesn't work). Antibiotics are not effective against cold and flu virus infections. And whatever temporary relief aspirin might afford, it can enhance viral replication. A short, liquid diet to eliminate excess mucous (and the toxins that go with it), diet improvement, outdoor exercise and supplementation with herbs are the most beneficial and quickest means of overcoming colds and flu. Herbal combinations can work with, or following, a mucous cleansing diet. They increase oxygen uptake in the lungs and tissues, encourage adrenal gland function, and allow better sleep while progress on the underlying causes is taking place.

Do You Have A Cold, or The Flu?

Colds and flu respond to different treatment. Colds and flu are distinct, separate upper respiratory infections, triggered by different viruses. (Outdoor environment, drafts, wetness, temperature changes, etc. do not cause either of these illnesses.) As noted above, colds are a natural way for the body to cleanse itself of toxic build-up. They increase elimination by sweating and mucous discharge. This elimination makes us unusually tired so that we rest. A cold automatically activates immune response. Most people feel much better after a cold because the body makes healing and environmental adjustments.

The flu is more serious, because it can spread to the lungs, and cause severe bronchitis or pneumonia. Initial symptoms for each condition may be similar because both colds and flu begin when viruses penetrate the body's protective barriers. Nose, eyes, and mouth are usually the sites of invasion for common cold viruses such as rhino-virus or corona virus. The most likely entry target for the flu virus is the respiratory tract.

A COLD PROFILE LOOKS LIKE THIS:
- Slow onset.
- No prostration.
- Rarely accompanied by fever and headache.
- Localized symptoms such as runny nose and sneezing.
- Mild fatigue and weakness from body cleansing.
- Mild to moderate chest discomfort, usually with a hacking cough.
- Sore throat common, especially at the beginning.

A FLU PROFILE LOOKS LIKE THIS:
- Swift, severe onset.
- Early and prominent prostration with flushed, hot, moist skin.
- Accompanied by high (102°-104°) fever, headache and sore eyes.
- General symptoms of chills, depression and body aches.
- Digestive symptoms of diarrhea and stomach soreness.
- Extreme fatigue, sometimes lasting 2-3 weeks.
- Acute chest discomfort, with severe hacking cough.

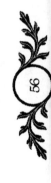

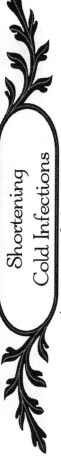

Shortening Cold Infections

INFECTIONS & INFLAMMATION

If you have a healthy, functioning immune system, a toxin-eliminating cold should not last more than four days. Herbs work with the body systems to reduce severity and duration of symptoms and enhance immune response. Herb teas, along with juices and broths are especially effective because they promote perspiration and cleansing, and help you get much needed rest. For a minor-misery cold, your best bet is to increase rest time, drink cleansing herbal teas, and take a natural immune activator to send you on your way with a cleansed system. Here's an effective herbal program to pursue when the first signs of a cold appear: •Take 15 to 30 drops ECHINACEA EXTRACT twice daily, along with the ZINC SOURCE extract drops below. •Take 2 to 3 cups daily of a warming tea, like chamomile or catnip tea, to help the body sweat and eliminate toxins faster. See HEALTHY HEALING 10th Edition for how to deal with more severe colds.

❧ ESSENTIAL CATEGORIES FOR COLD & FLU COMPOUNDS:

DECONGESTANT & EXPECTORANT HERBS	LYMPH CLEANSING HERBS	ANTIBACTERIAL HERBS	VITAMIN C/BIOFLAVONOID SOURCES	SWEATING/DIAPHORETIC HERBS	ENZYME THERAPY & DIGESTIVE HERBS
Elecampane	**Echinacea root**	**Garlic**	**Hawthorn bry., lf., flr.**	**Elder flower**	**Aloe vera**
Coltsfoot	**Goldenseal root**	**Echinacea root**	**Rose hips**	**White willow bark**	**Acidophilus pwdr.**
Ephedra	**Myrrh**	**Goldenseal root**	**Acerola cherry**	**White pine**	Chlorella/Spirulina
Boneset	**Elecampane**	Myrrh	**Ginkgo biloba**	Astragalus	Parsley root & lf.
Marshmallow root	Garlic	**Boneset**	**Bilberry**	Rose hips	**Peppermint**
Lobelia	Spirulina	Propolis	Cranberry powder	**Ginger root**	**Barley grass**
Pleurisy root	Bayberry bark	Aloe vera juice	Lemon peel	**Parsley root**	Bee pollen
Ginger root	Capsicum	Osha root	Hibiscus flower	Capsicum	**Ginger root**
Elder berry	**Turmeric**	**Pau d' arco**	Pau d' arco	Turmeric	**Garlic**

❧ ESSENTIAL HERBS FOR COLD & FLU COMPOUNDS:

PRIMARY HERBS	ASSISTING & COMPLEMENTARY HERBS	CATALYST & TRANSPORTING HERBS
Usnea	Yellow dock root	Capsicum
Rosehips	Alfalfa	Peppermint
Echinacea root	Ginkgo biloba	Rosemary
Hawthorn bry., lf., flr.	Mullein	Fennel seed
Garlic	Acerola cherry	Ginger root
Licorice root	White pine bark	Parsley root & lf.
Pau d' arco	Pleurisy root	Vitamin C powder
Chlorella	Osha root	White willow bark
Spirulina	Elder berry & flr.	Comfrey root

Astragalus	**Ephedra**	Aloe vera juice
Bee pollen	St. John's wort	**Lobelia**
Burdock rt.	Bilberry	Acidophilus pwdr.
Coltsfoot	Boneset	Cranberry powder
Barley grass	Myrrh	Turmeric
Marshmallow root	Propolis	Lemongrass
Dandelion root & lf.	Yarrow	Lemon peel
Goldenseal root	**Elecampane**	Calendula
Bayberry bark	Barberry bark	Hibiscus flr.

❧ EXAMPLE FORMULAS OF COLD & FLU COMPOUNDS:

A COLD SEASON DEFENSE COMPOUND			(PD - 1900)
Garlic	Parsley root	Boneset	
Acerola cherry	Ginger root	St. John's wort	
Bayberry bark	Rosemary	Echinacea root	
		Capsicum	

A COLD SEASON DEFENSE COMPOUND		A SORE THROAT, ZINC SOURCE COMPOUND	(PD - 4830)
Vitamin C pdwr.	Echinacea root	Peppermint	Alfalfa	Propolis
Acidophilus pdwr.	Spirulina	Bilberry	Barley grass	
Bee pollen	Gotu kola	Yellow dock rt.		

SEE PAGE 1 FOR FORMULATING INSTRUCTIONS.

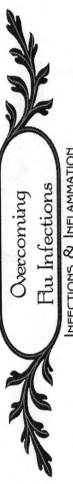

Overcoming Flu Infections

INFECTIONS & INFLAMMATION

Flu infections are longer-lasting and stronger than colds. Flu treatment programs work best in a series of stages. The ACUTE, or infective stage, includes aches, chills, prostration, fever, sore throat, etc., and usually lasts for 2 to 4 days. Sweating is effective at the first sign of infection. Heat de-activates viruses. • Take 1 cayenne capsule and 1 ginger capsule and a catnip enema. • Take a hot bath with 1 TBS. tea tree oil. • Go to bed for a long sleep; let the body concentrate on healing. The RECUPERATION, or healing stage, replenishes the body's natural resistance. • Take a hot sauna, spa, or bath to raise body temperature and increase circulation and a catnip enema to cleanse the intestinal tract. The IMMUNE SUPPORT stage, should be followed for two to three weeks, especially in high risk seasons. • Get a good massage therapy treatment to begin this phase. Recovery from flu is often slow, with a good deal of weakness.

❧ ESSENTIAL CATEGORIES FOR FLU COMPOUNDS:

ANTI-VIRAL HERBS	ENZYME THERAPY HERBS	CHLOROPHYLL-RICH DIGESTIVE TONIC HERBS	LIVER CLEANSING & SUPPORT HERBS	BETA CAROTENE SOURCES	PROTECTIVE & ANTIOXIDANT HERBS
St. John's wort	**Aloe vera**	**Chlorella/Spirulina**	**Milk thistle seed**	**Chlorella**	**White pine bark**
Lomatium	Peppermint	**Barley grass**	**Barberry bark**	**Pau d' arco**	Gotu kola
Myrrh	Bayberry bark	Nettles	**Red sage**	**Kelp sea plants**	Chlorella/Spirulina
Echinacea root	**Fennel seed**	Acidophilus pwdr.	Bupleurum	**Barley grass**	White willow bk.
Astragalus	**Spirulina**	**Alfalfa**	Ginkgo biloba	Hawthorn bry., lf., flr.	**Siberian ginseng**
Aloe vera	**Ginger root**	Fennel seed.	Burdock root	Watercress	**Garlic**
Garlic	**Chlorophyll-rich herbs**	Aloe vera juice	**Dandelion rt. & lf.**	Alfalfa	**Rosemary**
Boneset	Barberry bark	**Kelp & sea vegetables**	Buckthorn bark	Parsley root & lf.	**Fo-ti root**
Usnea	**Yellow dock root**	**Dandelion leaf**	**Oregon grape root**	Rosehips	Sarsaparilla root

❧ ESSENTIAL HERBS FOR FLU COMPOUNDS:

PRIMARY HERBS		ASSISTING & COMPLEMENTARY HERBS		CATALYST & TRANSPORTING HERBS	
Panax Ginseng	Kelp & sea vegetables	Yellow dock root	Nettles	Capsicum	Aloe vera juice
White pine bk.	Astragalus	Alfalfa	St. John's wort	Fennel seed	Bilberry
Echinacea root	Burdock root	Ginkgo biloba	Bilberry	Rosemary	Acerola cherry
Hawthorn bry., lf., flr.	White willow bk.	Gotu kola	Peppermint	Garlic	Acidophilus pwdr.
Siberian ginseng	Usnea barbata	Milk thistle seed	Myrrh	Ginger root	Orange peel
Licorice root	Barley grass/Spirulina	Bupleurum	Ginger root	Cloves	Parsley root & lf.
Pau d' arco	Sarsaparilla root	Red sage	Boneset	Vitamin C powder	Lemongrass
Chlorella	Japanese green tea	Oregon grape root	Fo-ti root	Cinnamon	Buckthorn bark
Bayberry bark	Reishi mushroom	Dandelion rt. & leaf	Barberry bark	Rosehips	Orange blossom

❧ EXAMPLE FORMULAS OF FLU COMPOUNDS:

FIRST AID EXTRACT & CAPSULE COMPOUNDS FOR OVERCOMING FLU			A GREEN TEA DAILY MORNING CLEANSER		(CD - 6400)
#1 Vit, C powder	White willow	#2 Usnea barbata	Japanese green tea	Gotu kola	Orange peel
Bayberry bark	Cloves		Kukicha twig	Fo-ti root	Orange blossom
Ginger root	Capsicum		Burdock root	Hawthorn lf. & flr.	Cinnamon

SEE PAGE 1 FOR FORMULATING INSTRUCTIONS.

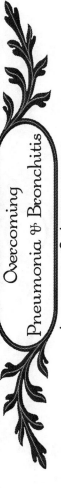

Overcoming
Pneumonia & Bronchitis

INFECTIONS & INFLAMMATION

Pneumonia and bronchitis are severe inflammatory lung diseases caused by a wide spectrum of micro-organisms. Acute pneumonia is still a leading cause of death in America, especially among the elderly. Low immune function and immuno-suppressive drugs are common denominators that allow pneumonia to take hold. **Bacterial pneumonia** is usually caused by staph, strep or pneumo-bacilli. It responds to antibiotics, both medical and herbal. **Viral pneumonia**, a systemic disease, is caused by a variety of virulent viruses, and does not respond to antibiotics. Herbal anti-virals have shown some success. **Chronic bronchitis** is a condition in which excessive mucous is secreted in the bronchi. The typical victim is forty or older, with lowered immunity from prolonged stress, fatigue or smoking. Chronic bronchitis usually develops slowly over a series of years, but will not go away on its own. Get a professional diagnosis if you think you have pneumonia or bronchitis.

❧ ESSENTIAL CATEGORIES FOR PNEUMONIA & BRONCHITIS COMPOUNDS:

DECONGESTANT & EXPECTORANT HERBS	ANTI-VIRAL HERBS	ANTIBACTERIAL HERBS	ANTI-INGFLAMMATORY HERBS	DIURETIC HERBS	ANTIOXIDANT HERBS
Elecampane	**St. John's wort**	**Garlic**	**St. John's wort**	**Cornsilk**	**White pine bark**
Coltsfoot	**Lomatium**	**Echinacea root**	**White willow bark**	**Juniper Berry**	Gotu kola
Ephedra	Myrrh	**Goldenseal root**	**Una da gato**	**Dandelion rt.**	Chlorella/Spirulina
Boneset	**Echinacea root**	Myrrh.	**Calendula**	Marshmallow rt.	Burdock rt.
Marshmallow root	**Astragalus**	**Boneset**	Marshmallow root	Goldenseal rt.	**Siberian ginseng**
Lobella	**Aloe vera**	Licorice root	Chamomile	**Uva ursi**	**Garlic**
Yarrow	Elderberry	Aloe vera juice	Alfalfa	**Parsley root & lf.**	**Rosemary**
Ginger root	Boneset	**Propolis**	Comfrey root	Ginger root	**Ginkgo biloba**
Bayberry bark	**Usnea**	Pau d' arco	**Turmeric**	Japanese green tea	Alfalfa

❧ ESSENTIAL HERBS FOR PNEUMONIA & BRONCHITIS COMPOUNDS:

PRIMARY HERBS		ASSISTING & COMPLEMENTARY HERBS		CATALYST & TRANSPORTING HERBS	
Usnea	Astragalus	St. John's wort	Elecampane	Capsicum	Aloe vera juice
Echinacea root	Propolis	Alfalfa	Pleurisy root	Peppermint	Acidophilus pwdr.
Hawthorn bry., lf., flr.	Burdock rt.	Ginkgo biloba	Boneset	Rosemary	Japanese green tea
White pine bark	White willow bark	Ephedra	Myrrh	Lobelia	Turmeric
Licorice root	Cornsilk	Gotu kola	Lomatium	Ginger root	Lemongrass
Pau d' arco	Marshmallow root	Garlic	Chamomile	Acerola cherry	Ephedra
Chlorella/Spirulina	Dandelion root & lf.	Rosehips	Parsley root & lf.	Vitamin C powder	Devil's claw
Goldenseal root	Bayberry bark	Coltsfoot	Uva ursi	Elder berry	Siberian ginseng
Una da gato	Juniper Berry	Yarrow	Bee pollen	Comfrey root	Calendula

❧ EXAMPLE FORMULAS OF PNEUMONIA & BRONCHITIS COMPOUNDS:

AN ANTI-INFLAMMATORY CAPSULE COMPOUND			(CO - 1180)
White willow	Gotu kola	Burdock root	Uva ursi
St John's wort	Red clover blsm	Dandelion root	Ginger root
Echinacea root	Devil's claw	Chamomile	Turmeric pwr.
White pine bk.	Alfalfa		Bromelain pwdr.

AN ANTI-INFLAMMATORY EXTRACT COMPOUND			(CD - 4700)
Cornsilk	Dandelion rt.	Goldenseal rt.	Parsley rt. & lf.
Juniper Berry	Marshmallow rt.	Ginger rt.	

A DIURETIC/ANTI-OXIDANT EXTRACT COMPOUND

SEE PAGE 1 FOR FORMULATING INSTRUCTIONS.

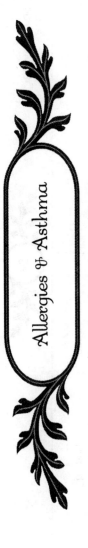

Allergies & Asthma

If it seems that your allergies are a lot worse in recent years, you may be right. Allergic reactions are multiplying, manifesting themselves not only as common symptoms of sneezing, headaches and rashes, but also as changes in personality and emotions. They are an unrecognized cause of many modern illnesses. The substances that cause allergies are called allergens. They can stem from almost anything, but the most common allergens are grass, pollen, dust, certain metals, some cosmetics, lanolin, hair and dander from some animals, insect bites or stings, some common drugs, some foods, and some chemicals found in soaps. Most allergens produce clogging and congestion as the body tries to seal them off from its regular processes, or tries to work around them. Extra mucous is formed as a shield around the offending substances, and we get the allergy symptoms of sinus clog, stuffiness, hayfever, headaches and watery, puffy eyes. Sometimes the body tries to throw this excess off through the skin, and rashes, fever blisters, abscesses or a scratchy sore throat occur. Allergies have a domino effect and they can affect any part of the body. Besides producing uncomfortable, unsightly symptoms, allergies can be imprisoning. They can make it impossible to go for a walk in the country, or even to go outside for fresh air. They restrict healthful aerobic exercise because congested sinuses lead to less efficient breathing and poor overall body function. They also limit friendships with friends that have pets (over 80% of the American population).

In times past, an allergy was defined as an inappropriate response by the immune system to a substance that is not normally harmful. While this definition is still true, there is no question that the harmful burden of toxic substances on our bodies is increasing. Impaired immune response from toxic overload is one of the primary causes of allergies. In modern times, it is hard to escape from the increasing exposure to chemicalized foods, polluted water, air and soil. Industrial chemicals, car exhaust, acid rain, and UV radiation allowed by the depletion of the earth's protective ozone layer. Compromised intestinal flora from over-reliance on antibiotic drugs, disturbance of infant immune systems through repeated immunizations, not to mention our stress-infused lifestyles, all result in reduced immune response and the inability of our bodies to cope with allergens.

In most allergic reactions, the immune system mis-identifies a substance, or can't identify a substance (usually a chemical), as an invader. Your white blood cells overreact in either case, and the allergic response becomes a disease in itself. Common responses are asthma, eczema, hayfever or severe headaches. Research on the immune system shows that allergy-prone people produce an over-abundance of certain complex proteins known as antibodies. These in turn, trigger special cells known as mast cells that release inflammation-causing chemicals throughout the body. These chemicals, called histamines and leukotrienes, must either be neutralized by a severe allergic reaction, such as an asthma attack or prevented through an optimal lifestyle therapy program.

Asthma is a life-threatening allergic reaction, but until recently, it was considered to be a mild condition that one got over or grew out of. However, new statistics show that 15 million Americans (3% Of the U.S. population, with perhaps many more undiagnosed) currently have asthma, compared to 6.8 million in 1980, an increase of 30% in the last decade alone. U.S. hospital admission rates due to asthma have almost quadrupled in the last two decades and reported deaths due to asthma have jumped 68% in the same period.

Drugs and over-the-counter medicines only relieve allergy and asthma symptoms. Drugs for allergies and asthma consist of antihistamines, steroids and desensitization shots. In obstinate cases, laser surgery may be used to vaporize mucus-forming nasal tissue. Yet most of these treatments do not work because they don't get to the cause of the problem. At best, they provide temporary symptom relief; at worst, they create side effects which may be worse than the problem itself.

❋ FORMULAS FOR OVERCOMING ALLERGIES & ASTHMA HELP IN THE FOLLOWING CONDITIONS:

•Respiratory Diseases •Bronchitis & Sinusitis •Seasonal Allergies •Chemical Sensitivites & Environmental Allergies •Asthma •Histamine Reactions •Taste & Smell Loss •Emphysema •Adrenal Exhaustion.

❋ COMPOUNDS FOR FORMULATION SHOULD INCLUDE:

•Managing seasonal allergies.
•Multiple chemical sensitivites and environmental illness.
•Controlling asthma.
•Rebuilding lung and respiratory strength.

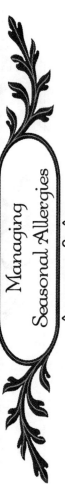

Managing Seasonal Allergies

ALLERGIES & ASTHMA

Seasonal allergies are Type 1 allergies, with symptoms called allergic rhinitis that we most associate with allergies - sinus congestion, itchy, watery nose and eyes, headaches, sneezing, coughing, scratchy throat, face swelling, insomnia, fatigue, skin itching and rashes. The most common causes of environmental allergies stem from: 1) allergic reactions to air pollutants such as asbestos, heavy metals, smoke and fumes; 2) allergic reactions to seasonal factors such as dust, pollen, spores and molds. This type of allergy most easily develops when the body already has an excess accumulation of mucous that harbors the allergen irritants.

Common drugstore medications for Type 1 allergies only mask symptoms, often cause undesirable drowsiness, and have a rebound effect. The more you use them the more you need them.

❧ ESSENTIAL CATEGORIES FOR MANAGING SEASONAL ALLERGIES:

ADRENAL ENHANCING HERBS	ALLERGEN CLEANSING HERBS	ANTIHISTAMINE LIVER SUPPORT HERBS	ANTI-INFLAMMATORY HERBS	DECONGESTANT HERBS	ANTIOXIDANT HERBS
Licorice root	Prickly ash bark	Burdock root	White willow bark	**Licorice root**	**White pine bark**
Sarsaparilla root	**Echinacea root**	Ephedra	St. John's wort	**Fennel seed**	**Rosemary**
Astragalus	**Goldenseal root**	**Aloe vera**	**Reishi mushroom**	Wild yam	**Bilberry**
Kelp/sea vegetables	**Kukicha Twig/Bancha**	**Kelp/sea vegetables**	**Echinacea root**	Garlic	**Barley grass**
Bilberry	Chlorella/Barley grass	**Red sage**	**Turmeric**	Eucalyptus	**Spirulina**
Bee pollen	Pau d' arco bark	**Spirulina/Chlorella**	**Burdock root**	Propolis	**Garlic**
Royal Jelly	Marshmallow root	Wild cherry bark	Una da gato	**Myrrh**	**Chlorella**
Hawthorn lf., bry., fl.	Yarrow	**Wild yam root**	Dandelion root	**Horehound**	**Kelp/sea vegetables**
Japanese green tea	Myrrh	Gotu kola	Calendula	**Ginger root**	Siberian ginseng

❧ ESSENTIAL HERBS FOR MANAGING SEASONAL ALLERGIES:

PRIMARY HERBS		ASSISTING & COMPLEMENTARY HERBS		CATALYST & TRANSPORTING HERBS	
Echinacea root	St. John's wort	Royal Jelly	Elder flower & bry.	Capsicum	Aloe vera juice
Goldenseal root	White pine bk.	Una da gato	Wild yam root	Lobelia	Yarrow
Licorice root	Kelp/sea vegetables	Rose hips	Dandelion rt.	Vitamin C powder	Eucalyptus
Spirulina/Chlorella	Hawthorn lf. flr. & bry.	Siberian ginseng rt.	Prickly ash bark	Acerola cherry	Rosemary
Burdock root	Astragalus	Mullein	Wild cherry bark	Ginger root	Parsley root & lf.
Pau d'arco bark	Ginkgo biloba	Red sage	Bilberry	Turmeric	Propolis
Myrrh	Green tea leaf	White willow bark	Barley grass	Fennel seed	Anise seed
Sarsaparilla root	Garlic	Gotu kola	Ephedra	Rosemary	Calendula
Marshmallow rt	Bee pollen	Horehound	Juniper bry.	Miso	Uva ursi

❧ EXAMPLE FORMULAS FOR MANAGING SEASONAL ALLERGIES:

AN ALLERGEN NEUTRALIZING COMPOUND		(B - 1060)	AN ANTIHISTAMINE CAPSULE COMPOUND		(B - 1200)
Marshmallow rt.	Ephedra	White pine bk.	Marshmallow rt.	Acerola cherry	Capsicum
Burdock rt.	Capsicum		Ephedra	Rosemary	Lobelia
Mullein	Rosemary		Bee pollen	Mullein	
			White pine bk.		

AN ALLERGEN NEUTRALIZING COMPOUND		
Goldenseal rt.	Goldenseal rt.	
Parsley rt. & lf.	Burdock rt.	
Acerola cherry	Juniper bry.	
	Parsley rt.	

SEE PAGE 1 FOR FORMULATING INSTRUCTIONS.

SEE PAGE 35 FOR A MUCOUS CLEANSE TO BEGIN THIS PROGRAM.

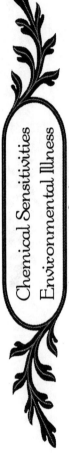

Chemical Sensitivities
Environmental Illness

ALLERGIES & ASTHMA

Allergic reactions to chemicals (Type 2 allergies) are usually a result of the body's attempt to isolate the dangerous substances from its functioning balance by storing them in fatty tissue. **The first allergic response occurs after the second exposure to the irritant**; the body's inflammatory response is alerted and histamines are produced. Repeated exposures to the irritant set off massive free-radical reactions as the body's contaminate toleration levels are reached, and a full allergic reaction sets in. Chemical hypersensitivity also initiates other forms of allergies, so that the sufferer becomes allergic to nearly everything else. Type 2 allergies are characterized by migraine headaches, hyperactivity (especially in children), depression, anxiety, mood swings, personality changes, confusion and memory loss. Symptoms may be both activated and aggravated by a combination of offending irritants.

➷ ESSENTIAL CATEGORIES FOR CHEMICAL/ENVIRONMENTAL SENSITIVITIES:

BLOOD CLEANSING & PURIFICATION	THYMUS & LYMPH STIMULATION	ANTI-INFLAMMATORY HERBS	BOOSTING LIVER PERFORMANCE	NEUTRALIZE TOXIC ALLERGENS	ANTIOXIDANT HERBS
Reishi mushroom	Prickly ash bark	White willow bark	Yellow dock root	Vitamin C powder	**White pine bark**
Green tea leaf	**Echinacea root**	St. John's wort	Ginger root	**Echinacea root**	**Rosemary**
Licorice root	**Goldenseal root**	**Reishi mushroom**	**Ginkgo biloba**	**Goldenseal root**	**Bilberry**
Kelp/sea vegetables	**Kukicha Twig/Bancha**	**Echinacea root**	**Burdock root**	**Kukicha Twig/Bancha**	**Barley grass**
Burdock root	Myrrh	**Turmeric**	**Milk thistle seed**	Chlorella/Barley grass	**Spirulina/Chlorella**
Sarsaparilla root	Licorice root	Gotu kola	**Dandelion rt.**	Pau d' arco bark	**Garlic**
Yellow dock root	Capsicum	Una da gato	Wild yam rt.	Prickly ash bark	Astragalus
Hawthorn lf., bry., fl.	Nettles	Dandelion root	Oregon grape root	Yarrow	**Kelp/sea vegetables**
Dandelion rt. & lf.	Ginger root	Calendula	Barberry bark	Royal Jelly/Bee pollen	Siberian ginseng

➷ ESSENTIAL HERBS FOR CHEMICAL/ENVIRONMENTAL SENSITIVITIES:

PRIMARY HERBS		ASSISTING & COMPLEMENTARY HERBS		CATALYST & TRANSPORTING HERBS	
Echinacea root	St. John's wort	Royal jelly	Reishi mushroom	Capsicum	Aloe vera juice
Goldenseal root	White pine bk.	Una de gato	Wild yam root	Lobelia	Barberry bk.
Licorice root	Kelp/sea vegetables	Yellow dock rt.	Dandelion rt.	Vitamin C powder	Calendula
Ginseng - all types	Hawthorn lf. flr. & bry.	Siberian ginseng rt.	Prickly ash bark	Acerola cherry	Rosemary
Burdock root	Astragalus	Spirulina/Chlorella	Wild cherry bark	Ginger root	Parsley root & lf.
Pau d'arco bark	Ginkgo biloba	Oregon grape rt.	Bilberry	Turmeric	Butcher's broom
Myrrh	Green tea leaf	White willow bark	Bee pollen	Fennel seed	Yarrow
Sarsaparilla root	Garlic	Gotu kola	Hyssop	Barberry bark	Lemon balm
Marshmallow rt	Barley grass/Alfalfa	Nettles	Milk thistle seed	Miso	Uva ursi

➷ EXAMPLE FORMULAS OF CHEMICAL/ENVIRONMENTAL SENSITIVITY COMPOUNDS:

A LIVER HEALTH CAPSULE COMPOUND		(CD - 3000)	A GREEN TEA DAILY MORNING CLEANSER COMPOUND		(CD - 6400)
Beet root.	Milk thistle seed	Wild cherry bk.	Ginger rt.	Japanese green tea	Gotu kola	Orange peel	Cinnamon
Oregon grape rt.	Yellow dock rt.	Licorice root	Barberry bk.	Kukicha twig	Fo-ti root	Orange blossom	
Dandelion rt.	Ginkgo biloba	Gotu kola		Burdock root	Hawthorn lf. & flr.		
Wild yam rt.							

SEE PAGE 1 FOR FORMULATING INSTRUCTIONS.
SEE PAGE 35 FOR A MUCOUS CLEANSE TO BEGIN THIS PROGRAM.

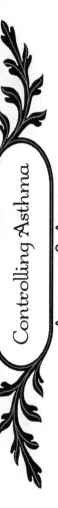

Controlling Asthma

ALLERGIES & ASTHMA

Asthma affects certain groups of people more than others. More children are affected by asthma than adults. It is the most frequent cause of missed school, and is now the leading serious, chronic illness among children under the age of ten, with a 2:1 ratio of boys to girls, and a death rate of about 5,000 kids yearly. Even if a child grows out of severe attacks he or she remains at risk. New studies show that the underlying inflammation of asthma never goes away. More adult males get asthma too, with a 2:1 ratio of men to women. Blacks are only slightly more likely to have asthma than whites but they are twice as likely to die from it. The greatest increase in asthma deaths has occurred in people 65 years old and over. Hospital costs for asthma treatment in 1995 were over 7.5 billion! Total mortality rates due to asthma have also increased more than 30% in the last decade, a trend being experienced in every industrialized nation. Traditional medicine has no cure.

❧ ESSENTIAL CATEGORIES FOR CONTROLLING ASTHMA SYMPTOMS:

ADRENAL STIMULATING TONICS	ANTI-INFLAMMATORY HERBS	RELAXING ANTISPASMODIC HERBS	BRONCHO-DILATING HERBS	DECONGESTANT HERBS	ANTIOXIDANT HERBS
Licorice root	White willow bark	**St. John's wort**	**Ginkgo biloba**	**Licorice root**	**Ginkgo biloba**
Sarsaparilla root	**St. John's wort**	**Lobelia**	**Fenugreek seed**	**Fennel seed**	**Rosemary**
Astragalus	**Reishi mushroom**	**Valerian rt.**	**Ephedra**	**Wild yam**	**Rose hips vitamin C**
Kelp/sea vegetables	Echinacea root	**Kava kava**	**Marshmallow root**	**Garlic**	Nettles
Bilberry	**Turmeric**	**Passionflower**	Turmeric	Bee pollen/Propolis	**Spirulina/Chlorella**
Bee pollen/Royal Jelly	Burdock root	Red raspberry	Garlic	Wild cherry bk.	**Garlic**
Mullein	Rose hips vit. C	Cramp bark	Bupleurum	Myrrh	Gotu kola
Hawthorn lf., bry., fl.	Dandelion root	Black haw	Angelica root	Japanese green tea	Kelp/sea vegetables
Pau d' arco bark	Calendula	Rosemary	Boneset	**Ginger root**	Burdock root

❧ ESSENTIAL HERBS FOR CONTROLLING ASTHMA SYMPTOMS:

PRIMARY HERBS	ASSISTING & COMPLEMENTARY HERBS	CATALYST & TRANSPORTING HERBS
Burdock root	Sarsaparilla root	Passionflower	Garlic	Hibiscus
Ginkgo biloba	Gotu kola	Wild yam rt.	**Royal Jelly**	Rosemary
Ginseng root	Wild cherry bk.	Rosehips vit. C	Turmeric	Lobelia
Astragalus	Fenugreek seed	Myrrh	Capsicum	Calendula
Bee pollen/Propolis	Angelica rt.	Black haw	Parsley root & lf.	Fennel
Marshmallow rt.	Red raspberry	Garlic	Ginger root	Bilberry
Kelp & sea vegetables	Sarsaparilla root	Ephedra	Carrot powder	Flax seed
Spirulina/Chlorella	Echinacea root	Valerian rt.	White willow bark	Boneset
Bupleurum	Passionflower	Mullein	Japanese green tea	Cinnamon

❧ EXAMPLE FORMULAS OF CONTROLLING ASTHMA FORMULAS:

A RELAXING, ANTI-SPASMODIC COMPOUND		(CO - 1250)	A CONGESTION REMOVING TEA COMPOUND		(B - 5010)
Kava kava	Wild yam rt.	Lobelia	Wild cherry bark	Rosemary	Cinnamon
Passionflower	St. John's wort	Valerian rt.	Ephedra	Angelica rt.	Lobelia
Red raspberry	Kelp		Ginkgo biloba	Passionflower	
Cramp bark			Marshmallow rt.		
Black haw			Fenugreek seed		
Rosemary			Mullein		

SEE PAGE 1 FOR FORMULATING INSTRUCTIONS.
SEE PAGE ** FOR A MUCOUS CLEANSE TO BEGIN THIS PROGRAM.

63

Strengthening
Respiratory Immunity

ALLERGIES & ASTHMA

Lifestyle changes help prevent allergies and asthma. Herbs help repair, rebuild and restore an exhausted immune system. Antioxidant-rich herbs are important in supporting the thymus control gland of the immune system - to help prevent thymic shrinking, and to encourage activation of immune-enhancing hormones that the thymus releases. Stress reduction techniques are pivotal, since stress and tension aggravate allergic reactions. Exercise is also important to increase oxygen uptake in the lungs and to enhance immune response. In fact, keeping normal immune response healthy is the key to overcoming all types of respiratory problems, because the things that depress immunity - air and water pollutants, toxic household substances, chemically treated foods, drugs, stress, and poor nutrition are the same things that cause respiratory problems. Providing immune-enhancement at the first sign of a respiratory infection vastly improves the body's defense shield.

✦ ESSENTIAL CATEGORIES FOR REBUILDING RESPIRATORY STRENGTH:

LIVER & BLOOD BUILDING HERBS	ENZYME THERAPY SOURCES	CHLOROPHYLL-RICH TONIC HERBS	IMMUNE STRENGTHENING HERBS	ADRENAL SUPPORT HERBS	PROTECTIVE ANTIOXIDANT HERBS
Alfalfa	**Garlic**	**Chlorella**	**Hawthorn bry., lf., flr.**	**Licorice root**	**White pine bark**
Chlorella & spirulina	**Nettles**	**Spirulina**	**Ginseng - all types**	**Sarsaparilla root**	**Gotu kola**
Barley grass	Reishi mushroom	**Barley grass**	Ashwagandha	**Kelp/Bladderwrack**	**Chlorella**
Siberian ginseng	**Chlorella**	Nettles	Astragalus	Astragalus	**Spirulina**
Milk thistle seed	**Dandelion root**	**Alfalfa**	**Ginkgo biloba**	Hawthorn bry., lf., flr.	**Siberian ginseng**
Yellow dock root	**Alfalfa**	Parsley lf.	Reishi mushroom	Ginger root	**Garlic**
Gotu kola	Myrrh	Aloe vera juice	**Royal Jelly/Bee pollen**	**Bee pollen**	**Rosemary**
Reishi mushroom	Barberry bark	**Kelp & sea vegetables**	Burdock rt.	**Royal Jelly**	**Pau d' arco bark**
Panax ginseng	**Turmeric**	**Dandelion leaf**	Japanese green tea	**Gotu kola**	**Alfalfa**

✦ ESSENTIAL HERBS FOR REBUILDING RESPIRATORY STRENGTH:

PRIMARY HERBS		ASSISTING & COMPLEMENTARY HERBS		CATALYST & TRANSPORTING HERBS	
Panax ginseng	Kelp & sea vegetables	Ginkgo biloba	Japanese green tea	Capsicum	Aloe vera juice
Barley grass	Astragalus	Alfalfa	St. John's wort	Fennel seed	Lobelia
Dandelion root/leaf	Ashwagandha	Chlorella	Bilberry	Rosemary	Acerola cherry
Hawthorn bry., lf., flr.	Burdock rt.	Gotu kola	Nettles	Garlic	Acidophilus pwdr.
Siberian ginseng	Yellow dock root	Dulse	Myrrh	Ginger root	Irish moss
Licorice root	Royal Jelly	White pine bark	Royal Jelly	Parsley root & lf.	Calendula
Pau d' arco	Sarsaparilla root	Red raspberry lf.	Wild cherry bk.	Vitamin C powder	Rice protein pwr.
Spirulina	Bee pollen	Rosehips vit. C	Marshmallow root	White willow bark	Valerian rt.
Milk thistle seed	Reishi mushroom	Mullein	Barberry bark	Uva ursi	Turmeric

✦ EXAMPLE FORMULAS FOR REBUILDING RESPIRATORY STRENGTH:

AN ADRENAL REBUILDING CAPSULE COMPOUND		(E - 1000)	A NORMALIZING GREEN CAPSULE COMPOUND		(SA - 2135)
Licorice rt.	Uva ursi	Ginger rt.	Capsicum	Barley grass	Spirulina	Acerola cherry	Gotu kola

AN ADRENAL REBUILDING CAPSULE COMPOUND (E - 1000)

Licorice rt.	Uva ursi	Ginger rt.	Capsicum
Sarsaparilla rt.	Irish moss	Astragalus	Vitamin C
Bladderwrack			Royal Jelly

A NORMALIZING GREEN CAPSULE COMPOUND (SA - 2135)

Barley grass	Spirulina	Acerola cherry	Gotu kola
Alfalfa	Siberian ginseng	Chlorella	Hawthorn berry
Bee pollen	Sarsaparilla rt.	Dulse	Licorice root
Rice protein pdwr.	Dandelion rt./lf.	Kelp	

SEE PAGE 1 FOR FORMULATING INSTRUCTIONS.
SEE PAGE 35 FOR A MUCOUS CLEANSE TO BEGIN THIS PROGRAM.

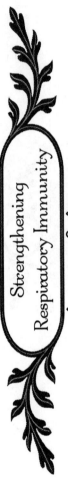

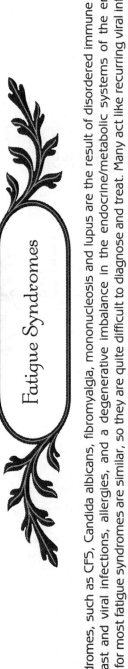

Fatigue Syndromes

Fatigue syndromes, such as CFS, Candida albicans, fibromyalgia, mononucleosis and lupus are the result of disordered immune dysfunction which allows chronic yeast and viral infections, allergies, and a degenerative imbalance in the endocrine/metabolic systems of the entire body. The outward symptoms for most fatigue syndromes are similar, so they are quite difficult to diagnose and treat. Many act like recurring viral infections that mimic colds and flu. A high stress lifestyle is often involved. A strong immune system is critical for dealing with fatigue syndromes, especially those that have that have severe allergic reactions as part of their symptomology.

While protocols vary, current thinking states that **chronic fatigue syndrome** is most often due to an infection from the Epstein Barr virus - a common, latent virus in humans that replicates and becomes active when normal immune response is compromised. Support and enhancement of immune system function is the key to reducing susceptibility and achieving resistance. A recent survey indicates that vitamins, minerals and other natural therapies are more helpful than prescription drugs in rebuilding immune response. Concentration should be on system detoxification, enhancing liver and adrenal functions and immune support.

Mononucleosis, also thought to be due to the EBV virus, attacks the respiratory and lymphatic systems with severe flu-like infection. Glands, lymph nodes, bronchial tubes, liver, spleen are all affected. The virus is virulent and highly infectious. Immune response is very weak. The whole body feels the symptoms of fever, sore throat, headache, swollen glands, jaundice, muscle aches and general long-term fatigue. Medical antibiotics are not effective for this virus. Liver, lymph and spleen systems are the main organs involved in healing. Three to six months of rebuilding are needed for restoration of strength.

Candidiasis is a state of imbalanced body ecology, not a germ, bug or disease. Candida albicans is a strain of yeasts commonly found in the gastro-intestinal and genito-urinary areas of the body. It is generally harmless, but when resistance and immunity are low, candida is able to multiply rapidly, feeding on sugars and carbohydrates in these tracts. It releases toxins into the bloodstream, and causes far-reaching problems. It is a stress-related condition, brought about because the body is severely out of balance and the immune system is seriously compromised. Repeated rounds of antibiotics, birth control pills or cortico-steroids, a nutritionally poor diet high in refined carbohydrates and alcohol, and a life-style short on rest encourage candida.

Fibromyalgia is a debilitating, often painful muscle disease, involving neuro-hormonal imbalances and impaired deep sleep. Generally considered an auto-immune condition, caused by nutrient deficiencies and environmental toxins, many symptoms mimic those of Chronic Fatigue Syndrome (CFS) and arthritis. Researchers now estimate that up to ten million Americans (mostly mid-life women) suffer from fibromyalgia. Although labeled untreatable and incurable, it may be vastly helped by natural therapies.

Lupus is a multi-system, auto-immune, inflammatory, viral disease affecting over half a million Americans, more than 80% black and Hispanic women. The immune system becomes disoriented and develops antibodies that attack its own connective tissue. Joints and blood vessels are affected producing arthritis-like symptoms. The kidneys and lymph nodes become inflamed, and in severe cases there is heart, brain and central nervous system degeneration. Orthodox treatment has not been very successful for lupus. Natural therapies help rebuild a stable immune system. Our experience shows that you feel worse for 1 or 2 months until toxins are neutralized. Then, suddenly, as a rule, you feel much better. Natural and herbal healing programs work, but require many months of healing.

See also MULTIPLE CHEMICAL SENSITIVITIES AND ENVIRONMENTAL ILLNESS for more on auto-immune diseases.

❖ FORMULAS FOR OVERCOMING FATIGUE SYNDROMES HELP IN THE FOLLOWING CONDITIONS:

•Chronic Viral Infections •Chronic Fatigue Syndrome •EBV Virus •Chronic Fatigue Syndromes •Fibromyalgia •Mononucleosis •Candidiasis (Candida Albicans) •Rheumatic Fever •Lupus •Eczema & Psoriasis •Cervical Dysplaysia & HPV •Environmental Illness •Toxic Shock Syndrome •Hepatitis •Herpes • Lyme Disease •Internal Parasites & Worms •Sexually Transmitted Diseases.

❖ COMPOUNDS FOR FORMULATION SHOULD INCLUDE:

•Purifying herbal compounds to detoxify from candida albicans.
•Rebuilding strength from chronic fatigue syndrome.
•Overcoming fibromyalgia.

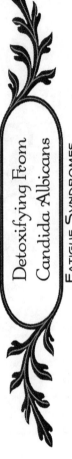

Detoxifying from Candida Albicans

FATIGUE SYNDROMES

Candida albicans is an opportunistic yeast strain that takes advantage of a reduced immune system to overrun the body. Healthy liver function and a strong immune system are the keys to lasting prevention and control of candida overgrowth. The healing/rebuilding process usually takes 3 to 6 months or more. The changes in diet and lifstyle habits are often radical. Some people feel better right away; others go through a rough "healing crisis". But most people with candida are feeling so bad anyway, that the treatment and the knowledge that they are getting better, pulls them through the hard times. A comprehensive protocol for overcoming candida includes: **Stage 1:** Kill the yeasts through diet change and supplement therapy. **Stage 2:** Cleanse the dead yeasts and waste cells from the body with an herbal cleanser. **Stage 3:** Strengthen the digestive system by enhancing its ability to assimilate nutrients. **Stage 4:** Rebuild the immune system.

✔ ESSENTIAL CATEGORIES FOR DETOXIFYING FROM CANDIDA ALBICANS:

COLON CLEANSING HERBS	ENZYME THERAPY TO STRENGTHEN DIGESTION	LIVER DETOXIFYING HERBS	THYROID SUPPORT & BALANCE	IMMUNE-ENHANCING HERBS	ANTIOXIDANT HERBS
Sarsaparilla root	Peppermint	Pau d' arco bark	**Dandelion rt. & lf.**	**Ashwagandha**	Kelp/ocean plants
Licorice root	**Goldenseal root**	**Milk thistle seed**	**Spirulina & Chlorella**	**Suma**	**Rosemary**
Pau d' arco bark	Thyme	**Oregon grape root**	Parsley rt. & lf.	**Ginseng - all types**	Siberian ginseng
Aloe vera juice	Ginkgo biloba	Yellow dock root	Nettles	**Pau d'arco bark**	**Barley grass**
Buckthorn bark	Veg. acidophilus	**Barberry bark**	**Barley grass**	**Chlorophyll-rich herbs**	**Spirulina & Chlorella**
Butternut bark	Barberry bark	**Red sage**	Borage seed	**Schizandra berry**	**Garlic**
Psyllium husks	**Chlorophyll-rich herbs**	Capsicum	**Kelp/sea vegetables**	Garlic	**Aloe vera juice**
Organic oat bran	**Kelp & sea vegetables**	Lobelia	**Sarsaparilla rt.**	Echinacea root	Parsley leaf
Organic flax seed	Fennel seed	**Gotu kola**	**Miso**	Burdock root	Ginsengs - all types

✔ ESSENTIAL HERBS FOR DETOXIFYING FROM CANDIDA ALBICANS:

PRIMARY HERBS	ASSISTING & COMPLEMENTARY HERBS	THYROID SUPPORT & BALANCE (CATALYST & TRANSPORTING HERBS)	
Echinacea root	Pau d'arco bark	Siberian ginseng rt.	Butternut bark
Garlic	Sarsaparilla root	Yellow dock root	Cranberry pwr.
Goldenseal root	Myrrh	Oregon grape root	Buckthorn bark
Alfalfa/Barley grass	Kelp/sea vegetables	Rosehips vit. C	Barberry bk.
Chlorella/Spirulina	Hawthorn lf. flr. & bry.	Dandelion root	Milk thistle seed
Ginkgo biloba	Astragalus	Gotu kola	Bilberry
Burdock root	Suma root	Nettles	Bee pollen
Licorice root	Ginseng - all types	Schizandra bry.	Psyllium husks
Ashwagandha	Veg. acidophilus	Fennel seed	Organic flax seed

CATALYST & TRANSPORTING HERBS

Capsicum	Aloe vera juice
Dong quai	Rosemary
Organic oat bran	Red sage
Lobelia	Thyme
Ginger root	Parsley rt & lf.
Acerola cherry	Borage seed
Peppermint	Apple pectin
Rosemary	Miso powder
Damiana	Guar gum

✔ EXAMPLE FORMULAS FOR DETOXIFYING FROM CANDIDA ALBICANS:

A FIBER TONE CLEANSING COMPOUND   (CD - 8100)

Organic oat bran	Guar gum	Fennel seed	Wild cherry bk.
Organic flax seed	Veg. acidophilus	Acerola cherry	
Psyllium husks	Apple pectin		

A CANDIDA DETOXIFYING COMPOUND   (CD - 1650)

Pau d' arco bk.	Barberry bk.	Rosemary
Veg. acidophilus	Spirulina	Dong quai
Black walnut hulls	Cranberry pwr.	Damiana
Garlic	Licorice root	Rosehips vit. C

A CANDIDA DETOXIFYING CAPSULE COMPOUND

Pau d' arco bk.	Burdock root
Veg. acidophilus	Echinacea root
Black walnut hulls	Peppermint
Garlic	Thyme

SEE PAGE 1 FOR FORMULATING INSTRUCTIONS.

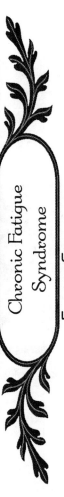

Chronic Fatigue Syndrome

FATIGUE SYNDROMES

Chronic fatigue syndrome is sometimes referred to as a condition without a cause. In reality, the opposite is true. There are a wealth of causative factors. CFS is a depressed immune response) to the ever-increasing mental, emotional and physical stresses in our environment. Susceptibility to chronic viral infections has become more and more prevalent in the last decades. As our immunity drops lower and lower, almost anything can be the final trigger for CFS. Onset is abrupt in almost 90% of cases. Over 85% of CFS victims are women, usually between 30 and 50, who are outgoing, productive, independent, active, overachievers. It affects close to 2 million people in America today. People who suffer from chronic fatigue need supernutrition. A good diet and lifestyle habits are paramount in keeping the body clear of toxic wastes and balancing the the lymphatic system.

✦ ESSENTIAL CATEGORIES FOR CHRONIC FATIGUE SYNDROME COMPOUNDS:

DEEP BODY ENERGIZING TONICS	ADRENAL SUPPORT HERBS	LIVER DETOXIFYING HERBS	IMMUNE STIMULATING HERBS	ANTI-VIRAL HERBS	THYROID SUPPORT HERBS
Ashwagandha	**Licorice root**	Pau d' arco bark	**Astragalus**	**St. John's wort**	**Dandelion rt. & lf.**
Gotu kola	**Sarsaparilla root**	**Milk thistle seed**	**Echinacea root**	**Propolis**	**Spirulina & Chlorella**
Damiana	**Kelp/Bladderwrack**	**Oregon grape root**	**Reishi mushroom**	**Echinacea root**	Parsley rt. & lf.
Burdock root	**Astragalus**	Yellow dock root	Myrrh	**Goldenseal root**	Nettles
Dong quai	Hawthorn bry., lf., flr.	**Barberry bark**	Siberian ginseng	**Pau d' arco**	**Barley grass**
Spirulina	Red clover	**Red sage**/White sage	Ginseng - all types	Myrrh	Black cohosh rt.
Licorice root	Bee pollen	Dandelion rt.	Garlic	Usnea	**Kelp/sea vegetables**
Ginseng - all types	Royal Jelly	Wild yam rt.	Alfalfa	Lomatium dissectum	**Sarsaparilla rt.**
Ginkgo biloba	Rosemary	Red raspberry	**Ashwagandha**	Garlic	Aloe vera juice

✦ ESSENTIAL HERBS FOR CHRONIC FATIGUE SYNDROME COMPOUNDS:

PRIMARY HERBS		ASSISTING & COMPLEMENTARY HERBS		CATALYST & TRANSPORTING HERBS	
Ashwagandha	Oregon grape rt.	Sarsaparilla root	Bee pollen/Royal jelly	Aloe vera juice	Thyme
Burdock root	Nettles	Gotu kola	White sage	Oatstraw	Rosemary
Ginseng - all types	Pau d' arco bark	Red sage	St. John's wort	Turmeric	Lobelia
Dong quai	Hawthorn lf. & bry.	Barberry bark	Myrrh	Capsicum	Damiana
Damiana	Milk thistle seed	Barley grass	Red clover	Peppermint	Calendula
Echinacea root	Dandelion rt. & lf.	Spirulina	Garlic	Rose hips vit. C	Propolis
Kelp & sea vegetables	Licorice root	Astragalus	Ginkgo biloba	Ginger root	Flax seed oil
Goldenseal root	Yellow dock rt.	Wild yam root	Red raspberry	Schizandra berry	Fennel
Chlorella/Alfalfa	Reishi mushroom	Usnea	Peony	Evening primrose oil	Parsley rt. & lf.

✦ EXAMPLE FORMULAS OF CHRONIC FATIGUE SYNDROME COMPOUNDS:

FOUR SPECIFIC CFS SUPPORT EXTRACT COMPOUNDS				A DEEP BODY NORMALIZING TOPICAL COMPOUND		(w - 7400)
#1 Ashwagandha	#2 Ginkgo biloba	#3 Panax ginseng	#4 Hawthorn	Aloe vera juice	Damiana	Sarsaparilla	Red clover
Damiana		Licorice root	lf., flwr., bry	Wild yam rt.	Licorice rt.	Red raspberry	Peony
Dong Quai				Panax ginseng	Black cohosh rt.	Dandelion rt.	Oatstraw
				Dong quai	Burdock root	Echinacea rt.	Vitamin C powder

SEE PAGE 1 FOR FORMULATING INSTRUCTIONS.

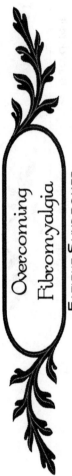

Overcoming Fibromyalgia

FATIGUE SYNDROMES

The profile for fibromyalgia is similar to other fatigue conditions; painful, tender, recurrent points aching all over the body, persistent, diffuse musculo-skeletal pain; fatigue, weakness, headaches, confusion, migraine headaches, chronic diarrhea and irritable bowel, poor sleep patterns and nervous symptoms like depression, and hypoglycemia - symptoms of mild cortisol deficiency. There are always stomach and digestive problems, with high uric acid. People who fall victim to fibromyalgia are generally not physically fit, and usually have allergies, arthritis-type stiffness, panic attacks, and an accompanying cardiovascular problem, such as mitral valve prolapse, palpitations or shortness of breath. No conventional medical treatment or drug on the market today has been able to help fibromyalgia; most hinder immune response and recovery.

ESSENTIAL CATEGORIES FOR OVERCOMING FIBROMYALGIA COMPOUNDS:

NERVE & TISSUE REBUILDERS	IMMUNE SUPPORT HERBS	ANTI-INFLAMMATORY HERBS	ANTI-DEPRESSANT HERBS	ADRENAL SUPPORT HERBS	PROTECTIVE ANTIOXIDANT HERBS
Alfalfa	**Astragalus**	**Burdock rt.**	**St. John's wort**	**Licorice root**	White pine bark
Chlorella/spirulina	**Echinacea root**	**Marshmallow root**	**Kava kava rt.**	**Sarsaparilla root**	Bilberry
Barley grass	**Reishi mushroom**	**St. John's wort**	Panax ginseng rt.	**Kelp/Bladderwrack**	Siberian ginseng
Kava kava rt.	Myrrh	**White willow bk.**	Black haw	**Astragalus**	**Garlic**
Ashwagandha	Eur. mistletoe	**Dandelion rt.**	**Fo-Ti root**	Hawthorn bry., lf., flr.	**Rosemary**
Black cohosh rt.	Ginseng - all types	Rose hips vitamin C	**Gotu kola**	Suma rt	Pau d' arco bark
Siberian ginseng	Garlic	Turmeric	**Siberian ginseng rt.**	Bee pollen	**Chlorophyll-rich herbs**
Dong qual	**Bupleurum**	**Kelp & sea vegetables**	**Wood betony**	Royal jelly	**Kelp/sea vegetables**
Hawthorn bry., lf., flr.	**Ashwagandha**	**Reishi mushroom**	Scullcap	Ginger rt.	Gotu kola

ESSENTIAL HERBS FOR OVERCOMING FIBROMYALGIA COMPOUNDS:

PRIMARY HERBS		ASSISTING & COMPLEMENTARY HERBS		CATALYST & TRANSPORTING HERBS	
Ginseng - all kinds	Kelp & sea vegetables	Black cohosh rt.	Nettles	Capsicum	Aloe vera juice
Barley grass	Astragalus	Fo-Ti root	Valerian rt.	Chlorella/spirulina	Rosehips vitamin C
Echinacea root	Ginkgo biloba	Scullcap	Royal jelly	Lobelia	Turmeric
Hawthorn bry., lf., flr.	Burdock rt.	Dong qual	Hops	Rosemary	Bilberry berry
Siberian ginseng	Gotu kola	Damiana	Myrrh	Garlic	Parsley root
Licorice root	Kava kava rt.	White pine bark	White willow bk.	Ginger root	Lemon peel
Pau d' arco	Sarsaparilla root	St. John's wort	Black haw	Suma rt	Acidophilus pwdr.
Alfalfa	Dandelion root & lf.	Bupleurum	Eur. Mistletoe	Anise seed	Heartsease
Ashwagandha	Reishi mushroom	Bee pollen	Wood Betony	Oatstraw	Calendula

EXAMPLE FORMULAS OF OVERCOMING FIBROMYALGIA COMPOUNDS:

A GINSENG INNER ENERGY CAPSULE COMPOUND		(н - 2127)	A NERVE-REBUILDING CAPSULE COMPOUND		(co - 3800)
Kava kava rt.	American ginseng	Fo-Ti root	Ginkgo biloba	Ashwagandha	Valerian rt.	Lobelia
Chinese ginseng	Dong qual	Gotu kola	Ashwagandha	Black cohosh rt.	Eur. mistletoe	Oatstraw
Siberian ginseng	Suma rt.	Prince ginseng		Scullcap	Hops	Wood Betony

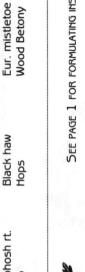

SEE PAGE 1 FOR FORMULATING INSTRUCTIONS.

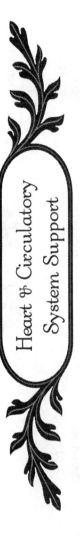

Heart & Circulatory System Support

Almost unknown at the turn of the twentieth century, two-thirds of Americans suffer from heart disease today. Cardiovascular disease remains the number one killer in civilized nations. The term heart disease covers all ailments of the heart from heart attacks to congenital defects. Cardiovascular disease refers to disorders of both the heart and circulatory system, including hypertension atherosclerosis, stroke, rheumatic heart disease, etc. Nutritional prevention measures and natural therapies are proving to reduce mortality far better than many aggressive medical intervention techniques, and also better than most advanced drugs. Indeed, some of the favored drugs for heart disease have serious side effects and can even shorten life. In recent tests on women, for instance, much to their surprise, researchers discovered that women had different problems of the heart than men. Heart attacks in women appear to be hormone related. Estrogen and hormone balance can be a major protective factor for women

Poor diet is the overriding cause of cardiovascular problems. Not one food or aspect of diet, but the whole array of high calorie, low nutrient foods and eating habits. Fried and high fat foods, refined, low fiber foods, pasteurized dairy products, too much salt, sugar, tobacco, red and processed meats all contribute to clogged arteries, LDL cholesterol, high blood pressure and heart attacks. The good news is that diet is also the single most influential factor for preventing these problems. Indeed, almost all circulatory problems can be treated or prevented with a better diet and specific herbal supplements. Your own lifestyle changes can improve your future far more than a lifetime of dependence on drugs, pacemakers, or multiple surgeries.

While lifestyle changes are not easy, and take time to accomplish, natural heart therapy is infinitely preferable for a better quality of life, and especially for there to be permanent results.

Without question, traditional, heroic medicine and its life-saving abilities should be used at once for any kind of a heart attack or stroke. But once the heart and circulation are stabilized, the heart disease victim is faced with a defining lifestyle choice as he or she considers how to live life after a heart attack. Recovering from a heart attack or major heart surgery is tough. Sticking to a new lifestyle that changes the way you eat, exercise, handle stress and the smallest details of your life is a challenge. Herbs can play a positive role in the rehabilitation of a healthier heart and arteries, and offer assurance about the fears felt in regard to recurrence.

Here are some HEALTHY HEART TIPS to blend into your lifestyle:

- ✔ Reduce the fat in your diet to 15% or less. Limit poly-unsaturates (margarine, oils) to 10%. Add mono-unsaturates (olive oil, nuts and seeds).
- ✔ Eat plenty of fish. Cold water fish oils are beneficial to blood viscosity and its propensity to clot, with preventive effects on arteriosclerosis and heart attacks.
- ✔ Reduce caffeine, nicotine and hard liquor stimulants to keep your heartbeat more stable
- ✔ Add exercise as a nutrient in your life; a brisk walk every day possible.
- ✔ Do deep breathing exercises every morning to stimulate the brain, reduce stress, and oxygenate the body for the day.
- ✔ Use dry skin brushing, alternating hot and cold hydrotherapy, and smaller meals with a little white wine, to increase circulation.
- ✔ Consciously add relaxation and a good daily laugh to your life. A positive mental outlook can do wonders for your heart and your well-being.

❧

❋ FORMULAS FOR HEART & CIRCULATORY PROBLEMS HELP IN THE FOLLOWING CONDITIONS:

•High or Low Blood Pressure   •Cholesterol Build-Up   •Reducing Risk of Congestive Heart Failure, Angina, a Coronary or Stroke   •Heart Arrhythmias - Palpitations, Tachycardia & Irregular Heartbeat   •Arterio- and Athero-sclerosis   •Mitral Valve Prolapse   •Alzheimer's Disease   •Poor Circulation   •Blood Clots, Phlebitis & Embolism   •Excessive Bleeding   •Easy Bruising   •Stress & Tension.

❋ COMPOUNDS FOR FORMULATION SHOULD INCLUDE:

•Managing high blood pressure.
•Reducing cholesterol and harmful blood fats to reduce the instance of atherosclerosis.
•A cardiotonic combination to regulate and strengthen heartbeat.

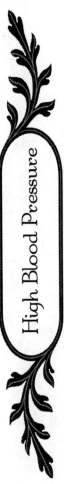

High Blood Pressure

HEART & CIRCULATORY PROBLEMS

High blood pressure is a major problem in today's high-stress world. It is a silent disease that steals health and is a precursor to serious cardiovascular disease that can steal life. Most cases of high blood pressure can be brought under control by improvement in diet and lifestyle. In fact, recent clinical studies show that people with hypertension who make the necessary lifestyle changes actually fare much better than those on anti-hypertensive prescription drugs. (Many of these drugs have such unpleasant side effects that 45% of high blood pressure patients either stop taking them altogether or take them erratically.) High blood pressure symptoms include chronic headaches and respiratory problems, irritability, dizziness, ringing in the ears, flushed complexion, red eye streaks, unusual fatigue, bloating, frequent urination, heart arrhythmia. High blood pressure and hypertension are caused by clogging arterial fats, calcium/fiber deficiency, poor sugar metabolism, obesity, and lack of exercise.

ESSENTIAL CATEGORIES FOR MANAGING HIGH BLOOD PRESSURE:

CARDIOTONIC HERBS	STRESS & TENSION RELIEVING HERBS	ADRENAL STIMULATING HERBS	ARTERY-CLEANSING HERBS	EDEMA CLEARING HERBS	ANTIOXIDANT HERBS
Hawthorn br., lf., flr.	**Valerian root**	**Kelp/sea vegetables**	**Garlic**	Uva ursi	**Alfalfa**
Ginkgo biloba	Oatstraw	**Evening primrose**	**Hawthorn lf., bry., & fl.**	Parsley rt. & lf.	**Ginkgo biloba**
Capsicum	Scullcap	**Licorice root**	**Butcher's broom**	**Dandelion rt. & lf.**	**Rosemary**
Kelp/sea vegetables	European mistletoe	**Sarsaparilla root**	Ginger root	Juniper bry.	**Siberian ginseng**
Motherwort	**Wood betony**	Astragalus	**Capsicum**	Cornsilk	**Pau d' arco**
Ginger root	Black cohosh	Irish moss	**Chlorella/Spirulina**	Cleavers	Chlorella
Heartsease	**Passionflower**	Watercress	Japanese green tea	Poria mushroom	Hawthorn lf., bry. & fl.
Bayberry bark	Pau d' arco	Rose hips	**Barley grass**	Cranberry pwr.	Goldenseal root
Siberian ginseng	Siberian ginseng	**Bilberry**	Red sage	Buchu lf.	Kelp/sea vegetables

ESSENTIAL HERBS FOR MANAGING HIGH BLOOD PRESSURE:

PRIMARY HERBS		ASSISTING & COMPLEMENTARY HERBS		CATALYST & TRANSPORTING HERBS	
Hawthorn lf., bry. & fl.	Pau d'arco bark	Dandelion root	Butternut bark	Capsicum	Chaparral
Kelp/sea vegetables	Sarsaparilla root	Marshmallow root	Cranberry pwr.	Poria mushroom	Acerola cherry
Ginkgo biloba	Bee pollen/royal jelly	Licorice root	Buckthorn bark	Ginger root	Irish moss
Siberian ginseng	Chlorella/Spirulina	Rosemary	Japanese green tea	Red sage	Lecithin
Butcher's broom	Barley grass	Wood betony	Bilberry	Oatstraw	Cornsilk
Motherwort	Alfalfa	European mistletoe	Buchu lf.	Hibiscus	Soy powder.
Evening primrose	Astragalus	Bayberry bark	Uva ursi	Aloe vera juice	Watercress
Garlic	Scullcap	Goldenseal root	Heartsease	Apple pectin	Veg. acidophilus pwr.
Ginseng - all types	Valerian root	Rosehips	Cleavers	Miso powder	Psyllium husks

EXAMPLE FORMULAS FOR MANAGING HIGH BLOOD PRESSURE:

A HIGH BLOOD PRESSURE CAPSULE COMPOUND			(H - 2750)
Garlic	Dandelion rt.	Heartsease	Bilberry
Hawthorn lf., flr., bry.	Parsley rt.	Goldenseal rt.	
Siberian ginseng	Ginger rt.		
	Capsicum		

A HIGH BLOOD PRESSURE TEA COMPOUND			(H - 5600)
Hawthorn lf., flr., bry.	Dandelion rt., lf.	Valerian root	Rose hips
Scullcap	Ginseng root	Hibiscus	
	Heartsease	Ginger root	

SEE PAGE 1 FOR FORMULATING INSTRUCTIONS.

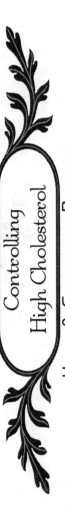

Controlling High Cholesterol

HEART & CIRCULATORY PROBLEMS

Cholesterol is a naturally-occurring, fat-related substance needed for many nerve, hormone, and cell functions. However, abnormal metabolism and over-indulgence in high cholesterol foods leads to serious deposits on arterial linings, and to gallstones. HDL, high density lipo-protein, is regarded as good cholesterol, LDL and VLDL (low density and very low density lipo-proteins), are seen as bad cholesterol. (Triglycerides are a related type of blood fat that travels with cholesterol and isinvolved with sugar metabolism.) Ideal cholesterol levels should be from 140 to 165 mg/dl, with LDL cholesterol from 30 to 50 mg/dl, and HDL cholesterol from 80 to 90 mg/dl. (Over 244 is a classic heart attack victim; 210 is the average American level.) Ideal triglyceride levels are 200 to 240 mg/dl. Harmful cholesterol and triglyceride deposits can be reduced by increasing intake of fibrous plants and herbs that dissolve, cleanse or otherwise render these harmful lipids unabsorbable in the bloodstream.

➔ ESSENTIAL CATEGORIES FOR HIGH CHOLESTEROL REDUCING COMPOUNDS:

LIVER SUPPORT HERBS	CIRCULATION SUPPORT HERBS	FIBER SUPPORT SOURCES	BIOFLAVONOID-RICH HERBS	ENZYME THERAPY COLON SUPPORT HERBS	DIGESTIVE FLORA SUPPORT
Red sage	**Ginkgo biloba**	**Apple pectin**	**Hawthorn lf., bry., fl.**	Fennel seed	**Acidophilus powder**
Milk thistle seed	**Green tea lf.**	**Brewer's yeast**	**Bilberry**	Butternut bark	**Barley grass/Spirulina**
Oregon grape root	**Gotu kola**	Kelp/sea vegetables	**Rose hips**	Kelp/sea vegetables	Peppermint
Dandelion rt.	**Butcher's broom**	**Psyllium husks**	Alfalfa	Ginger root	Licorice root
Bee pollen	**Siberian ginseng**	Chlorella	Lemon peel	Irish moss	**Ginger root**
Goldenseal rt.	Garlic	Spirulina	Parsley root & lf.	**Rhubarb root**	Apple pectin powder
Watercress	Capsicum	Garlic	Red raspberry	**Nettles**	**Calendula**
Lecithin	Ginger root	**Oat bran**	**Acerola cherry**	Papaya	**Fennel seed**
Pau d' arco bk.	Evening primrose oil	**Lecithin**	**Kelp/sea vegetables**	Brewer's yeast	Aloe vera juice

➔ ESSENTIAL HERBS FOR HIGH CHOLESTEROL REDUCING COMPOUNDS:

PRIMARY HERBS		ASSISTING & COMPLEMENTARY HERBS		CATALYST & TRANSPORTING HERBS	
Hawthorn lf., bry., fl.	Green tea lf.	Sarsaparilla root	Evening primrose oil	Aloe vera juice	Heartsease
Burdock root	Nettles	Parsley root & lf.	White sage	Cinnamon	Rosemary
Ginseng - all types	Pau d' arco bark	Red sage	Rose hips vit. C	Lecithin	Apple pectin pwr.
Barley grass	Bilberry	Barberry bark	**Rhubarb root**	Capsicum	Acidophilus powder
Butcher's broom	Milk thistle seed	Watercress	Oregon grape rt.	Peppermint	**Irish moss**
Alfalfa	Dandelion rt. & lf.	Spirulina	Garlic	Vitamin C powder	Fennel seed
Kelp & sea vegetables	Licorice root	**Psyllium husks**	Ginkgo biloba	Ginger root	Flax seed
Goldenseal root	Siberian ginseng	Acerola cherry	Red raspberry	Papaya	Brewer's yeast
Chlorella	Gotu kola	Bee pollen	Butternut bark	Lemon peel	Oat bran

➔ EXAMPLE FORMULAS OF HIGH CHOLESTEROL REDUCING COMPOUNDS:

A CIRCULATION CLEANSING TEA COMPOUNDS		(w - 5100)	A CHOLESTEROL LOWERING FIBER CAPSULE COMPOUND		(w - 1800)
Hawthorn lf. & bry.	Red sage	Yellow dock rt.	Hawthorn lf. & bry.	Psyllium husks	Fenugreek seed	Barley grass
Bilberry	Licorice root	Peppermint	Lecithin	Apple pectin pwr.	Acidophilus pwr.	Heartsease
Green tea leaf	White sage	Astragalus rt.	Rose hips vit. C	Plantain	Siberian ginseng	
	Calendula				Capsicum	

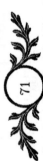

SEE PAGE 1 FOR FORMULATING INSTRUCTIONS.

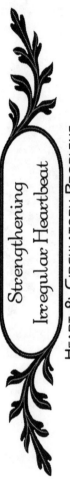

Strengthening Irregular Heartbeat

HEART & CIRCULATORY PROBLEMS

Cardiotonic herbal combinations can help regulate heartbeat by strengthening both heart muscle and vascular system. Sluggish circulation is one of the causes of arrhythmias. Herbs can invigorate blood circulation throughout the body, and help keep the artery/venous structure toned and elastic. Cardiotonic herbs may be taken over several months to strengthen the heart. **Arrhythmia:** Electrical disruptions that affect the natural rhythm of the heart. **Palpitations:** the heart beating out of sequence. **Atrial fibrillation:** episodic heart flutter, shortness of breath and the uncomfortable awareness of the racing of the heart, sometimes accompanied by dizziness or fainting; may predispose a person to having a stroke. **Atrial tachycardia:** too rapid contractions of the heart coming on in sudden attacks; usually associated with coronary artery disease. May increase the risk of congestive heart failure.

❧ ESSENTIAL CATEGORIES FOR STRENGTHENING HEARTBEAT COMPOUNDS:

CARDIOTONIC HERBS	STRESS REDUCING HERBS	FLAVONOID-RICH HERBS	MINERAL-RICH HERBS	CALMING SOOTHING HERBS	PROTECTIVE ANTIOXIDANT HERBS
Hawthorn lf., bry., fl.	**Suma root**	**Hawthorn lf., bry., fl**	**Kelp/sea vegetables**	**European mistletoe**	White pine bark
Ginkgo biloba	Fo-Ti root	**Bilberry**	**Chlorophyll-rich herbs**	**Passionflower**	Bilberry
Kelp/sea vegetables	Kelp & sea vegetables	Garlic	**Pau d' arco bark**	Ashwagandha root	Astragalus
Siberian ginseng	Bee pollen/ royal jelly	Horsetail	**Horsetail**	Oatstraw	**Garlic**
Capsicum	**Ashwagandha**	Milk thistle seed	**Nettles**	**Scullcap**	**Rosemary**
Ginger root	**Ginseng - all types**	**Ginkgo biloba**	**Alfalfa**	**Valerian root**	Capsicum
Licorice root	**Evening primrose**	**Lemon peel**	Dandelion root & lf.	**Kava kava root**	**Chlorophyll-rich herbs**
Dong quai	Borage seed	Butcher's broom	**Parsley lf. & root**	Hops	**Kelp/sea vegetables**
Ginseng - all types	Black cohosh root	**Rose hips**	**Watercress**	Wood betony	Gotu kola

❧ ESSENTIAL HERBS FOR STRENGTHENING HEARTBEAT COMPOUNDS:

PRIMARY HERBS		ASSISTING & COMPLEMENTARY HERBS		CATALYST & TRANSPORTING HERBS	
Ginseng - all kinds	Kelp & sea vegetables	Black cohosh rt.	Nettles	Capsicum	Aloe vera juice
Chlorophyll-rich herbs	Astragalus	Butcher's broom	Valerian rt.	Horsetail	Bilberry berry
Evening primrose	Ginkgo biloba	Scullcap	Royal jelly	Lobelia	Parsley root
Hawthorn bry., lf., flr.	Burdock rt.	Dong quai	Milk thistle seed	Rosemary	Lemon peel
Siberian ginseng	Gotu kola	Passionflower	Fo-Ti root	Garlic	Dulse
Licorice root	Kava kava rt.	White pine bark	Watercress	Ginger root	Rose hips
Pau d' arco	Oatstraw	St. John's wort	Prince ginseng	Lecithin	Horsetail
Alfalfa	Dandelion root & lf.	Borage seed	Eur. Mistletoe	Chlorophyll-rich herbs	Heartsease
Ashwagandha	Suma root	Bee pollen	Wood Betony	Oatstraw	Calendula

❧ EXAMPLE FORMULAS OF STRENGTHENING HEARTBEAT COMPOUNDS:

A HEART-STRENGTHENING CAPSULE COMPOUND			(H - 1700)
Hawthorn bry., lf., flr.	Bilberry	Lecithin	Heartsease
Motherwort	Capsicum	Ginkgo biloba	Ginger root
Siberian ginseng	Astragaluss		

A HEART REGULATING POTASSIUM CAPSULE COMPOUND			(SA - 2875)
Kelp	Dandelion rt.	Barley grass	Borage seed
Alfalfa	Dulse	Nettles	Watercress
	Spirulina		

SEE PAGE 1 FOR FORMULATING INSTRUCTIONS.

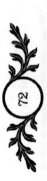

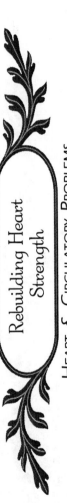

Rebuilding Heart Strength

HEART & CIRCULATORY PROBLEMS

If you've had a heart attack, you know. Rebuilding your strength after such a traumatic body experience is tough work. **Heart attacks** result from damage to the arteries that carry blood to the heart. When these arteries become clogged with fats, blood flow to the heart is cut off or diminished. When there is not adequate blood flow to the heart, its muscles can no longer function and die from lack of nourishment, resulting in heart attacks. **Congestive heart failure,** marked by extreme fatigue and water retention, occurs when the heart is unable to efficiently pump blood. High iron stores after menopause may put a woman at CHF risk. On this page, we will explore herbal combinations to strengthen the heart after a heart attack or if you have congestive heart failure. Remember, if you think you are having a heart attack, seek medical attention immediately.

❧ ESSENTIAL CATEGORIES FOR REBUILDING YOUR HEART COMPOUNDS:

MAGNESIUM RICH HERBS	ANTIOXIDANT SOURCE HERBS	CARDIOTONIC HERBS	LIVER SUPPORT DIURETIC HERBS	VASODILATING HERBS	RELAXING HERBS
Horsetail	**Gingko biloba**	**Hawthorn**	**Red Sage**	**Bilberry**	**Valerian**
Pau d'Arco	**Ginger**	**Arjuna**	Dandelion	Rosemary	Passionflowers
Alfalfa	**Bilberry**	**Motherwort**	Capsicum	**Ginseng-all kinds**	**Scullcap**
Nettles	Garlic	Panax ginseng	Oregon grape	Ginkgo biloba	Eur. Mistletoe
Valerian	Hawthorn	Eur. mistletoe	**Heartsease**	Ginger	Ashwagandha
Parsley	White pine bark	**Night blooming cereus**	**Juniper Berries**	**Cayenne**	Kava Kava
Carrot	**Rosemary**	Black cohosh	Ginger	Evening Primrose	Oatstraw
Watercress	Astragalus	Capsicum	Poria cocus	Red Sage	Hops
Kelp/sea vegetables	Maitake mushroom	Suma	Uva Ursi	Garlic	Wood Betony

❧ ESSENTIAL HERBS FOR REBUILDING YOUR HEART COMPOUNDS:

PRIMARY HERBS	ASSISTING & COMPLEMENTARY HERBS	CATALYST & TRANSPORTING HERBS
Hawthorn	Astragalus	Cayenne	Olive Leaf	Carrot
Arjuna	Dong Quai	White Pine	Heartsease	Lobelia
Motherwort	Nettles	Pau d'Arco	Juniper Berries	Chamomile
Ginkgo biloba	Eur. mistletoe	Horsetail	Parsley	Lemon Balm
Ashwagandha	Red Sage	Valerian	Poria cocos	Butcher's Broom
Night Blooming Cereus	Scullcap	Dandelion	Uva Ursi	Hibiscus
Kelp/sea vegatbles	Black Cohosh	Evening primrose	Wood Betony	Fennel seed
Gotu Kola	Wild Yam	Passionflowers	Peppermint	Aloe Vera

(Primary Herbs second column:) Garlic, Siberian Ginseng, Ginseng-all kinds, Ho-Shou-Wu, Suma, Alfalfa, Bilberry, Kava Kava

❧ EXAMPLE FORMULAS OF REBUILDING YOUR HEART COMPOUNDS:

A HEART-STRENGTHENING FORMULA FOR WOMEN	A TONIC FORMULA TO REGENERATE THE HEART
Hawthorn bry, lf, flr.	Ashwagandha	Poria Cocos	Valerian	Hawthorn lf.& flr.	Ginkgo Biloba	Astragalus	Poria Cocus Mushroom
Motherwort	Dong Quai	Red Sage	Ginger	Siberian Ginseng	Bilberry	Heartsease	Uva Ursi
	Ginkgo Biloba	Scullcap					

SEE PAGE 1 FOR FORMULATING INSTRUCTIONS.

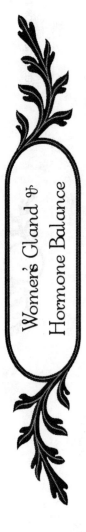

Women's Gland & Hormone Balance

The intricacies of a woman's body are extraordinarily tuned and balanced. When health imbalances occur in a woman, they not only affect her physical state, but cause a lack of union between her mind and body. When she loses the accustomed oneness with herself, both physiological and emotional problems result. From time immemorial women have been close to the Earth as part of the creative process. Herbs, important nutrients of the Earth and its regenerating design, are primarily body balancers - and so work amazingly well with a woman's system. A healthy endocrine system is a must for solving female problems... Hormones, incredibly potent glandular secretions, seem to be at the root of most women's problems. Some hormones have almost immediate effects, some a long-delayed reaction. Even in tiny amounts they have, as any woman can tell you, dramatic effects.

Drugs, chemicals and synthetic medicines, standing outside the body's natural cycle, often do not bring positive results for women at deep body levels like glands and hormones. Women with hysterectomies are only beginning to see the harm that removing delicate glands, or treating fragile hormones with drugs can do. Other women are acquainted with the unpleasant side effects of contraceptive and hormone replacement drugs. A wide range of female problems are caused by too much estrogen production. Breast and uterine fibroids, endometriosis, PMS, and heavy, painful menstrual periods are good examples. Some research shows that these problems and perhaps even breast cancer may be caused from overstimulation of the glands by synthetically reproduced hormones.

Herbs work, instead, with a woman's own hormone action for body balance. Herbal therapy supports in a broad spectrum, like the female essence itself, and a woman's body responds to it easily without side effects. Plant or phyto-hormones are remarkably similar to human hormones. They can be accepted by hormone receptor sites in our bodies. At $1/_{400th}$ to $1/_{50,000th}$ the strength of circulating hormones, they are gentle and safe, exerting a tonic effect rather than drug-like activity. Recent studies on soy foods and herbs such as ginseng, black cohosh and wild yam clearly show hormone-normalizing effects.

What about environmental estrogens and a woman's glandular health? Only in the last five years has anyone realized how common environmental estrogens are in our society. Pesticides, herbicides and many other new chemicals contain man-made estrogens. Estrogens and other hormones are common today in meats, dairy products, and drugs such as hormone replacement therapies. Science is just beginning to accept, although naturopaths have known for some time, that man-made estrogens can stack the deck against women by increasing their estrogen levels hundreds of times.

There is a link between pesticides and breast cancer. Pesticides, like other pollutants, are stored in body fat areas like breast tissue. Some pesticides including PCB's and DDT compromise immune function, overwork the liver and affect the glands and hormones the way too much estrogen does. One study shows 50 to 60% more dichloro-diphenyl-ethylene (DDE) and polychlorinated bi-phenols, (PCB's) in women who have breast cancer than in those who don't. The dramatic rise in breast cancer is consistent with the accumulation of organo-chlorine residues in the environment.

Good nutrition and herbal therapy for the glands can "change the world" for a woman. Using herbal therapy to rebalance hormone ratios gently harmonizes your body, rather than regulating hormone levels by injection. Women can have a great deal of confidence that herbal therapy will work for them. Herbs are in the forefront of modern science today with the proven value of ancient wisdom that women prize. We have found that most women know their own bodies better than anyone else, and can instinctively pinpoint foods within a diet range that are right for their personal renewal and balance. Relief, and response time are often quite gratifying.

✤ FORMULAS FOR FEMALE GLAND & HORMONE PROBLEMS HELP IN THE FOLLOWING CONDITIONS:

•Hormone & Gland Imbalances •Breast & Uterine Fibroids •Adrenal Exhaustion •Endometriosis •Frigidity •Infertility •PMS, Cramps & Other Menstrual Difficulties •Menopausal Symptoms •Post-Menopausal Bone Loss & Osteoporosis •Vaginal Dryness •Cysts, Polyps & Benign Tumors •Chronic Yeast Infections

✤ COMPOUNDS FOR FORMULATION SHOULD INCLUDE:

•Managing PMS and menstrual difficulties.
•Overcoming breast and uterine fibroids and ovarian cysts.
•Normalizing menopause symptoms.
•Rebalancing the body against chronic yeast infections.

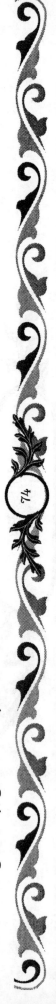

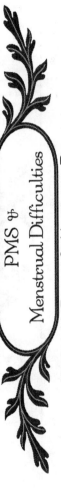

PMS & Menstrual Difficulties

WOMEN'S GLAND & HORMONE PROBLEMS

It is estimated that **90%** of women between the ages of 20 and 50 experience one or more symptoms of PMS. Symptoms increase in the late thirties and beyond, after taking birth control pills and after pregnancy, but with over 150 documented symptoms affecting every system of the body, there is clearly no one cause and no one treatment. Traditional medicines have not been able to address PMS. A holistic approach has shown far more successful results, because self care can tailor treatment to individual needs. A program including a nutritious diet, herbal compounds, and daily exercise encourage the body to do its own work, providing more permanent balance. A natural therapy program for PMS takes at least two months as the body works through both ovary cycles. However, PMS is complex. Numerous body functions are tied into hormone secretions and glandular cycles. Some women need 6 months or more to gently coax the glands and hormones into balance.

❧ ESSENTIAL CATEGORIES FOR PMS AND MENSTRUAL DIFFICULTY COMPOUNDS:

HORMONE BALANCING HERBS	ANTISPASMODIC HERBS	BODY CHEMISTRY BALANCERS	MINERAL-RICH HERBS	MOOD-STABILIZING NERVINES	ANTIOXIDANTS & EFAs
Wild yam root	**Black haw**	**Kelp/sea vegetables**	**Kelp/sea vegetables**	**Valerian root**	**Evening primrose oil**
Licorice root	**Cramp bark**	**Evening primrose**	**Nettles**	**Oatstraw**	**Borage seed**
Dong qual root	**Kava kava**	**Licorice root**	**Dandelion root**	**Scullcap**	**Barley grass**
Burdock root	**Red raspberry**	**Sarsaparilla root**	**Alfalfa**	Lemongrass	**Spirulina**
Damiana	**Chamomile**	Hawthorn lf., flr. bry.	Watercress	**Wood betony**	**Kelp/sea vegetables**
Sarsaparilla root	Wild yam root	Alfalfa	**Horsetail**	Black cohosh	Flax seed
Ashwagandha	Peony root	Dandelion root	**Oatstraw**	**Passionflower**	Black currant
Red raspberry	Angelica root	Strawberry	Spirulina	Valerian root	Fennel seed
Squaw vine	False unicorn root	Rose hips	Yellow dock root	**Rosemary**	Rosemary

❧ ESSENTIAL HERBS FOR PMS AND MENSTRUAL DIFFICULTY COMPOUNDS:

PRIMARY HERBS		ASSISTING & COMPLEMENTARY HERBS	
Hawthorn lf., bry. & fl.	Chamomile	Dandelion root	Angelica rt.
Kelp/sea vegetables	Sarsaparilla root	Scullcap	Yellow dock rt.
Ginkgo biloba	Wild yam root	Nettles	Oatstraw
Licorice root	Black cohosh	Lemon grass	Squaw vine
Burdock rt.	Ashwagandha root	Parsley rt. & lf.	Bilberry
Dong qual rt.	Kava kava	Alfalfa	Wood betony
Evening primrose	Royal Jelly	False unicorn root	Horsetail
Damiana	Red raspberry	Goldenseal root	Peony rt.
Ginseng - all types	Cramp bark	Spirulina/Barley grass	Rose hips

❧ EXAMPLE FORMULAS OF PMS AND MENSTRUAL DIFFICULTY COMPOUNDS:

A FEMALE HARMONY TEA COMPOUND		(w - 5360)	A FEMALE HARMONY CAPSULE COMPOUND		(w - 2290)
Red raspberry	Spearmint	Lemongrass	Burdock root	Dong qual	Ashwagandha	Yellowdock rt.
Licorice root	Rose hips	Strawberry	Rosebuds	Damiana	Hawthorn lf., bry.., flr.	Dandelion rt.
Nettles		Sarsaparilla root		Burdock root	Licorice root	Peony rt.	Fennel
				Nettles	Sarsaparilla root	Angelica root	Rose hips
					Red raspberry		
					Oatstraw		

SEE PAGE 1 FOR FORMULATING INSTRUCTIONS.

75

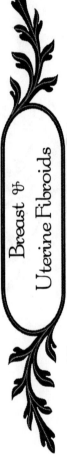

Breast & Uterine Fibroids

Women's Gland & Hormone Problems

Disheartening statistics show 1 out of every 1500 American women between the ages of 35 and 49 have fibroid growths; and the risk of getting them increases dramatically with age. Hormone imbalances, primarily too much estrogen and an under active thyroid are the usual cause. Customary medical protocol prescribes regular mammograms for early detection, surgical biopsies and then fibroid removal. Yet there is a very real risk in receiving regular doses of radiation through mammograms, even though X-ray dosage is decreasing. Breast tissue is so sensitive that sometimes the time between a having a mammogram and getting a fibroid growth may be as little as three months. Since fibroids are not cancer, and have little chance of becoming cancerous, many women are turning to alternative methods to reduce them. Natural therapies focus on improving lifestyle habits for prevention, and herbal supplementation to rebalance gland and hormone activity.

❧ ESSENTIAL CATEGORIES FOR BREAST & UTERINE FIBROID COMPOUNDS:

TUMOR GROWTH DETERRENTS	HORMONE BALANCING HERBS	BODY CHEMISTRY BALANCERS	IODINE-RICH HERBS FOR THYROID BALANCE	BIOFLAVONOID & CAROTENE SOURCES	ANTIOXIDANT SUPPORT
Echinacea root	**Dong qual root**	**Kelp/sea vegetables**	**Watercress**	**Alfalfa**	Chlorophyll sources
Panax ginseng	**Sarsaparilla root**	**Alfalfa/Chlorella**	**Kelp/sea vegetables**	**Barley grass**	Ginseng - all types
Pau d'arco bark	**Wild yam root**	Squaw vine	**Spirulina**	**Kelp/sea vegetables**	Parsley rt. & lf.
Licorice root	**Burdock root**	**Aloe vera**	**Borage seed**	Chlorella	Ginkgo biloba
Kelp/sea vegetables	Licorice root	**Astragalus**	**Ginger root**	**Bilberry**	Rosemary
Chamomile	**False unicorn root**	Dandelion root	**Capsicum**	**Spirulina**	Licorice root
Garlic	**Peony root**	Cramp bark	Nettles	Aloe vera	Alfalfa
Goldenseal root	**Black cohosh root**	Ashwagandha root	Alfalfa	Lemongrass	Pau d'arco bark
Evening primrose oil	**Red raspberry**	**Ginseng - all types**	Irish moss	Hawthorn lf., bry., fl.	Ginger root

❧ ESSENTIAL HERBS FOR BREAST & UTERINE FIBROID COMPOUNDS:

PRIMARY HERBS		ASSISTING & COMPLEMENTARY HERBS		CATALYST & TRANSPORTING HERBS	
Hawthorn lf., bry., fl.	Black cohosh root	Sarsaparilla root	Evening primrose oil	Aloe vera juice	Heartsease
Burdock root	Nettles	False unicorn	White sage	Acerola cherry	Rosemary
Ginseng - all types	Pau d'arco bark	Barley grass	Rose hips vit. C	Irish moss	Blessed thistle
Dong qual root	Bilberry	Parsley rt. & lf.	Borage seed	Capsicum	Horsetail
Ashwagandha root	Wild yam root	Watercress	Oregon grape rt.	Peppermint	Calendula
Alfalfa	Dandelion rt. & lf.	Spirulina	Garlic	Vitamin C powder	Fennel seed
Kelp & sea vegetables	Licorice root	Astragalus	Ginkgo biloba	Ginger root	Flax seed
Goldenseal root	Red raspberry	Yellow dock root	Peony root	Lobelia	Brewer's yeast
Chlorella	Cramp bark	Echinacea root	Squaw vine	Rehmannia root	Uva ursi

❧ EXAMPLE FORMULAS OF BREAST & UTERINE FIBROID COMPOUNDS:

A WOMAN'S BALANCE FIBROID CAPSULE COMPOUND		(w - 4345)
Pau d'arco bark	Ashwagandha	Ginger root.
Burdock root	Dong qual root	Astragalus rt.
Goldenseal root	Red raspberry	
Licorice root		
Dandelion rt. & lf.		
Yellow dock root		

A WOMAN'S BEST FRIEND CAPSULE COMPOUND		(w - 4350)
Goldenseal root	Rose hips	Ginger root
Cramp bark	Dong qual root	Rehmannia root
Squaw vine	False unicorn	Lobelia
Red raspberry	Sarsaparilla root	
	Peony root	
	Uva ursi	
	Blessed thistle	

SEE PAGE 1 FOR FORMULATING INSTRUCTIONS.

Normalizing Menopause Symptoms

WOMEN'S GLAND & HORMONE PROBLEMS

Phyto-hormone containing herbs have effective, antioxidant and hormone balancing properties that make them a first choice to address the imbalances and discomforts of menopause. They have a safety record of centuries, and offer a gentle, effective way to stimulate a woman's own body to produce amounts of estrogen and progesterone that are in the right proportion for her needs as menopause progresses. They can help control hot flashes, tighten sagging tissue, lubricate a dry vagina, enhance circulation, and generally keep the female system very female. Herbs are taken in by the body as foods through the enzyme system, not as drugs working outside the system. At only ¹/₄₀₀ₜₕ the potency of synthetic estrogen, phyto-estrogens do not have the unpleasant side effects of increased appetite, fluid retention and cellulite deposits caused by synthetic hormones, yet they still offer symptom control and osteoporosis deterrence.

✒ ESSENTIAL CATEGORIES FOR NORMALIZING MENOPAUSE COMPOUNDS:

ESTROGEN-BALANCING HERBS	PHYTO-HORMONE CONTAINING HERBS	CALMING, SOOTHING NERVINES	IODINE & MINERAL-RICH HERBS	GLAND & TISSUE STRENGTHENERS	ALKALIZING HERBS
Black cohosh root	**Sarsaparilla root**	**Black cohosh**	**Kelp/sea vegetables**	**Royal jelly**	**Marshmallow root**
Dong qual root	**Wild yam root**	**Rosemary**	**Spirulina/chlorella**	**Gotu kola**	**Alfalfa**
Licorice root	**Licorice root**	**Cramp bark**	Barley grass	**Evening primrose oil**	Chlorella
Sarsaparilla root	Bee pollen/ royal jelly	**Valerian root**	Watercress	**Hawthorn lf., bry., fl.**	Barley grass
False unicorn root	**Ashwagandha**	**Scullcap**	Parsley leaf & root	Wild yam root	Dandelion root
Panax ginseng/Suma	Panax ginseng root	**Passionflower**	**Alfalfa**	Ginkgo biloba	**Aloe vera**
Squaw vine	Evening primrose	Peppermint	**Oatstraw**	Red raspberry	**Calendula**
Blessed thistle	**Damiana**	Kava kava rt.	**Nettles**	Borage seed	Yellow dock root
Ashwagandha	**Burdock root**	**Chamomile**	Horsetail	**Bilberry**	**Pau d'arco bark**

✒ ESSENTIAL HERBS FOR NORMALIZING MENOPAUSE COMPOUNDS:

PRIMARY HERBS		ASSISTING & COMPLEMENTARY HERBS		CATALYST & TRANSPORTING HERBS	
Ginseng - all kinds	Kelp & sea vegetables	False unicorn	Nettles	Capsicum	Aloe vera juice
Barley grass	Wild yam root	Spirulina	Valerian rt.	Angelica root	Bilberry berry
Evening primrose	Ginkgo biloba	Scullcap	Royal jelly	Lobelia	Parsley root & lf.
Hawthorn bry., lf., flr.	Oatstraw	Marshmallow root	Kava kava rt.	Rosemary	Watercress
Black cohosh rt.	Gotu kola	Barley grass/Chlorella	Passionflower	Garlic	Dulse
Licorice root	Squaw vine	Chamomile	Cramp bark	Ginger root	Pennyroyal
Dong qual	Sarsaparilla root	Horsetail	Red raspberry	Yellow dock root	Blessed thistle
Burdock root	Dandelion root & lf.	Borage seed	Damiana	Peppermint	Calendula
Ashwagandha	Suma root	Bee pollen	Alfalfa	Pau d'arco bk.	Cinnamon

✒ EXAMPLE FORMULAS OF NORMALIZING MENOPAUSE COMPOUNDS:

AN EASY CHANGE CAPSULE COMPOUND			(w - 2100)	AN EASY CHANGE TEA COMPOUND			(w - 5280)
Black cohosh rt.	False unicorn	Uva ursi	Ginger root	Burdock root	Dong quai root	Red raspberry	Ginger root
Scullcap	Sarsaparilla root	Red raspberry	Rosemary	Licorice root	Damiana	Sarsaparilla rt.	Bayberry bk.
Damiana	Dong quai	Bayberry bk.	Pennyroyal	Black cohosh root	Scullcap	Ginkgo biloba	
Ashwagandha	Squaw vine	Cramp bark	Blessed thistle				

SEE PAGE 1 FOR FORMULATING INSTRUCTIONS.

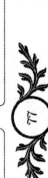

85

Chronic Yeast Infections

WOMEN'S GLAND & HORMONE PROBLEMS

Vaginal yeast infections are a scourge of modern times as women are more exposed to water and environmental pollutants, long courses of antibiotics or cortico-steroid drugs and frequent use of spermicidal preparations. These things weaken immunity, and throw off the chemistry of the vagina's delicate acid mantle. Most yeast infections are a condition of pH imbalance rather than a disease. Natural therapies abate vaginal yeast infections, but long-term cure is not likely unless dietary and lifestyle changes are made. Common yeast infections are: **trichomonas** - a parasitic infection contracted through intercourse, severe itchiness and a thin, foamy, foul discharge; **gardnerella** - a bacterial infection transmitted through sexual contact, with a foul, fishy odor, white discharge, and itchiness; **leukorrhea** - a condition occurring when normal vaginal acidity is disrupted, with itching, irritation and inflammation of the vaginal tissues, foul odor, "cottage cheese" discharge, and painful intercourse.

❧ ESSENTIAL CATEGORIES FOR YEAST INFECTIONS COMPOUNDS:

ANTIBACTERIAL HERBS	BODY CHEMISTRY BALANCING HERBS	TISSUE SOOTHING HERBS	ASTRINGENT HERBS	IMMUNE SUPPORT HERBS	ANTI-FUNGAL SUPPORT
Echinacea root	**Dong qual root**	**Marshmallow root**	**Witch hazel bk. & lf.**	**Chlorophyll-rich herbs**	**Black walnut hulls**
Black walnut hulls	**Acidophilus powder**	Parsley root	**White oak bark**	St. John's wort	**Acidophilus powder**
Goldenseal root	**Alfalfa/Nettles**	**Slippery elm bark**	**Bayberry bark**	**Reishi mushroom**	**Tea tree oil**
Chaparral	**Kelp & sea vegetables**	Dandelion root	**Cranesbill**	**Kelp/sea vegetables**	**Gentian root**
Myrrh	Barley grass/Chlorella	**Aloe vera**	Plantain	**Bee pollen/royal jelly**	**Chaparral**
Garlic	Red raspberry	Red raspberry	Red raspberry	Alfalfa	Garlic
Ginger root	**Spirulina**	**Plantain lf.**	Sage	Barley grass	Myrrh
Pau d'arco bark	**Ashwagandha**	**Calendula**	St. John's wort	Lemongrass	Juniper bry.
Yarrow	Squaw vine	**Irish moss**	Buchu lf.	Vitamin C powder	Goldenseal root

❧ ESSENTIAL HERBS FOR YEAST INFECTIONS COMPOUNDS:

PRIMARY HERBS	ASSISTING & COMPLEMENTARY HERBS	CATALYST & TRANSPORTING HERBS
Reishi mushroom	Barley grass	Aloe vera juice
Burdock root	Parsley root & lf.	Garlic
Ginseng - all types	Gentian	Ashwaganda
Bayberry	Barberry bark	Capsicum
Myrrh	Uva ursi	Lemongrass
Alfalfa	Spirulina	Vitamin C powder
Kelp & sea vegetables	Chaparral lf.	Ginger root
Goldenseal root	Buchu lf.	Cranesbill
Chlorella	Echinacea root	Dong qual root
Juniper bry.	Tea tree oil	Acidophilus powder
Nettles	Squaw vine	Rosemary
Pau d' arco bark	St. John's wort	Rose hips vit. C
Black walnut	Slippery elm bark	Calendula
Bee pollen/royal jelly	Marshmallow root	Fennel seed
Dandelion rt. & lf.	Yarrow	Flax seed
Licorice root	White oak bk	Irish moss
Witch hazel lf. & bk.	Red raspberry	Brewer's yeast
Plantain lf.	Comfrey rt	Sage

❧ EXAMPLE FORMULAS OF YEAST INFECTIONS COMPOUNDS:

A YEAST INFECTION DOUCHE COMPOUND		(w - 7750)
Witch hazel lf. & bk.	Juniper bry.	Pau d'arco bark	White oak bk.
Comfrey rt.	Myrrh	Buchu lf.	Acidophilus pdwr.
	Goldenseal root	Squaw vine	

A YEAST INFECTION CLEANSING CAPSULE COMPOUND		(w - 4310)
Burdock root	Squaw vine	Parsley root & lf.	Black walnut
Juniper bry.	Bayberry	Dandelion rt. & lf.	Uva ursi
		Gentian	

SEE PAGE 1 FOR FORMULATING INSTRUCTIONS.

78

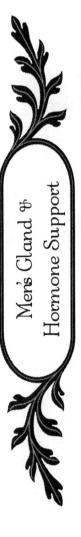

Men's Gland &
Hormone Support

Today's fast paced, high stress lifestyle seems to demand that men be "supermen." A man must be strong physically during workouts and sports, supportive emotionally in relationships, balanced under stress, mentally creative and quick, and sexually keen and virile. Diet and exercise are the pillars supporting a man's health and energy. But both are woefully deficient in the modern American man's life. Chemical-laden farming methods and foods have made us one of the earth's most nutritionally deficient nations. Our hectic, yet sedentary lives don't readily allow for exercise unless a conscious effort is made. In addition, women aren't the only ones endangered by the estrogen-imitating effects of chemicals and pesticides. There is substantial evidence that supports the role played by man-made estrogens in hormone imbalances that threaten male health and fertility, too. The most alarming statistics relate to sperm count (which have fallen by almost half since 1940), and hormone-driven cancers which have risen dramatically.

Men tend to keep a health problem to themselves until it becomes a medical crisis. To a man, illness is more than just physical pain or discomfort. It exposes vulnerability and weakness, opens him up to the unwelcome intimacy of a body exam, and is a source of embarrassment for not being able to handle the problem himself. No one likes to go to a doctor or undergo medical treatment, but the whole male ego/personality profile becomes threatened during illness. Men grow up knowing very little information about their bodies except in the context of sexual function or sports performance, so they rarely see the need to take disease prevention measures or seek understanding about health maintenance.

HERBS CAN BE A VALUABLE ANSWER FOR MEN'S CHRONIC HEALTH PROBLEMS, A KIND OF NATURAL INSURANCE POLICY FOR MANY MALE NEEDS.

•Information about how to use herbs safely and effectively is readily available for a man wishing to take more responsibility for his health. Before the industrial-ized/heroic medicine era most families knew how to use herbs for health. Men, generally, were the more respected herbalists, with a long tradition of understanding the relationship between mind/body/health connection.

•Herbs provide men with an effective way to deal with the greatest underlying cause of their health problems - stress. Because they are reluctant to admit setbacks, have a tendency to deny problems rather than deal with them, and hold their feelings in, men are far more susceptible than women to stress-related illnesses, such as hypertension, heart attack and fatigue.

•Herbs are strong enough to benefit the male system without the side effects of drugs. They have broad range activity for long term results. They work quickly through the body's own enzyme structure, and act cumulatively to rebalance body chemistry.

•Herbal supplements provide concentrated nutrients to reproduce new cells and tissue and to increase male strength and physique. They can overcome nutrient depletions, especially body building minerals, and tonify the body for extra energy and endurance. Herbal formulas are valuable at all levels of an active lifestyle. They are a proven adjunct to muscle growth, and speed healing from sports-related injuries.

•Herbs can add more energy to the reproductive system, a major area of male strength and longevity, thus making the whole body healthier.

•Herbs are easy. A man doesn't have to relinquish his strong, self-reliant perspective to use herbs for many health problems successfully.

✥ FORMULAS FOR MALE GLAND & HORMONE PROBLEMS HELP IN THE FOLLOWING CONDITIONS :

•Prostate Enlargement & Inflammation •High Blood Pressure •Male Infertility •Reducing Risk of Congestive Heart Failure, Angina, a Coronary or Stroke •Heart Arrhythmias - Male Circulatory Health •Arterio- and Atherosclerosis & Cholesterol Build-up •Hemorrhoids & Colon Health •Adrenal Exhaustion •Weight Control •Improving Endurance & Stamina •Stress & Tension.

✥ COMPOUNDS FOR FORMULATION SHOULD INCLUDE:

•Overcoming prostate enlargement and inflammation
•Deep level gland balance and revitalization of the male system.

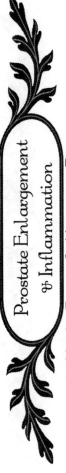

Prostate Enlargement & Inflammation

MEN'S GLAND & HORMONE PROBLEMS

A man's prostate can be his worst friend. The little doughnut-shaped gland that lies below a man's bladder is a source of big problems to many men. The prostate's job in life is to secrete a fluid/enzyme mixture for sperm health and motility. Almost 60% of men between the ages of 45 and 70 have BPH (benign prostatic hyperplasia). As middle age approaches, the prostate often enlarges, strangling the urethra, and causing symptoms of frequent urination, trouble starting urination, weak flow and the feeling that the bladder isn't empty afterwards. While BPH is not cancer, an enlarged prostate can eventually completely block the flow of urine, an obviously life-threatening condition. Research indicates that prostate enlargement is caused by an enzyme, testosterone reductase, which produces di-hydro-testosterone, a hormone form that also affects male pattern baldness. BPH usually reponds to nutritional and herbal support, especially in the early stages.

❧ ESSENTIAL CATEGORIES FOR MANAGING PROSTATE ENLARGEMENT:

ANTIBIOTIC/TUMOR DETERRENT HERBS	CHLOROPHYLL SOURCE HERBS	GLAND & HORMONE BALANCING HERBS	DIURETIC/SEDIMENT DISSOLVING HERBS	ANTI-INFLAMMATORY HERBS	IODINE THERAPY HERBS
Echinacea root	**Chlorella**	**Muira pauma**	**Hydrangea root**	**White willow bark**	**Kelp/sea vegetables**
Pau d' arco bark	Barley grass	**Damiana**	Uva ursi	**St. John's wort**	**Nettles**
Capsicum	Nettles	**Licorice root**	**Juniper berry**	**Chamomile**	**Borage seed**
Goldenseal root	**Spirulina**	**Sarsaparilla root**	Ginger root	**Dandelion root**	**Garlic**
Myrrh	**Alfalfa**	**Evening primrose oil**	Cornsilk	**White oak bark**	Alfalfa
Chaparral	Watercress	**Bee pollen/royal jelly**	**Yarrow**	Marshmallow root	Irish moss
Butternut bark	Parsley leaf	**Saw palmetto berry**	Gravel root	Eur. Mistletoe	Dulse
Panax ginseng	**Kelp/sea vegetables**	Flax seed	Poria mushroom	Ginger root	Spirulina
Licorice root	**Aloe vera**	**Pygeum Africanum**	**Parsley lf. & rt.**	Turmeric	Watercress

❧ ESSENTIAL HERBS FOR MANAGING PROSTATE ENLARGEMENT:

PRIMARY HERBS		ASSISTING & COMPLEMENTARY HERBS		CATALYST & TRANSPORTING HERBS	
Saw palmetto bry.	Pau d'arco bark	Dandelion root	Butternut bark	Capsicum	Borage seed
Kelp/sea vegetables	Sarsaparilla root	Marshmallow root	Barley grass	Chamomile	Vitamin E pdwr.
Ginkgo biloba	Damiana	Poria mushroom	Uva ursi	Ginger root	Parsley rt & lf.
Siberian ginseng	Wild yam	Spirulina	White oak bk.	Irish moss	Yarrow
Licorice root	Hawthorn lf. flr. & bry.	Oregon grape	Echinacea root	Rosemary	Calendula flr
Muira pauma/Ptncy.wd.	Panax ginseng	Chlorella	Myrrh	Flax seed	Chaparral
Evening primrose	Gravel root	St. John's wort	Bee pollen	Aloe vera juice	Nettles
Garlic	Goldenseal root	Eur. Mistletoe	Royal Jelly	Watercress	Turmeric
Ginseng - all types	Pygeum africanum	Juniper berry	Hydrangea	Miso broth powder	Cornsilk

❧ EXAMPLE FORMULAS OF COMPOUNDS FOR PROSTATE ENLARGEMENT:

AN ANTI-INFLAMMATORY PROSTATE CAPSULE COMPOUND   (M - 3760)

Saw palmetto bry.	Juniper berry	Hydrangea
Kelp/sea vegetables	Parsley rt.	Capsicum
Ginkgo biloba	Potency wood	Vitamin E
Siberian ginseng	Goldenseal root	
Licorice root	Uva ursi	
Muira pauma/Ptncy.wd.	Marshmallow rt.	
Evening primrose	Ginger root	
Garlic		
Ginseng - all types		

A HORMONE-BALANCING TOPICAL PROSTATE GEL COMPOUND (M - 7430)

Saw palmetto bry.	Aloe vera juice	Goldenseal root	Oregon grape
Licorice root	Wild yam	Pau d'arco bk.	Eur. Mistletoe
Gravel root	Panax ginseng	Licorice root	Marshmallow rt.
Pygeum africanum	Pygeum Afric.	Echinacea root	Burdock root	Uva ursi

SEE PAGE 1 FOR FORMULATING INSTRUCTIONS.

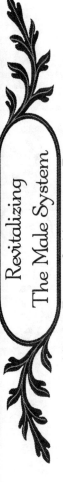

Revitalizing
The Male System

MEN'S GLAND & HORMONE PROBLEMS

Herbs are a good choice for re-energizing male physical energy and combating fatigue and stress. Herbs work at the deepest level of the body processes, stimulating and supporting without depleting the adrenals and other glands. They are valuable for improving hormone function and balance, and add more energy to the reproductive system. Male reproductive energy does far more than just create offspring. It makes the whole male body healthier, with the solid foundation energy stimulants a man's system needs to reproduce new cells and tissues, to increase vitality and tonify sexual organs for potency and sperm production. Herbs are strong enough to specifically benefit the male system without the side effects of drugs, and they have broad spectrum activity for long term results. Very few foods are able to offer either the strength or the specific nutrients with the rapid results of herbal combinations.

❧ ESSENTIAL CATEGORIES FOR REVITALIZING THE MALE SYSTEM COMPOUNDS:

GLANDULAR REGENERATIVE HERBS	CHLOROPHYLL & AMINO ACID SUPPORT	BIOFLAVONOID & CAROTENE SOURCES	MINERAL-RICH HERBS	HORMONE BALANCING & EFA SOURCES	BODY CHEMISTRY BALANCING HERBS
Bee pollen/royal jelly	**Chlorella**	**Chlorella**	**Oatstraw**	**Damiana**	**Ginkgo biloba**
Damiana	**Barley grass**	**Barley grass**	**Kelp/sea vegetables**	**Saw palmetto bry.**	**Garlic**
Sarsaparilla root	**Alfalfa**	**Kelp/sea vegetables**	**Yellow dock root**	**Muira pauma**	**Suma root**
Wild yam root	**Nettles**	**Bilberry**	**Nettles**	**Wild yam root**	Burdock root
Fo-Ti-root	**Spirulina**	Hawthorn bry., lf., fl.	**Horsetail**	**Panax ginseng**	**Ginger root**
Panax ginseng	**Kelp/sea vegetables**	**Bee pollen/royal jelly**	**Pau d'arco bark**	**Sarsaparilla root**	Goldenseal root
Siberian ginseng	Bee pollen/royal jelly	**Spirulina**	Borage seed	**Licorice root**	**Astragalus**
White oak bark	Watercress	**Aloe vera**	Dandelion root	**Evening primrose oil**	**Echinacea root**
Saw palmetto berry	Parsley leaf	Dandelion root	Chlorophyll-rich herbs	**Flax seed**	Capsicum

❧ ESSENTIAL HERBS FOR REVITALIZING THE MALE SYSTEM COMPOUNDS:

PRIMARY HERBS			ASSISTING & COMPLEMENTARY HERBS			CATALYST & TRANSPORTING HERBS	
Saw palmetto bry.	Potency wood		Parsley root & lf.	Evening primrose oil		Aloe vera juice	St. John's wort
Burdock root	Fo-Ti root		Hawthorn bry., lf., fl.	Alfalfa		Coriander	Rosemary
Ginseng - all types	Pau d'arco bark		Marshmallow root	White oak bark		Lecithin	Watercress
Sarsaparilla root	Gotu kola		Nettles	Yellow dock rt.		Capsicum	Oatstraw
Damiana	Royal jelly		Spirulina	Bilberry		Peppermint	Calendula
Licorice root	Dandelion rt. & lf.		Astragalus	Garlic		Vitamin C powder	Fennel seed
Kelp & sea vegetables	Suma root		Barley grass	Ginkgo biloba		Ginger root	Flax seed
Goldenseal root	Siberian ginseng		Echinacea root	Wild yam root		Rose hips	Turmeric
Chlorella	Panax ginseng		Bee pollen	Hawthorn bry., lf., fl.		Chamomile	Horsetail

❧ EXAMPLE FORMULAS OF REVITALIZING THE MALE SYSTEM COMPOUNDS:

A MALE PERFORMANCE CAPSULE COMPOUNDS		(M - 3150)	A GINSENG BODY TONIC EXTRACT COMPOUND		(M - 4438)
Saw palmetto bry.	Royal jelly	Wild yam root	Fo-Ti root	Panax ginseng rt.	Ginkgo biloba	Saw palmetto bry.	Capsicum
Damiana	Potency wood	Licorice root	Yellow dock rt.	Damiana	Potency wood	Ginger rt.
Siberian ginseng	Gotu kola	Dandelion root	Capsicum		Gotu kola
Sarsaparilla root		Panax ginseng		

SEE PAGE 1 FOR FORMULATING INSTRUCTIONS.

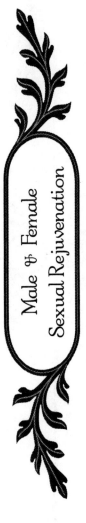

Male & Female
Sexual Rejuvenation

Herbs have been associated with love potions and sexuality for thousands of years. Is there some herbal smoke behind the fires of passion? Can certain herbs really enhance libido and sexual performance? Recent studies are showing that, once again, science is validating herbal tradition. In fact, it turns out that certain herbal nutrients may have a great deal of influence on several aspects of sexual response and performance in human beings. Herbs don't turn men into supermen, or make women love slaves, but herbs can be a good remedy choice when there are sexual function problems. They can help awaken libido, boost sexual vigor and performance stamina, and heighten sexual excitement for both partners. We tend to think that our modern era is the only one beset with libido-lowering elements. Certainly there is no question that our nutrient-poor, high-fat diets, over-use of drugs, and high-pressure lifestyles lead to low energy and lack of time for love. But the reality is that humanity in every era has felt the need for help in the sexual and reproductive area. After all, this part of our lives is at the most elemental center of our being.

Many people wonder whether there really are aphrodisiac herbs. There are indeed herbs that stimulate gland and hormone activity and increase body energy. Herbal "aphrodisiacs" offer both men and women nutrients that help build up sexual energy and vitality; the kind of energy that turns thoughts and mood to love. A good herbal formula for sexual energy will help improve blood supply, enhance nerve stimulation, and glandular activity.

Herbs can help maximize personal potential for more rewarding sexuality and a happier love life. They promote clearer skin, a more even temperament, fewer allergies, sweeter breath, softer hair, brighter eyes and a more pleasing body shape. Better sex naturally emerges from a healthier body. Herbs also help increase stamina, vitality, and libido by encouraging gland and hormone activity. Effectiveness can be quite specific to the system of both sexes. If there are psychological or stress-related problems impeding sexuality, (up to 80% of sexual dysfunction is of mental or emotional origin), herbs can help overcome them by turning the attention to love-making, and stimulating short term energy against impotence or frigidity. For the 20% of physiological factors causing sexual problems, the most common are diabetes, the use of certain prescription or pleasure drugs and poor circulation. Aging is not a cause of impotence or lack of libido for either a man or a woman. Normal sexual function requires healthy organs, and balanced glands to produce necessary sex hormones. Herbs, as superior body balancers that work through the glands, are uniquely qualified to help us achieve better gland response and overcome body deficiencies for a healthier sex life. But they can do even more than that. There are also herbal constituents that help combat disorders associated with sex, such as impotence, difficulty achieving orgasm, menstrual and menopausal complaints, prostate problems and herpes. Herbs can work quite specifically, and often quite quickly to remedy sexual problems and enrich the sexual experience.

HERBS WORK DIFFERENTLY IN MEN AND WOMEN FOR SEXUAL ENHANCEMENT.

They can be a valuable answer for male sexual health. The most sexually stimulating herbs contain substances that support male gland and nerve systems in a direct way. 1) Herbs increase energy to the male reproductive system. 2) Herbs supply highly absorbable nutrients, such as minerals that can help give the male body solid foundation nourishment it needs to favorably affect potency and sperm production. We know that zinc, for instance, is concentrated in semen, thus frequent ejaculation may diminish body zinc stores. If a zinc deficiency exists, the body may respond by reducing sexual drive. Herbs can be a primary source of absorbable, safe zinc for men. 3) Herbs are strong enough to benefit the male system without the side effects of drugs. They can act quickly, but are also cumulative in the system to build a strong nutritional base.

For women, it all comes down to hormones - those incredibly important, potent substances that seem to be at the root of most women's problems. Hormones are secreted into the bloodstream by the glands, and are carried throughout the body to stimulate specific functions. Even in the tiniest amounts, they have, as any woman can tell you, dramatic effects. Plant hormones from herbal sources nourish and tone and improve blood flow to the female glands and organs. Since many women are more conscious of what turns them off than what turns them on, the qualities of plant hormones make them useful in a broad range of female conditions such as low sexual desire and function, dry vagina, and moodiness.

⬧FORMULAS FOR SEXUAL REJUVENATION HELP IN THE FOLLOWING CONDITIONS:
•Low Libido & Lack of Sexual Energy   •Impotence   •Male Infertility   •Frigidity   •Sterility   •Pituitary & Pineal Gland Health

⬧COMPOUNDS FOR FORMULATION SHOULD INCLUDE:
•Formulas for male sexual rejuvenation.
•Formulas for female sexual rejuvenation.

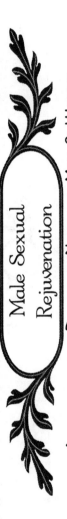

Male Sexual Rejuvenation

ADDRESSING THE DIFFERENT NEEDS OF MEN & WOMEN

What about ginseng and sexual vigor? Ginseng has been used around the world for thousands of years to enhance sexuality. There are many kinds of ginseng. In fact, every major healing culture has a ginseng or ginseng-like plant in its healing tradition. Ginseng doesn't make a man a "super man," but it has several undeniable qualities that validate its reputation. 1) As an adaptogenic herb, ginseng helps the body deal with stress, increasing energy levels and decreasing fatigue, all of which indirectly affect libido. 2) Ginseng is an effective precursor for the male hormone testosterone, and is the only known herb to have this property. A wild Manchurian variety found in China has a particularly stimulating effect on the endocrine glands - increasing testosterone production and encouraging a rejuvenation even greater than testosterone injections. 3) Japanese studies show that ginseng increases the weight of the seminal vesicles, the prostate gland, and sperm count, which all increase fertility.

ESSENTIAL CATEGORIES FOR MALE SEXUAL REJUVENATION COMPOUNDS:

REPRODUCTIVE GLAND REGENERATORS	CHLOROPHYLL & AMINO ACID SOURCES	GLAND & HORMONE BALANCING HERBS	MINERAL-RICH HERBS	ESSENTIAL FATTY ACID SOURCES	LIBIDO & ENERGY STIMULANTS
Bee pollen/royal jelly	**Chlorella**	**Muira pauma**	**Kelp/sea vegetables**	**Borage seed**	**Sarsaparilla root**
Panax ginseng	Barley grass	**Damiana**	Hawthorn lf. flr. & bry	**Spirulina**	**Damiana**
Kelp/sea vegetables	Nettles	**Licorice root**	Dandelion root	**Evening primrose oil**	**Kola nut**
Licorice root	**Spirulina**	**Sarsaparilla root**	White oak bk.	**Schizandra bry.**	**Guarana seed**
Damiana	**Alfalfa**	**Evening primrose oil**	Nettles	Flax seed	**Panax ginseng**
Siberian ginseng	Watercress	**Bee pollen/royal jelly**	Alfalfa	Black currant	**Ginseng - all types**
Sarsaparilla root	Parsley leaf	**Saw palmetto berry**	**Yellow dock root**	**Pumpkin seed**	Kava kava
Gotu kola	**Kelp/sea vegetables**	Burdock root	**Oats/oatstraw**	Fennel seed	Yohimbe
Fo-Ti root	**Aloe vera**	Pygeum Africanum	**Parsley rt. & lf.**	Sage	Suma root

ESSENTIAL HERBS FOR MALE SEXUAL REJUVENATION COMPOUNDS:

PRIMARY HERBS		ASSISTING & COMPLEMENTARY HERBS		CATALYST & TRANSPORTING HERBS	
Damiana	Pau d'arco bark	Saw palmetto bry.	Schizandra bry.	Capsicum	Fennel seed
Bee pollen	Sarsaparilla root	Kava kava root	Suma root	Chamomile	Vitamin E pwr.
Ginkgo biloba	Dandelion root	Pumpkin seed	Kola nut	Ginger root	Pygeum Africanum
Siberian ginseng	Kelp/sea vegetables	Barley grass	White oak bk.	Ginkgo biloba	Yarrow
Licorice root	Hawthorn lf. flr. & bry.	Parsley rt. & lf.	Chlorella	Rosemary	Borage seed
Potency wood	Panax ginseng	Marshmallow root	Alfalfa	Flax seed	Yohimbe bark
Evening primrose	Wild oats	Wild yam	Kirin ginseng root	Aloe vera juice	Nettles
Gotu kola	Spirulina	Burdock root	Royal jelly	Ma huang	Yellow dock root
Ginseng - all types	Guarana seed	Fo-Ti root	Horsetail	Oats/oatstraw	Watercress

EXAMPLE FORMULAS OF MALE SEXUAL REJUVENATION COMPOUNDS:

A MALE, "LOVING MOOD" EXTRACT COMPOUND		(M - 4900)
Damiana	Licorice root	Capsicum
Siberian ginseng rt.	Wild oats	Yohimbe bark
	Dandelion root	

A LOVE MALE CAPSULE COMPOUND		(M - 3100)
Bee pollen	Potency wood	Wild yam root
Siberian ginseng	Gotu kola	Ginger root
Sarsaparilla root	Suma root	
Yohimbe bark		
Guarana seed		
Damiana		
Saw palmetto bry.		
Kava kava root		

SEE PAGE 1 FOR FORMULATING INSTRUCTIONS.

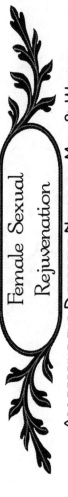

Female Sexual Rejuvenation

Addressing the Different Needs of Men & Women

Reduced or inhibited sexual desire in women can stem from many reasons, both psychological and physical. For many of us these days, lack of time to turn our attention to our partners and our thoughts to love seems to be the biggest problem. Physically, both women and men today are overwhelmed with important career responsibilities, family and home care, sports and other activities that require all our energy, leaving us only able to collapse at the end of the day. Psychologically, women who are dissatisfied with their looks or their life often feel inhibited toward spontaneous love-making, emotional problems at home and work hold a larger place and sometimes crowd out thoughts of love, childhood abuse or relationship experiences have a long reach, and finally a poor diet and lack of exercise take their toll in a loss of well-being. Herbs are a good choice for women who want to rejuvenate their sexual energy

❧ ESSENTIAL CATEGORIES FOR SEXUAL WELL-BEING COMPOUNDS FOR WOMEN:

Phytohormone Containing Herbs	Circulation Enhancers	Libido & Energy Stimulants	Ginseng & Ginseng Type Supports	Mineral-Rich Herbs	Mood-Stabilizing Nerve Supports
Sarsaparilla root	**Ginkgo biloba**	**Ashwagandha**	**Panax ginseng**	Oatstraw	**Gotu kola**
Wild yam root	**Green tea lf.**	**Ginkgo biloba**	**Dong qual root**	Yellow dock root	**Barley grass**
Licorice root	**Gotu kola**	Siberian ginseng	**Ashwagandha**	Kelp/sea vegetables	Scullcap
Bee pollen/ royal jelly	**Butcher's broom**	**Gotu kola**	**Gotu kola**	Alfalfa	Spirulina
Ashwagandha	**Siberian ginseng**	Kola nut	Fo-Ti root	**Barley grass**	**Black cohosh root**
Panax ginseng root	Evening primrose	Guarana seed	Kirin ginseng	**Spirulina**	Alfalfa
Dong qual root	Capsicum	Bee pollen	Angelica root	**Nettles**	**Bayberry bark**
Damiana	Ginger root	**Licorice root**	**Siberian ginseng**	Schizandra berry	Hawthorn lf., bry., fl.
Burdock root	Cinnamon	**Panax ginseng**	**Suma root**	Horsetail	Kava kava

❧ ESSENTIAL HERBS FOR SEXUAL WELL-BEING COMPOUNDS FOR WOMEN:

Primary Herbs		Assisting & Complementary Herbs		Catalyst & Transporting Herbs	
Licorice root	Gotu kola	Sarsaparilla root	Kola nut	Aloe vera juice	Garlic
Burdock root	Nettles	Parsley root & lf.	Schizandra berry	Cinnamon	Evening primrose
Ginseng - all types	Bee pollen/Royal Jelly	Suma root	Horsetail	Lecithin	Rosemary
Dong qual root	Ginkgo biloba	Angelica root	Kola nut	Capsicum	Bayberry bark
Damiana	Black cohosh root	Wild yam root	Hawthorn lf., bry., fl.	Peppermint	Calendula
Alfalfa	Dandelion rt. & lf.	Spirulina	Kava kava	Suma root	Fennel seed
Kelp & sea vegetables	Fo-Ti root	Barley grass	Scullcap	Ginger root	Flax seed
Ashwagandha	Siberian ginseng	Guarana seed	Red raspberry	Butcher's broom	White willow bark
Ginkgo biloba	Bayberry bark	Green tea lf.	Spirulina	Lemon peel	Oatstraw

❧ EXAMPLE FORMULAS OF SEXUAL WELL-BEING COMPOUNDS FOR WOMEN:

TWO FEMININE SUPPORT EXTRACT COMPOUNDS (w - 4808, 4765)			A LOVE FEMALE CAPSULE COMPOUND (w - 3050)		
#1 Licorice root	#2 Ashwagandha	Damiana	Dong qual root	Kola nut	Parsley
Dendrobium	Dong qual root		Damiana	Gotu kola	Ginger root
			Licorice root	Sarsaparilla root	
			Burdock root		
			Guarana seed		
			Ashwagandha		

SEE PAGE 1 FOR FORMULATING INSTRUCTIONS.

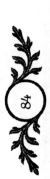

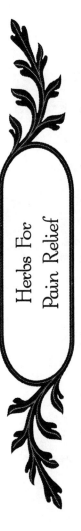

Herbs For Pain Relief

Pain is a mechanism our bodies use to draw attention to a problem that the autonomic system cannot handle by itself. Pain signals us to consciously address the underlying cause. Pain is almost completely individual. It can stem from large centers that control the main pain blocks of the body, and also from specific local areas that demand exact pinpointed action. Even mental trauma will eventually manifest itself as physical pain. There are different kinds of pain - physical, emotional, chronic, local, intermittent, throbbing, dull, spasmodic, sharp, shooting, etc. Add to this the fact that every person feels and reacts differently to pain, and you have some idea of how difficult it is to make or find a universal analgesic or pain killer.

Pain can be your body's best friend. It alerts you when something is wrong and needs your attention. It identifies the location, severity, and type of problem, so that you can treat the right area. But pain can also be your body's worst enemy. Continuous, constant body trauma saps strength and spirit, causes irrational acts and decisions, and alters personality. This is the reason pain killers are useful. They allow you to think clearly, work and live, while addressing the cause of the problem. Other than injury or degenerative disease, chronic pain is based in lifestyle habits. Poor nutrition (to most people's surprise), plays a big role in back and muscle pain. For instance, a lack of green vegetables and calcium-rich foods may be the underlying cause. A stressful lifestyle exhausts adrenal and pituitary glands resulting in physical pain. An over-acid diet can eat away protective mucous membranes and nerve sheathing, so improving body chemistry through a better diet and herbal supplements affords long term nerve and stress relief. Being seriously overweight puts strain and pain on body parts from feet to shoulders.

Chemical pain-killing drugs, while strong, afford relief by masking pain, or deadening certain body mechanisms so that they cannot function. Herbal pain relievers are more subtle and work at a deeper level, to relax, soothe, ease and calm the distressed area. They allow you to use the pain for information about the state of your body, yet not be overwhelmed by the trauma to body and spirit that unrelieved pain can bring.

THERE ARE FOUR BASIC PAIN CENTERS IN THE BODY:

1) the cerebro-spinal area, controlling neural affliction, lower back pain and cramping;
2) the frontal lobe area, involved in earaches, toothaches, and headaches over the eyes;
3) the base of the brain, involved in migraines and tension headaches;
4) the abdominal area, affecting spasmodic menstrual cramping, digestive and elimination pain.

Note: See the section in this book on ARTHRITIC & JOINT PAIN for herbs to relieve these symptoms.

Herbal analgesic combinations are effective for each of the pain areas. For many people, natural therapies and herbs are superior to pharmaceutical drugs and their side effects. Herbs may be used topically or taken orally. They work by soothing membranes, relaxing muscles and spasms, calming the mind, and providing oxygen or heat for relief. All of them allow your body full function and communication while it is healing. Relaxation techniques like chiropractic adjustment, shiatsu massage, biofeedback, acupuncture, and massage therapy are excellent methods to use along with pain relieving herbs for the best results in controlling pain.

✦ FORMULAS FOR PAIN CONTROL AND RELIEF HELP IN THE FOLLOWING CONDITIONS:

•Chronic Headaches & Tension Headaches •Migraines & Cluster Headaches •Earaches & Ear Infections •Toothaches •Menstrual Cramps •Digestive & Eliminative Pain •Neuritis & Neuralgia •Spine & Lower Back Pain •Spasmodic Pain •Tendonitis •Stress, Tension & Muscle Cramping

✦ COMPOUNDS FOR FORMULATION TO HELP PAIN CONTROL AND RELIEF SHOULD INCLUDE:

•Relieving frontal Lobe headaches, sinus pain, over-the-eyes pain, toothaches and earaches.
•Relieving migraine and cluster headaches.
•Relieving neuritis and neuralgia.
•Relieving lower back pain.
•Relieving spasmodic, throbbing pain.

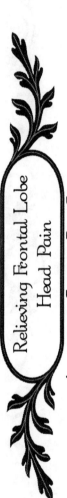

Relieving Frontal Lobe Head Pain

ADDRESSING SPECIFIC PAIN CENTERS

Frontal lobe pain is one of the body's most insistent mechanisms for drawing attention to a health problem. Earaches, toothaches, face twinges, sinus pressure and over-the-eyes headaches all signal us to address the trouble right away. The frontal lobe pain center occurs roughly from the ear line forward, and includes all parts of the face and skull. This type of up-front pain is usually caused by the pressure of swelling and inflammation, and is characterized by throbbing or sharp shooting twinges. Frontal lobe pain is frequent in children, who seem to be more plagued than adults with toothaches, earaches and headaches caused by asthma or allergy attacks. Fortunately, most underlying origins for frontal lobe pain can be addressed easily and successfully with herbal analgesics or anodynes, that are safe and gentle for children as well as effective for adults.

❧ ESSENTIAL CATEGORIES FOR FRONTAL HEAD PAIN COMPOUNDS:

ANALGESIC HERBS	CALMING, NERVINE HERBS	BODY CHEMISTRY BALANCERS	MINERAL-RICH HERBS	ANTI-INFLAMMATORY HERBS	DECONGESTANT & CIRCULATION AIDS
White willow bark	**European mistletoe**	**Ashwagandha**	**Kelp/sea vegetables**	**St. John's wort**	**Nettles**
St. John's wort	**Scullcap**	**Lemon balm**	**Horsetail**	**Chamomile**	**Ginkgo biloba**
Kava kava	**Gotu kola**	**Dandelion root**	**Yellow dock root**	**White willow bark**	**Ephedra**
Wintergreen	**Ashwagandha**	Chamomile	**Pau d' arco bark**	**Marshmallow root**	**Marshmallow root**
Wild lettuce	Valerian root	Ginger root	Black cohosh root	Yarrow	**Wild cherry bark**
Wood betony	Passion flower	Parsley lf. & rt.	Dandelion root	Calendula	**Mullein**
Blue violet	Catnip	**Chlorella/Barley grass**	Spirulina	Blue vervain	Elecampane
Black cohosh root	Hops	Slippery elm	Nettles	Bilberry	Hyssop
Valerian root	**Wood betony**	Licorice root	Oatstraw	Peppermint	Slippery elm

❧ ESSENTIAL HERBS FOR FRONTAL HEAD PAIN COMPOUNDS:

PRIMARY HERBS	ASSISTING & COMPLEMENTARY HERBS	CATALYST & TRANSPORTING HERBS	
White willow bark	Chamomile	Dandelion root	Echinacea root	Capsicum	Wild cherry bark
St. John's wort	Sarsaparilla root	Marshmallow root	Yellow dock rt.	Lobelia	Yarrow
Ginkgo biloba	Black cohosh root	Nettles	Oatstraw	Ginger root	Hyssop
Licorice rt.	Pau d' arco bark	Alfalfa leaf	Heartsease	Blue violet	Horsetail
Burdock rt.	Chlorella/Barley grass	Slippery elm	Bilberry	Rosemary	Mullein
Gotu kola	Kava kava	Wild lettuce	White pine bark	Parsley root & lf.	Wintergreen
Valerian root	Wood betony	Slippery elm	Elecampane	Peppermint	Kelp/sea vegetables
Ashwagandha	Red raspberry	Blue vervain	Devil's claw root	Mullein	Uva ursi
Eur. mistletoe	Cramp bark	Scullcap	Passionflower	Ephedra	Hops

❧ EXAMPLE FORMULAS OF FRONTAL HEAD PAIN COMPOUNDS:

AN ANTI-INFLAMMATORY CAPSULE COMPOUND		(co - 1180)
White willow bark	Devil's claw root	Dandelion root
St. John's wort	Alfalfa leaf	Chamomile
Echinacea root	Burdock rt.	Uva ursi
		Ginger rt.

AN "ASPIR-SOURCE" CAPSULE COMPOUND		(co - 1350)
White willow bark	Heartsease	Blue vervain
Rosemary	Scullcap	Eur. mistletoe
Wood betony	Valerian root	

SEE PAGE 1 FOR FORMULATING INSTRUCTIONS.

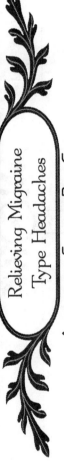

Relieving Migraine Type Headaches

ADDRESSING SPECIFIC PAIN CENTERS

Vascular headaches like migraines and cluster headaches appear to be disorders of the brain, indicating vascular instability, cranial artery constriction and inadequate brain blood supply. There is neurologic inflammation and a drop in estrogen levels. Migraines affect 15% of American men and 30% of American women. Chronic stress is a potentiator of migraines. Platelet aggregation, build-up of histamine and serotonin levels are common, resulting in inflammation, vasodilation, serotonin release and histamine reactions. Migraines can be helped with herbal methods. Sometimes herbs work when nothing else does. Cluster headaches, characterized by two or more sudden, extremely painful headaches in a day, come in cycles for several days, and recur every few months. They also respond to herbal pain relievers. Herbs act as relaxants for neural pain in the neck, face and base of the brain. They encourage body chemistry balance by providing brain and nerve nutrient support.

✦ ESSENTIAL CATEGORIES FOR VASCULAR HEADACHE COMPOUNDS:

LIVER CLEANSING & SUPPORT	CIRCULATION STIMULANT HERBS	BODY CHEMISTRY BALANCERS	ADRENAL & DEEP GLAND SUPPORT	ANTI-SPASMODIC NERVINE HERBS	ANTIOXIDANT SUPPORT
Licorice root	**Capsicum**	**Aloe vera**	**Licorice root**	**Valerian root**	**White pine bark**
Oregon grape root	**Feverfew fl.**	**Gotu kola**	**Kelp/sea vegetables**	**Chamomile**	**Gotu kola**
Milk thistle seed	**Butcher's broom**	**Evening primrose oil**	Ginger root	**Wild lettuce**	**Ginkgo biloba**
Dandelion root	**Ginkgo biloba**	**Ginseng - all types**	**Gotu kola**	**Scullcap**	**Chlorella**
Bupleurum	Hawthorn bry., lf., fl.	**Ashwagandha**	**Bee pollen/royal jelly**	**Passion flower**	**Spirulina**
Yellow dock root	Fenugreek seed	**St. John's wort**	Hawthorn bry., lf., fl.	Lobelia	Siberian ginseng
Gentian root	**Kelp/sea vegetables**	Peppermint	Bayberry bark	Hops	Garlic
Fennel seed	**Ginger root**	Garlic	Rose hips	Catnip	**Rosemary**
Wild yam root	Siberian ginseng root	**Kelp/sea vegetables**	**Sarsaparilla root**	Marshmallow root	Bilberry

✦ ESSENTIAL HERBS FOR VASCULAR HEADACHE COMPOUNDS:

PRIMARY HERBS	ASSISTING & COMPLEMENTARY HERBS	CATALYST & TRANSPORTING HERBS
Feverfew	Sarsaparilla root	Aloe vera juice	Hops
Capsicum	European mistletoe	Gentian root	Garlic
Ashwagandha	Bee pollen/royal jelly	Marshmallow root	Rose hips
Ginkgo biloba	Siberian ginseng	Capsicum	Horsetail
Chamomile	Catnip	Peppermint	Calendula
St. John's wort	Spirulina	Vitamin C powder	Fennel seed
Gotu kola	White pine bark	Ginger root	Flax seed
Hawthorn bry., lf., fl.	Yellow dock root	Lobelia	Fenugreek seed
Chlorella	Ginseng - all types	Bayberry bark	Uva ursi

Black cohosh root, Garlic, Milk thistle seed, Bilberry, Valerian root, Dandelion rt. & lf., Licorice root, Wild lettuce, Cramp bark
Evening primrose oil, Kelp/sea vegetables, Rosemary, Goldenseal root., Butcher's broom, Wild yam root, Scullcap, Oregon grape root, Bupleurum

✦ EXAMPLE FORMULAS OF VASCULAR HEADACHE COMPOUNDS:

A MIGRAINE RELIEF CAPSULE COMPOUND		(co - 3400)
Feverfew	Rosemary	European mistletoe	Ginger root.
Valerian root	Catnip	Ginkgo biloba	Licorice root
Wild lettuce			

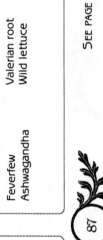

A CLUSTER HEADACHE RELIEF CAPSULE COMPOUND		(co - 1870)
Feverfew	Valerian root	Ginkgo biloba	Capsicum
Ashwagandha	Wild lettuce	Goldenseal root	

SEE PAGE 1 FOR FORMULATING INSTRUCTIONS.

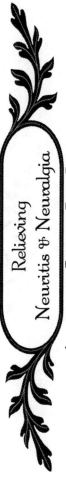

Relieving Neuritis & Neuralgia

ADDRESSING SPECIFIC PAIN CENTERS

Neuritis (peripheral neuropathy) is an inflammation of a nerve or nerves characterized by a burning or tingling sensation in the muscles or nerve area, culminating in numbness of the nerve area. It is usually a degenerative process, and often part of a degenerative illness, such as diabetes or leukemia. **Trigeminal neuralgia** is sudden, sharp, severe pains shooting along the course of a nerve - often because of pressure on the nerve trunks, or poor nerve nutrition and an over-acid condition. Herbal healing compounds are a good choice because they act as both tonics and sedatives, boosting circulation while calming and soothing, relieving pain while helping to rebuild nerve and muscle strength with mineral-rich nutrients. Herbs should be combined with stress management techniques, such as massage therapy, or shiatsu for best results.

❧ ESSENTIAL CATEGORIES FOR NEURITIS AND NEURALGIA COMPOUNDS:

HERBAL PAIN RELIEVERS	NERVE REBUILDERS & RESTORERS	RELAXING, SOOTHING NERVINES	CIRCULATION STIMULANT HERBS	BIOFLAVONOID-RICH TISSUE TONERS	HERBAL ALKALIZERS & NOURISHERS
Wild yam root	**Ashwagandha**	Lobelia	**Kelp/sea vegetables**	**Royal Jelly/Bee pollen**	**Marshmallow root**
Kava kava	**Hawthorn bry., lf., flr.**	Hops	**Ginkgo biloba**	**Gotu kola**	**Alfalfa**
Passionflower	Licorice root	**Gotu kola**	Ginger root	**Evening primrose oil**	Chlorella/Spirulina
Wood betony	**Siberian ginseng**	**Valerian root**	Red raspberry	**Hawthorn lf., bry., fl.**	Barley grass
Valerian root	Nettles	**Scullcap**	Parsley leaf & root	Wild yam root	**Dandelion root**
Black haw	**Panax ginseng**	**Passionflower**	**Alfalfa**	**Ginkgo biloba**	**Aloe vera**
Rosemary	**Oatstraw**	Peppermint	Hawthorn bry., lf., flr.	Red raspberry	**Calendula**
Cramp bark	**Gotu kola**	Cramp bark	Peppermint	**Horsetail**	Lecithin
St. John's wort	**European mistletoe**	**Chamomile**	Lobelia	**Bilberry**	**Borage seed**

❧ ESSENTIAL HERBS FOR NEURITIS AND NEURALGIA COMPOUNDS:

PRIMARY HERBS		ASSISTING & COMPLEMENTARY HERBS		CATALYST & TRANSPORTING HERBS	
Kava kava rt	Kelp & sea vegetables	Wild yam root	Nettles	Capsicum	Aloe vera
Gotu kola	Siberian ginseng	Spirulina	Passionflower	Chlorella	Bilberry berry
Evening primrose	Ginkgo biloba	Black haw	Royal Jelly	Lobelia	Parsley root & lf.
Hawthorn bry., lf., flr.	Oatstraw	European mistletoe	Hops	Rosemary	Alfalfa
Black cohosh rt.	Alfalfa	Barley grass	Horsetail	Garlic	Marshmallow root
Licorice root	Scullcap	Chamomile	Cramp bark	Ginger root	Chaste tree berry
Valerian root	St. John's wort	Black cohosh rt.	Red raspberry	Lecithin	Calendula
Burdock root	Dandelion root & lf.	Borage seed	Wood betony	Peppermint	Carrot powder
Ashwagandha	Watercress	Bee pollen	Panax ginseng	Pau d' arco bk.	Suma root

❧ EXAMPLE FORMULAS OF NEURITIS AND NEURALGIA COMPOUNDS:

A NERVE RELAXING CAPSULE COMPOUND		(RX - 3800)
Ashwagandha	Kava kava rt.	Wood betony
Black cohosh rt.	Black haw	Lobelia
Scullcap	Hops	Oatstraw
Valerian root	European mistletoe	

A CALCIUM-SOURCE, MUSCLE-RELAXING EXTRACT COMPOUND (SA - 4800)		
Watercress	Oatstraw	Dandelion lf.	Alfalfa
	Rosemary	Borage seed	Horsetail

SEE PAGE 1 FOR FORMULATING INSTRUCTIONS.

Relieving Lower Back Pain

ADDRESSING SPECIFIC PAIN CENTERS

The spine is the major seat of human nerve structure, and as such manifests many of the body's emotional, psychological and physical stresses. Eighty percent of Americans suffer from back pain at some point in their lives and almost 40% wind up with crippling back pain. Back pain is second only to childbirth as a reason for hospitalization, and it can last for months. Causes for back pain can be as far apart as a slipped disc and family financial problems. In fact, lower back pain is a far more complex problem than once thought. High stress lifestyles and poor dietary habits inhibit mineral absorption needed for strong back muscle structure. Organically grown foods, sea plants, herbs and outdoor exercise for vitamin D are good habits to consider for healing. Major back surgery, like removing discs may do more harm than good. Diet improvement, supplementation, and a good chiropractor or massage therapist who treats more than just the physical problem, is often the best answer.

❧ ESSENTIAL CATEGORIES FOR LOWER BACK PAIN COMPOUNDS:

MUSCLE RELAXING HERBS	MINERAL-RICH HERBS	KIDNEY & DIURETIC SUPPORT	ALKALIZING HERBS	ANTI-SPASMODIC NERVINE HERBS	PAIN-KILLING HERBS
Wild lettuce lf.	**Oatstraw**	**Uva ursi**	**Lemon balm**	**Valerian root**	**White willow bark**
Valerian rt.	**Dandelion rt. & lf.**	**Parsley root & lf.**	**Dandelion root**	Chamomile	**St. John's wort**
Passionflower	**Horsetail**	Mullein	**Alfalfa**	**Wild lettuce**	**Passionflower**
Kava kava root	**Kelp & sea vegetables**	**Dandelion root**	**Ginger root**	**Scullcap**	**Wild lettuce**
Scullcap	Barley grass	Burdock root	**Parsley root & lf.**	**Passionflower**	**Kava kava root**
Chamomile	Nettles	Juniper berry	Chlorella/Barley grass	Gotu kola	Turmeric
Hops	**Spirulina/Chlorella**	**Plantain lf.**	Panax ginseng	Peppermint	Wood betony
Wood betony	Marshmallow root	Calendula	Pau d' arco bark	Lemongrass	European mistletoe
Black haw	Licorice root	Yarrow	Lobelia	St. John's wort	Yarrow

❧ ESSENTIAL HERBS FOR LOWER BACK PAIN COMPOUNDS:

PRIMARY HERBS		ASSISTING & COMPLEMENTARY HERBS		CATALYST & TRANSPORTING HERBS	
White willow bark	Wild lettuce lf.	Barley grass	Lobelia	Aloe vera juice	Mullein
Burdock root	Nettles	Passion flower	Cramp bark	Garlic	Rosemary
White pine bark	Pau d' arco bark	Black haw	Panax ginseng	Lemongrass	Red raspberry
St. John's wort	Scullcap	Turmeric	European mistletoe	Capsicum	Calendula
Valerian rt.	Gotu kola	Uva ursi	Marshmallow root	Uva ursi	Oatstraw
Alfalfa	Dandelion rt. & lf.	Spirulina	Parsley root & lf.	Lemon balm	Hops
Kelp & sea vegetables	Licorice root	Wood betony lf.	Ashwagandha	Ginger root	Yarrow
Kava kava root	Black cohosh rt.	Chamomile	Red clover	Horsetail	Juniper berry
Chlorella	Ginkgo biloba	Turmeric	Catnip	Peppermint	Carrot powder

❧ EXAMPLE FORMULAS OF LOWER BACK PAIN COMPOUNDS:

A BACK TO RELIEF CAPSULE COMPOUND		(co - 1380)
Wild lettuce lf.	White willow bark	Capsicum	Kava kava root
Valerian rt.	St. John's wort		

A STRESS RELIEVING EXTRACT COMPOUND		(w - 4978)
Black cohosh rt.	Black haw	Kava kava root	Carrot powder
Scullcap	Wood betony lf.		

SEE PAGE 1 FOR FORMULATING INSTRUCTIONS.

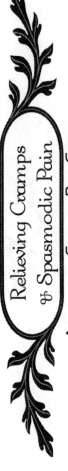

Relieving Cramps & Spasmodic Pain

ADDRESSING SPECIFIC PAIN CENTERS

Spasmodic pain occurs in a wide variety of body reactions - from menstrual cramping to a spastic colon to whooping cough. Herbal relaxants, with their complex ability to address disparate problems with similar symptoms, are effective for all types of spasmodic pain. For instance, a spastic colon spasms because food allergens or a stress reaction inflames colon tissue, menstrual cramping may be the result of hormone or prostaglandin imbalance, a spastic cough is evidence of throat irritation, and stomach cramps occur from indigestion. A wide variety of origins indeed; and yet the body is able to use the pain-killing, muscle-relaxing properties of herbs to help relieve all of them. In addition to herbal support, treat yourself to a good massage, sauna or shiatsu session if you have chronic, spasmodic pain, to cleanse the system and improve circulation.

❧ ESSENTIAL CATEGORIES FOR LOWER BACK PAIN COMPOUNDS:

Antispasmodic Herbs	Muscle & Nerve Relaxers	Essential Fatty Acid Support	Circulation Degongestant Herbs	Kidney Support Diuretic Herbs	Gland Balancing Herbs
Valerian root	**Wild lettuce**	**Chlorella**	**Capsicum**	**Uva ursi**	**Licorice root**
Cramp bark	**Gotu kola**	**Evening primrose oil**	**Hawthorn lf., bry., fl.**	Buchu lf.	**Wild yam root**
Wild lettuce	**Valerian root**	Spirulina	Butcher's broom	**Parsley root & leaf**	Black cohosh rt.
Scullcap	**Passionflower**	Fennel seed	**Ginkgo biloba**	Plantain	**Burdock root**
Passionflower	**Kava kava**	Alfalfa	**Gotu kola**	Cornsilk	Siberian ginseng
St. John's wort	**European mistletoe**	**Flax seed**	Kelp/sea vegetables	**Juniper berry**	**Bee pollen/royal jelly**
Hops	Scullcap	**Barley grass**	Ginger root	Dandelion rt. & lf.	**Sarsaparilla root**
Chamomile	Wild yam root	**Borage seed**	**Siberian ginseng root**	Mullein	**Ashwagandha**
Black haw	Lobelia	Red raspberry	**Fo-Ti root**	Cleavers	**Gotu kola**

❧ ESSENTIAL HERBS FOR LOWER BACK PAIN COMPOUNDS:

Primary Herbs		Assisting & Complementary Herbs	Catalyst & Transporting Herbs	
White willow bark	Wild lettuce lf.	Barley grass	Aloe vera juice	Mullein
Cramp bark	Wild yam root	Passionflower	Borage seed	Rosemary
Hawthorn lf., bry., fl.	Black haw	Red raspberry	Bee pollen/royal jelly	Cleavers
St. John's wort	Scullcap	Plantain	Evening primrose oil	Calendula
Valerian rt.	Gotu kola	Uva ursi	Flax seed	Oatstraw
Alfalfa	Dandelion rt. & lf.	Spirulina	Butcher's broom	Hops
Kelp & sea vegetables	Licorice root	Wood betony lf.	Ginger root	Yarrow
Kava kava root	Black cohosh rt.	Chamomile	Horsetail	Orange peel
Chlorella	Ginkgo biloba	Sarsaparilla root	Fennel seed	Fo-Ti root

❧ EXAMPLE FORMULAS OF LOWER BACK PAIN COMPOUNDS:

AN ANTI-SPASMODIC CAPSULE COMPOUND		(co - 1250)
Kava kava	St. John's wort	Lobelia
Passionflower	Kelp	Valerian
Red raspberry		

AN ANTI-SPASMODIC EXTRACT COMPOUND		(co - 4740)
Cramp bark	St. John's wort	Orange peel
Black haw	Kelp	
Rosemary		

A CRAMP CONTROL EXTRACT COMPOUND		(co - 4740)
Black haw	Kava kava	Lobelia
Cramp bark	Rosemary	Peppermint

See page 1 for formulating instructions.

98

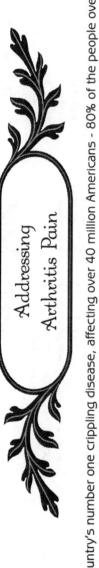

Addressing Arthritis Pain

Arthritis is the country's number one crippling disease, affecting over 40 million Americans - 80% of the people over 50. The term arthritis, meaning joint inflammation, refers to over 100 rheumatic diseases that attack joints and connective tissue. Over 40 million Americans are afflicted by one or more of these crippling rheumatic conditions. Other degenerative joint diseases include gout, lupus erythematosus, ankylosing spondylitis (arthritic spine), psoriatic arthritis (skin and nail arthritis), infective arthritis (bacterial joint infection) and rheumatism. Arthritis is not a simple disease in any form, affecting not only the bones and joints, but also the blood vessels, kidneys, skin, eyes and brain.

OSTEOARTHRITIS, degenerative joint disease, is the most common form of arthritis. It most often appears in the weight-bearing joints like the knees, hips and spine, and in the hands, where there is much cartilage destruction followed by hardening and the formation of large bone spurs on the joints. The first signs of osteoarthritis show up as morning stiffness especially in damp weather, then pain in motion that worsens with prolonged activity. Osteoarthritis is a condition of age, (we see it in the creaking and cracking of joints on movement), because decades of use lead to degenerative changes in joints, and the decreasing ability of the body to repair itself. Although osteoarthritis affects more women than men, a man who is more than 20 pounds overweight doubles his risk of knee and hip arthritis. Repair ability can be greatly increased with body chemistry improvement. Food allergies almost always contribute to osteoarthritis symptoms, so a good body detox followed by a diet with plenty of fresh vegetables is the first place to start.

RHEUMATOID ARTHRITIS affects more than 6 million Americans, the vast majority of them women. RA is a chronic, auto-immune, inflammatory disease whose primary target is the joint lining synovial membrane. When this connective membrane becomes inflamed, it invades and damages nearby bone and cartilage, resulting in pain, stiffness, loss of movement, and eventually destruction of multiple joints. Damage goes even further, because RA also causes inflammation of the blood vessels and the outer lining of the heart and lungs. Most RA sufferers also have digestive problems, fatigue, anemia, ulcerative colitis, chronic lung and bronchial congestion, and liver malfunction. Common causes include calcium depletion, gland and hormone imbalance (especially adrenal exhaustion), prolonged use of aspirin or cortico-steroid drugs, that eventually impair the body's own healing powers, poor diet, with few fresh vegetables, and high in mucous-forming foods; food allergens; auto-toxemia from constipation; inability to relax; resentments and a negative attitude toward life that locks up the body's healing ability.

Because its causes are rooted in lifestyle habits and wear-and-tear effects, conventional medicine has been able to address arthritis with only a small degree of success. In fact, not only is there little improvement from current arthritis drugs, many patients who receive drug therapy become progressively worse and may suffer serious side effects. Cortico-steroid drugs, often medically prescribed for arthritic conditions, sometimes depress the immune system so dramatically that even minor infections can become life-threatening. Steroidal type drugs also cause calcium depletion, bone weakening, and adrenal gland depression, one of the primary cause of arthritis in the first place. Herbal therapies, along with lifestyle changes, however, do work extremely well, addressing the causes of arthritis while reducing pain and discomfort. Herbs can be primary help for detoxification and improving body biochemistry, both necessary procedures for success with arthritis. The herb suggestions in this section promote body detoxification, dissolve and flush out inorganic mineral deposits, and help replace them with non-mucous-forming nutrients. Herbs are alkalizing, anti-inflammatory, and effective for over-acid conditions. Herbs are especially helpful for adrenal gland nourishment because arthritic inflammation is evidence that the body is not producing enough natural cortisone.

❋ FORMULAS FOR ARTHRITIS ALSO HELP IN THE FOLLOWING CONDITIONS:
- Joint Inflammation & Pain •Rheumatism •Bursitis •Gout •Bone Spurs •Chronic Constipation •Corns, Callouses & Carbuncles •Shingles & Hives •Acidosis •Canker Sores & Fever Blisters

❋ COMPOUNDS FOR FORMULATION SHOULD INCLUDE:
- A formula to reduce inflammation and restore joint flexibility
- A formula to help restore normal cartilage and tissue

91

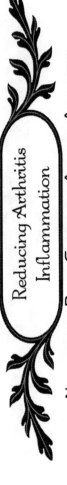

Reducing Arthritis Inflammation

NORMALIZING BODY CHEMISTRY AGAINST ARTHRITIS

Herbs are effective for symptomatic relief and for normalizing body dysfunctions that lie at the cause of arthritis. Over-acidity in the body tissues is one of the basic causes of arthritic diseases. Diet suggestions include avoiding nightshade plants, such as potatoes, tomatoes, chillies, peppers, eggplant, and tobacco, that impair calcium absorption; adding vitamin C-rich foods or supplements for connective tissue formation, adrenal health and detoxification; and adding fiber foods, such as fresh vegetables and whole grains for digestive/elimination regulation. Emphasize a diet low in animal proteins and dairy products to reduce uric acids and mucous formation, and add vegetable fiber foods to keep the body free flowing and alkaline. Other beneficial actions might include hot and cold hydrotherapy, and early morning sunbaths for vitamin D and better calcium use.

❧ ESSENTIAL CATEGORIES FOR ADDRESSING ARTHRITIS INFLAMMATION & PAIN:

ANALGESIC PAIN REDUCERS	HERBS TO DISSOLVE INORGANIC DEPOSITS	ACID/ALKALINE BALANCING HERBS	BIOFLAVONOID-RICH TISSUE TONING HERBS	ANTI-INFLAMMATORY SOURCES	ANTI-OXIDANT HERBS
White willow bark	**Devil's claw root**	**Aloe vera**	**Bilberry**	Licorice root	**Ginkgo biloba**
Kava kava	**Hydrangea**	**Barley grass/chlorella**	**Ginkgo biloba**	**St. John's wort**	**Siberian ginseng**
St. John's wort	Turmeric	Kelp/sea vegetables	Bee pollen/royal jelly	**Yarrow**	Pau d' arco bark
Aloe vera	**Slippery elm**	**Marshmallow root**	**Chlorella/baerley grass**	Alfalfa	**Hawthorn lf., br., fl.**
Turmeric	**Buckthorn bk.**	Parsley root & lf.	**Hawthorn bry., lf., fl.**	Evening primrose oil	**Garlic**
Wintergreen	Kelp/sea vegetables	**Chamomile**	Lemon peel	**Turmeric**	**Royal Jelly**
Capsicum	Uva ursi	Wild yam	Fo-Ti root	**Chamomile**	**Rosemary**
Ginger root	**Horsetail**	Black cohosh rt.	**Dandelion root**		Chlorophyll rich herbs
Devil's claw rt.	**Aloe vera**	Sarsaparilla root	**Rose hips**		Panax ginseng

❧ ESSENTIAL HERBS FOR ADDRESSING ARTHRITIS INFLAMMATION & PAIN:

PRIMARY HERBS		ASSISTING & COMPLEMENTARY HERBS		CATALYST & TRANSPORTING HERBS	
Alfalfa lf. & sd.	Pau d'arco bark	Slippery elm	Astragalus	Capsicum	Japanese green tea
Yucca root	Sarsaparilla root	Kava kava root	Bee pollen/royal jelly	Chamomile	Vitamin C pwdr.
Ginkgo biloba	Dandelion lf. & root	Uva ursi	Goldenseal root	Ginger root	Garlic
Siberian ginseng	Kelp/sea vegetables	White willow bark	Barley grass	Wintergreen	Yarrow
Licorice root	Hawthorn lf. flr. & bry.	Parsley rt. & lf.	Chlorella	Rosemary	Horsetail
Burdock rt.	Panax ginseng	Marshmallow root	Bilberry	Flax seed	Poria mushroom
Evening primrose	Devil's claw	Wild yam	Hydrangea root	Aloe vera juice	Echinacea root
St. John's wort	Spirulina	Black cohosh rt.	Royal Jelly	Irish moss	Turmeric
Ginseng - all types	Buckthorn bk.	Fo-Ti root	Rose hips	Oats/oatstraw	Watercress

❧ EXAMPLE FORMULAS OF ARTHRITIS INFLAMMATION & PAIN COMPOUNDS:

AN ARTHRITIS PAIN RELIEF CAPSULE COMPOUND			(CO - 1330)
Yucca root	Dandelion lf. & root	Black cohosh rt.	Yarrow
Alfalfa lf. & sd.	Bilberry	Rose hips	Licorice rt.
Devil's claw	Parsley rt.	Slippery elm	Hawthorn bry.
Buckthorn bk.	Burdock rt.	St. John's wort	Turmeric

AN ADRENAL ACTIVE SUPPORT CAPSULE COMPOUND			(E - 1000)
Licorice rt.	Uva ursi	Ginger rt.	Capsicum
Sarsaparilla rt.	Irish moss	Astragalus	Rose hips
Bladderwrack			Vitamin C pwr.

SEE PAGE 1 FOR FORMULATING INSTRUCTIONS.

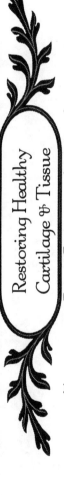

Restoring Healthy Cartilage & Tissue

NORMALIZING BODY CHEMISTRY AGAINST ARTHRITIS

Herbs have a unique place in arthritis treatment programs, because arthritis develops at such a deep level of the body system, and herbs naturally work at the deepest levels of the body processes. A long term program for restoring healthy tissue and cartilage should focus on nutritional changes that help dissolve inorganic mineral deposits in the joints, so they can be removed by the body's elimination system. Adding chlorophyll-rich superfoods and herbs for proper blood balance, and high vitamin C sources for better connective tissue can relieve symptoms. Improve assimilation of organic calcium and other minerals, encourage cortex formation, and alkalize for better body pH balance. Symptoms stemming from adrenal exhaustion, faulty elimination, long held resentments, overuse of prescription drugs and metabolic disorders brought on by stress may also be addressed successfully with herbal therapies..

❧ ESSENTIAL CATEGORIES FOR RESTORING HEALTHY CARTILAGE COMPOUNDS:

CONNECTIVE TISSUE SUPPORT	ORGANIC MINERAL SOURCES	ENZYME STIMULATING BODY BALANCERS	GLAND & ORGAN REBUILDERS	ADRENAL SUPPORT HERBS	JOINT & NERVE REBUILDERS
Horsetail	**Kelp/sea vegetables**	**Kelp & sea vegetables**	**Barley grass/chlorella**	**Licorice root**	**Scullcap**
Gotu kola	Yellow dock root	**Barley grass/chlorella**	**Bee pollen/royal jelly**	**Sarsaparilla root**	Burdock root
Chlorella/barley grass	**Alfalfa**	**Alfalfa/**Spirulina	**Evening primrose oil**	**Kelp/Bladderwrack**	**Ashwagandha**
Royal Jelly	**Dandelion root & lf.**	Garlic	Flax seed	**Astragalus**	**Hawthorn lf., bry., fl.**
Marshmallow root	Chlorella/barley grass	Capsicum	**Red raspberry**	Panax ginseng	**Siberian ginseng**
Licorice root	Parsley root & lf.	**Ginger root**	Dong quai root	Siberian ginseng	**European mistletoe**
Hawthorn bry., lf., fl.	**Oats/Oatstraw**	Peppermint	Damiana lf.	Ginkgo biloba	Chamomile
Oatstraw	Comfrey root	**Green tea**	Borage seed	**Bee pollen/royal jelly**	**Gotu kola**
Black cohosh rt.	Watercress	Ginseng - all types	Wild yam root	Ginger root	Passionflower

❧ ESSENTIAL HERBS FOR RESTORING HEALTHY CARTILAGE COMPOUNDS:

PRIMARY HERBS		ASSISTING & COMPLEMENTARY HERBS		CATALYST & TRANSPORTING HERBS	
Licorice root	Gotu kola	Sarsaparilla root	Evening primrose oil	Aloe vera juice	Black currant
Burdock root	Horsetail	Parsley root & lf.	Marshmallow root	Uva ursi	Borage seed
Panax ginseng	Bee pollen/ royal jelly	European mistletoe	Garlic	Comfrey root	Rosemary
Dong quai root	Ginkgo biloba	Bayberry bk.	Yellow dock rt.	Capsicum	Lemon peel
Wild yam rt.	Black cohosh root	Damiana lf.	Hawthorn lf., bry., fl.	Peppermint	Fennel seed
Alfalfa	Dandelion rt. & lf.	Spirulina	Kava kava	White willow bark	Flax seed
Kelp & sea vegetables	Evening primrose	Barley grass	Scullcap	Ginger root	Watercress
Ashwagandha	Siberian ginseng	Astragalus	Red raspberry	Acerola cherry	Oatstraw
Chlorella	Green tea leaf	Chamomile	Ma huang	Peony rt.	Dulse

❧ EXAMPLE FORMULAS OF RESTORING HEALTHY CARTILAGE COMPOUNDS:

A ROLL-ON BODY BALANCING COMPOUND		(W - 7410)		AN ENERGY GREEN DRINK COMPOUND		(SA - 8150)
Aloe vera	Dong quai rt.	Sarsaparilla rt.	Ginkgo biloba	Barley grass	Acerola cherry	Oats/Oatstraw
Wild yam rt.	Damiana lf.	Burdock rt.	Dandelion rt.	Alfalfa	Sarsaparilla rt.	Lemon peel
Panax ginseng	Black cohosh rt.	Alfalfa	Uva ursi	Bee pollen	Chlorella	
Licorice rt.	Scullcap	Peony rt.	Bayberry bk.	Siberian ginseng	Dulse	
					Dandelion lf.	
					Gotu kola	
					Licorice rt.	
					Dandelion rt.	

SEE PAGE 1 FOR FORMULATING INSTRUCTIONS.

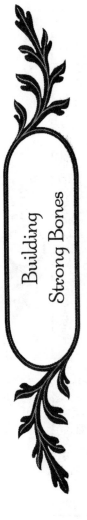

Building Strong Bones

Bone and cartilage are an ever-changing, ever-growing infrastructure of the body. Bone is living tissue, and like other body systems requires a wide variety of nutrients. Healthy bones both use and store the body's minerals, acting as reservoirs for its extra mineral needs. Minerals and trace minerals are the building block of the cells, the most basic elements needed for proper metabolism. They are the bonding agents between the body and food. Without them the body cannot absorb nutrients or utilize them for growth. Minerals regulate acid/alkaline balance, transport body oxygen, and control electrolytic movement between cells, nerves and tissue. They play a key role in heart health, sugar and blood pressure regulation and degenerative disease prevention. Even small mineral deficiencies can produce stress on the body, because imbalances mobilize the needed element(s) out of the various body "reservoirs" to compensate. Our bodies often feel the immediate effects of this process as irritability, nervousness, emotional tension, and depression. A mineral-poor diet can mean osteoporosis, premature aging, hair loss, brittle nails, dry, cracked skin, forgetfulness, food intolerances, back pain, P.M.S., poor motor coordination, joint deformity, difficult pregnancy, taste and smell loss, slow learning, poor attention span, and the inability to heal quickly. And this is only a partial list. **MINERALS ARE IMPORTANT!**

Minerals are not made by the body. They must be taken in through food, drink or mineral baths. Unfortunately, years of pesticides, non-organic fertilizers, and chemical sprays used in agri-business have leached good mineral quantity or quality out of the soil. So it's no longer easy to get them from foods we eat. Over a third of our population, and more than 50% of American women, suffer from calcium deficiency alone. Mineral needs increase as the body ages because digestive systems need more hydrochloric acid and enzyme help.

Osteoporosis is far more complex than was thought even just 5 years ago. Excessive meat consumption, over-refined foods, lack of vitamin D from sunlight, and too little exercise, are involved in bone porosity and poor mineral absorption. Steroid and excessive antibiotic use, tobacco, and too much alcohol, all contribute to mineral depletion and weakening of bone structure. Osteoporosis is partially a result of reduced nutrient (particularly mineral) absorption, which is highly bound to enzyme activity. High levels of phosphorous in meat, soft drinks and other common processed foods deprive the body of calcium. High stress life styles and habits also inhibit mineral absorption.

What about calcium? Calcium is the most abundant mineral in the body, and 98% of all calcium is stored in the bones. But osteoporosis is the result of much more than a calcium deficiency. It involves both mineral and non-mineral components of bone. Calcium supplements, while playing a role in preventing bone loss, can't stand on their own as a viable treatment. In fact, bone strength is best enhanced when calcium is used with other nutrients, such as B vitamins, magnesium, silica, manganese and boron. **How do you know if you have a calcium deficiency?** Calcium deficiencies show up pre-menstrually as back pain, cramping, or tooth pain. Taking a natural calcium supplement before your period can let you know if this is your problem, because supplementation should help these symptoms disappear. **There is a clear relationship between high protein consumption and osteoporosis, too.** As amino acids from excess protein enter the kidneys they cause loss of water and large amounts of minerals, especially calcium, which is released from bone material in order to neutralize the acidity of the protein amino acids. Excess protein from animal sources is an even bigger danger for osteoporosis. Studies of vegetarians and nonvegetarians from age 60 through 90, reveal that the mineral content in meat eater's bones decreased 35% over time, while mineral content of a vegetarian's bones decreased only 18%. Vegetarians traditionally have denser, better-formed bones, because the most usable minerals come from green vegetables, sprouts, whole grains, soy foods, eggs, and vegetable complex carbohydrates.

There is, however, no question that a solid mineral base is of prime importance to bone health. Organically grown foods, sea plants and herbs are becoming the best way to get them. These foods are used by the body's own enzyme action, as a whole, not as an extracted substance, and that is a key to their effectiveness.

❋ FORMULAS FOR STRENGTHENING BONES ALSO HELP IN THE FOLLOWING CONDITIONS:

• Osteoporosis & Brittle Bones • Back Pain • Nerve & Muscle Pain • Hypothyroidism • Menstrual Difficulties • Low Energy Levels • Skin, Hair & Nail Health • Stress & Tension • Tendonitis • Easy Bruising • Cramping & Body Aches

❋ COMPOUNDS FOR FORMULATION SHOULD INCLUDE:

• A formula with mineral-rich herbs for bone building
• A formula to help prevent osteoporosis

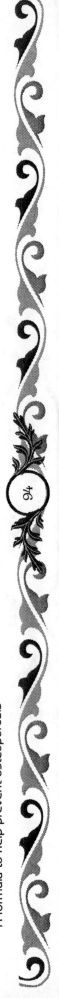

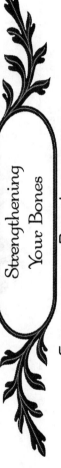

Strengthening Your Bones

STRENGTHENING BODY INFRASTRUCTURE

Minerals are essential to body balance and bone strength. The typical American diet has become increasingly sparse in mineral micronutrients, so most of us need more minerals than our nutritional habits provide. (Skin pallor and chronic fatigue are almost certain signs that the body isn't getting enough minerals.) Scientists, in fact, admit that the American diet is not supplying the minerals needed to build healthy bones over a lifetime. Minerals from plants are higher quality and more absorbable than other sources. They work optimally with enzyme production for nutrient assimilation. Plant minerals from herbs are an excellent choice to address nutrient density deficiencies against bone weakness. Calcium, magnesium, silica and trace minerals from herbal sources are superior in absorption and benefits to isolated sources. They help insure uptake by the body for optimum bone, and cartilage nutrition.

❧ ESSENTIAL CATEGORIES FOR BONE STRENGTHENING COMPOUNDS:

Calcium & Magnesium Sources	Connective Tissue Stimulants	Phyto-hormone Source Herbs	Vitamin A & D Sources	Enzyme-Producing Sources	Silica Source Herbs
Horsetail	**Bee pollen/royal jelly**	**Black cohosh**	**Kelp/sea vegetables**	**Alfalfa**	**Horsetail**
St. John's wort	**Horsetail**	**Panax ginseng**	**Chlorophyll-rich herbs**	Aloe vera juice	**Dulse**
Nettles	**White oak bk.**	**Dong quai**	**Dandelion root**	**Chlorella**	**Nettles**
Dandelion root	**Rose hips**	**Sarsaparilla root**	**Gotu kola**	**Spirulina**	**White willow bark**
Oatstraw	**Bilberry**	**Licorice root**	Soy powder	**Barley grass**	Marshmallow root
Kelp/sea vegetables	Ginkgo biloba	**Ashwagandha**	Burdock root	**Comfrey root**	Black cohosh
Pau d' arco	Evening primrose	**Saw palmetto**	Alfalfa	**Fennel seed**	Alfalfa
Gotu kola	Comfrey root	**Burdock rt.**	Yellow dock	Parsley rt. & lf.	Kelp/sea vegetables
Ginger root	Lobelia	**Alfalfa**	Capsicum	Barberry bk.	Borage seed

❧ ESSENTIAL HERBS FOR BONE STRENGTHENING COMPOUNDS:

Primary Herbs		Assisting & Complementary Herbs		Catalyst & Transporting Herbs	
Alfalfa lf. & sd.	Pau d'arco bark	Nettles	Dulse	Capsicum	Japanese green tea
Royal Jelly/Bee pollen	Sarsaparilla root	Yellow dock rt.	Oats/oatstraw	Dong quai	Vitamin C pwr.
Ginkgo biloba	Dandelion lf. & root	Red raspberry	White willow bark	Ginger root	Garlic
Chlorophyll-rich herbs	Kelp/sea vegetables	Fennel seed	Gotu kola	Lobella	Yarrow
Licorice root	Hawthorn lf. flr. & bry.	Parsley rt. & lf.	Chlorella	Comfrey root	Borage seed
Burdock rt.	Panax ginseng	Marshmallow root	Bilberry	Flax seed	Carrot powder
Evening primrose	Barley grass	Wild yam	White oak bk.	Aloe vera juice	Ashwagandha
St. John's wort	Spirulina	Black cohosh rt.	Saw palmetto	Irish moss	Goldenseal root
Ginseng - all types	Horsetail	Barberry bk.	Rose hips	Soy powder	Watercress

❧ EXAMPLE FORMULAS OF BONE STRENGTHENING COMPOUNDS:

A BODY & BONE BUILDING CAPSULE COMPOUND		(SA - 1450)		A FULL SPECTRUM MINERAL CAPSULE COMPOUND		(SA - 3200)	
Spirulina	Vitamin C powder	Siberian ginseng	Wild cherry	Nettles	Yellow dock rt.	Kelp	Borage seed
Bee pollen	Hawthorn lf. flr. & bry.	Sarsaparilla root	Chlorella	Irish moss	Dandelion rt. & lf.	Parsley rt. & lf.	Dulse
Alfalfa	Barley grass	Red raspberry	Goldenseal rt.	Watercress	Barley grass		
Rose hips	Carrot powder	Kelp	Mullein				

SEE PAGE 1 FOR FORMULATING INSTRUCTIONS.

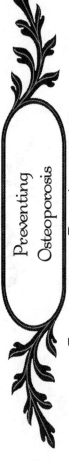

Preventing Osteoporosis

STRENGTHENING BODY INFRASTRUCTURE

Herbal therapy is a good choice for both treatment and prevention of osteoporosis because they offer the broadest base of protection against the widest array of factors. Phytohormones from herbs can be a key element in promoting bone marrow development. Phytohormones in plants are remarkably similar to those in humans, and work by encouraging the body's own hormone balance. For women, osteoporosis involves progesterone/estrogen balance, not just estrogen supply. Progesterone is a key factor in laying down and strengthening bone. Thyroid malfunction, and poor collagen protein development also contribute to osteoporosis. The mineral riches in phyto-estrogen plants stimulate proper cell growth and replacement. The naturally-occurring flavonoids in phyto-hormone rich herbs exert a similar balancing effect on hormone secretions. A broad range herbal formula containing estrogen and progesterone-stimulating substances as well as bioflavonoids and bone-building minerals is a good health choice.

ESSENTIAL CATEGORIES FOR OSTEOPOROSIS PREVENTION COMPOUNDS:

CALCIUM/MAGNESIUM-SOURCE HERBS	SILICA-RICH HERBS	BIOFLAVONOID-RICH SOURCES	HORMONE BALANCING HERBS	CHLOROPHYLL-RICH HERBS	VEGETABLE PROTEIN SOURCES
Oatstraw	**Kelp/sea vegetables**	Bilberry	Black cohosh root	Spirulina	Miso powder
Kelp/sea vegetables	**Burdock root**	Chlorophyll sources	Licorice root	Nettles	Alfalfa
Watercress	**Horsetail**	Garlic	Sarsaparilla root	Chlorella	Barley grass
White oak bark	Eyebright	Hawthorn lf., bry., fl.	Dong qual root	Watercress	Chlorella
Pau d' arco bark	Goldenseal root	Alfalfa	Wild yam root	Barley grass	Spirulina
Nettles	Echinacea root	**Kelp/sea vegetables**	Dandelion root	Alfalfa	Fo Ti root
Gotu kola	**Oatstraw**	Cranberry powder	Alfalfa	**Kelp/sea vegetables**	**Soy powder**
Peppermint	**Comfrey root**	Capsicum	**Vitex**	**Comfrey leaf**	**Oats/oatstraw**
Alfalfa	**Watercress**	Rose hips	**Ginsengs - all types**	**Parsley leaf**	**Brewer's yeast**

ESSENTIAL HERBS FOR OSTEOPOROSIS PREVENTION COMPOUNDS:

PRIMARY HERBS		ASSISTING & COMPLEMENTARY HERBS		CATALYST & TRANSPORTING HERBS	
Licorice root	Gotu kola	Sarsaparilla root	Rose hips	Dulse	Garlic
Burdock root	Horsetail	Parsley root & lf.	Fo Ti root	Uva ursi	Borage seed
Panax ginseng	Bee pollen/ royal jelly	Echinacea root	Nettles	Goldenseal root	Rosemary
Dong qual root	Ginkgo biloba	Bayberry bk.	Yellow dock rt.	Capsicum	Lemon peel
Wild yam rt.	Black cohosh root	Damiana lf.	Hawthorn lf., bry., fl.	Peppermint	Eyebright
Alfalfa	Dandelion rt. & lf.	Spirulina	Oats/Oatstraw	Cranberry powder	White oak bark
Kelp & sea vegetables	Evening primrose	Barley grass	Vitex	Ginger root	Miso powder
Ashwagandha	Siberian ginseng	Bilberry	Pau d' arco bark	Acerola cherry	Soy powder
Chlorella	Aloe vera juice	Comfrey leaf	Watercress	Peony rt.	Brewer's yeast

EXAMPLE FORMULAS OF OSTEOPOROSIS PREVENTION COMPOUNDS:

A ROLL-ON BODY BALANCING COMPOUND		(W - 7410)		AN ENERGY GREEN DRINK COMPOUND		(SA - 8150)	
Aloe vera	Dong quai rt.	Sarsaparilla rt.	Ginkgo biloba	Barley grass	Acerola cherry	Dandelion lf.	Oats/Oatstraw
Wild yam rt.	Damiana lf.	Burdock rt.	Dandelion rt.	Alfalfa	Sarsaparilla rt.	Gotu kola	Lemon peel
Panax ginseng	Black cohosh rt.	Alfalfa	Uva ursi	Bee pollen	Chlorella	Licorice rt.	
Licorice rt.	Scullcap	Peony rt.	Bayberry bk.	Siberian ginseng	Dulse	Dandelion rt.	

SEE PAGE 1 FOR FORMULATING INSTRUCTIONS.

Boosting Physical & Mental Energy

There's so much to do. Where can we get the energy to do it all? Most of us today want to increase our energy - to handle an extra job, to meet financial obligations, to maintain an exercise program, to take advantage of opportunities to learn and create in our lives, or even just to cope better. Americans live hurried, high pressure lives, often with continuing personal or emotional stress, in challenging environments with high noise and air pollution levels. Threatening surroundings sap both body and brain of oxygen and nutrients that provide us with fuel for work and productivity.

Although we might take in more food to fuel more energy, just eating more food (even good food), is not always the best choice for the time we want to spend or the weight we want to maintain. And it's hard to get quick energy from most foods, since nutrients necessarily follow slow, circuitous routes through the digestive system. Another answer could be chemical stimulants - drugs or caffeine. But, they're a dead end for energy and oxygen needs. After a short period of stimulation, these substances constrict rather than open up blood flow, especially to the brain. Most are harmful to the liver and other vital organs, and most are addictive.

Herbs are a good answer for the energy question. They are not addictive or habit-forming, but are powerful agents that work at the deepest levels of the body processes, nourishing as well as stimulating the body to use its own stores of energy. Herbs are a good source of absorbable food minerals for foundation energy. They help improve strength and endurance, and to help build tissue while maintaining low body fat. Many, like rosemary and ginkgo biloba, are excellent antioxidants.

Start from the inside out. The best way to build energy is at the gland and deep tissue level. The endocrine system with its all-important hormone secretions works at the deepest and most powerful level of the body. Herbs help revitalize gland functions and extend cell life, by working through the glands to ameliorate insufficiencies and dysfunctions. Minerals and trace minerals, so often lacking in today's diet, are critical to gland health. Herbs and sea vegetables are concentrated, highly absorbable sources of plant minerals. Endocrine health thrives on vegetable protein. Superfood plants, such as sea vegetables, spirulina, and alfalfa can supply needed protein without the density or accompanying fats of animal proteins.

Are your adrenals always fighting a rear guard action? Nourishing tired adrenal glands is one of the primary actions to take in combatting fatigue and low energy. Daily, ever-increasing stress for most Americans means many of us have exhausted adrenal glands. We find ourselves overly anxious, overly allergic and overly acidic, with diminished stamina and reduced alertness, yet without the ability to relax or sleep well. Adrenal support herbs provide tonic and toning activity for better energy use. Herbs for the adrenals encourage adrenal cortex secretion, which relieves other conditions, from skin problems to respiratory health. A formula like the one on the next page helps regulate metabolic activity and, through adrenalin regulation, helps control histamine reactions in allergy and asthma conditions

Thyroid health is primary to metabolic energy. The thyroid gland produces hormones to help keep energy-producing and energy-using processes in balance, and also influences the balance of hormones such as estrogen and progesterone. The thyroid needs iodine to produce its wide array of hormone secretions. Herbal supplements help balance thyroid activity with nutrients containing naturally-occurring iodine to strengthen the thyroid and help regulate metabolism. Minerals activate digestion to keep food available for fuel and energy. An herbal formula for thyroid support can enhance kidney, gallbladder and pancreatic functions, promoting vitality as it encourages a lazy thyroid. Many people use thyroid support herbs as part of a weight control program for middle age spread.

Tired blood can use an energy boost from herbs, too. Mineral-rich herbs offer easily assimilated, non-constipating iron along with other minerals that help in iron uptake to energizing oxygen for both blood and brain. Herbs can stimulate sluggish circulation to counteract fatigue and wake up a "tired brain."

❊FORMULAS FOR REVITALIZING BODY ENERGY ALSO HELP IN THE FOLLOWING CONDITIONS:

•Energy For Endurance & Stamina •Energy to Overcome Everyday Fatigue •Faster Healing of Injuries •Hormone & Metabolic Stimulation •Stress & Nervous Tension •Exhaustion & Mental Burn-Out •Hypothyroidism •Adrenal Exhaustion •Weight Control

❊COMPOUNDS FOR FORMULATION SHOULD INCLUDE:

•Energy for daily fatigue
•Nervous system and metabolic enhancement
•Mental and creative energy

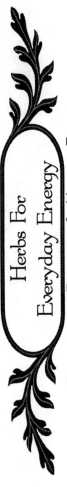

Herbs For Everyday Energy

OVERCOMING PHYSICAL & MENTAL FATIGUE

Fatigue and lack of daily energy are common complaints in America today. If there is no serious disease, the causes can be simple, like poor nutrition or not enough sleep. Most of us lead very busy lives - time for sleep and proper nutrition often get the short end of the stick. Even if you lead a "normal" life without obvious stress, life in the nineties is difficult. Daily stress takes its toll in blood pressure, hormone, heart and breathing changes. These changes make you feel really tired and burned out for no apparent reason. Herbs can help enhance your daily energy needs. Extremely high or low blood sugar is a common cause of energy loss. Studies show that people suffering from yo-yo blood sugar reactions have headaches, mental confusion, temper outbursts and depression because they have so little energy to cope with daily stresses. While everyone with blood sugar irregularities should consult a health care professional, diet improvement and specific herbal formulas can help in energy return.

ESSENTIAL CATEGORIES FOR DAILY ENERGY BOOSTING COMPOUNDS:

BLOOD SUGAR BALANCERS	CHLOROPHYLL SOURCE HERBS	SYSTEM STRENGTHENING HERBS	STRESS RELIEVING HERBS	ADRENAL GLAND SUPPORT HERBS	TONIC HERBS
Licorice root	**Chlorella**	**Panax ginseng**	**Siberian ginseng root**	**Kelp/sea vegetables**	**Kelp/sea vegetables**
Barley grass	Barley grass	**Damiana**	**Kava kava rt.**	**Sarsaparilla**	**Damiana**
Spirulina	Nettles	**Licorice root**	**Gotu kola**	**Astragalus**	**Hawthorn lf. flr. & bry.**
Gotu kola	**Spirulina**	Spirulina	**Ashwagandha**	**Dandelion root**	**Ginseng - all types**
Wild yam rt.	**Alfalfa**	Evening primrose oil	Peppermint	Uva ursi	**Gotu kola**
Suma rt	Watercress	**Bee pollen/royal jelly**	**Yarrow**	**Licorice root**	**Ginkgo biloba**
Nutritional yeast	Parsley leaf	**Suma root**	**St. John's wort**	Capsicum	Nettles
Panax ginseng	**Kelp/sea vegetables**	Pau d'arco bark	Red raspberry	Schizandra bry.	Spirulina
Dandelion root	**Aloe vera**	Yellow dock rt.	Fo-Ti root	**Ginkgo biloba**	Licorice root

ESSENTIAL HERBS FOR DAILY ENERGY BOOSTING COMPOUNDS:

PRIMARY HERBS		ASSISTING & COMPLEMENTARY HERBS		CATALYST & TRANSPORTING HERBS	
Bee pollen	Pau d'arco bark	Dandelion root	Aralia root	Capsicum	Red raspberry
Kelp/sea vegetables	Sarsaparilla root	Barley grass	Wild cherry bk.	Cloves	Nutritional yeast pwr.
Ginkgo biloba	Damiana	Chlorella	Prince ginseng rt.	St. John's wort	Parsley rt & lf.
Siberian ginseng	Nutritional yeast	Kava kava rt.	Goldenseal root	Aloe vera	Yarrow
Licorice root	Hawthorn lf. flr. & bry.	Peppermint	Echinacea root	Rosemary	Uva ursi
Barley grass	Panax ginseng	Ashwagandha	Nettles	Red clover	Rice protein pwr.
Fo-Ti root	Gotu kola	Wild yam rt.	Black cohosh	Irish moss	Juniper bry.
Suma rt	Spirulina	Astragalus	Royal jelly	Watercress	Evening primrose oil
Ginseng - all types	Yellow dock rt.	Alfalfa	Schizandra bry.	Miso broth powder	Horsetail

EXAMPLE FORMULAS OF COMPOUNDS FOR DAILY ENERGY:

A HIGH ENERGY TEA COMPOUND			(ε - 5570)
Gotu kola	Red clover	Prince ginseng rt.	Aralia root
Peppermint	Cloves	Kava kava rt.	Red raspberry
Damiana			

A FEEL GREAT BODY TONIC CAPSULE COMPOUND			(ε - 2250)
Bee pollen	Licorice root	Alfalfa	Goldenseal rt.
Siberian ginseng rt.	Suma rt.	Wild Cherry	Nutritional yeast
Gotu kola	Schizandra bry.	Black cohosh	Hawthorn bry.
Sarsaparilla rt.	Rice protein pwdr.	Kelp	Spirulina

SEE PAGE 1 FOR FORMULATING INSTRUCTIONS.

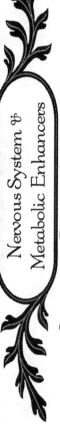

Nervous System & Metabolic Enhancers

OVERCOMING PHYSICAL & MENTAL FATIGUE

Nervous system stimulants act by affecting the cerebral cortex and the medulla of the brain. Most contain either natural xanthines, like kola nut, or stimulants like ephedra, or certain free-form amino acids like those in green superfoods. These substances promote alertness, energy, and a more rapid, clearer flow of thought. **Metabolic enhancers** improve the performance of biochemical pathways. They do not stress or deplete the body. Examples include co-enzyme factors like B vitamins such as those found in sea plants and superfoods, fat mobilizers from thermogenic herbs like green tea, electron transporters such as enzyme CoQ_{10}, and tissue oxygenators like ginkgo biloba and garlic. **Adaptogens** are body chemistry regulators, like ginsengs, that help the body handle stress and maintain vitality. They are rich sources of important strengthening nutrients like germanium for long term revitalization rather than immediate energy.

❧ ESSENTIAL CATEGORIES FOR REVITALIZING DEEP BODY ENERGY COMPOUNDS:

NERVOUS SYSTEM ENHANCERS	METABOLIC ENERGY SUPPORT	CIRCULATION TONIC HERBS	MINERAL-RICH HERBS	ADRENAL SUPPORT SOURCES	THYROID SUPPORT HERBS
Ginkgo biloba	**Ginger root**	**Capsicum**	**Horsetail**	**Royal jelly**	Kelp/sea vegetables
Damiana	**Rosemary**	**Ginger root**	**Kelp/sea vegetables**	**Bee pollen**	**Horsetail**
Green tea	**Green tea**	**Kelp/sea vegetables**	**Yellow dock root**	**Kelp/sea vegetables**	**Spirulina**
Yerba mate	**Royal Jelly/Bee pollen**	Red clover	**Nettles**	**Borage seed**	Burdock root
Guarana	Suma root	Hawthorn bry., lf., fl.	**Alfalfa**	**Panax ginseng**	Chlorella
Gotu kola	**Ginseng - all types**	**Bee pollen/royal jelly**	**Pau d' arco bark**	**Sarsaparilla root**	Watercress
Siberian ginseng	Capsicum	**Spirulina**	Oats/Oatstraw	**Licorice root**	**Garlic**
Kola nut	Chlorophyll-rich herbs	**Licorice root**	Siberian ginseng root	**Evening primrose oil**	Parsley root & lf.
Ephedra	Peppermint	**Ginkgo biloba**	Chlorophyll-rich herbs	Fo-Ti root	Green tea

❧ ESSENTIAL HERBS FOR REVITALIZING DEEP BODY ENERGY COMPOUNDS:

PRIMARY HERBS		ASSISTING & COMPLEMENTARY HERBS		CATALYST & TRANSPORTING HERBS	
Gotu kola	Guarana seed	Parsley root & lf.	Evening primrose oil	Watercress	Horsetail
Red clover	Fo-Ti root	Alfalfa	Nettles	Burdock root	Rosemary
Ginseng - all types	Ginkgo biloba	Green tea	White oak bark	Irish moss	Watercress
Sarsaparilla root	Astragalus	Pau d' arco bark	Yellow dock rt.	Capsicum	Yerba mate
Damiana	Royal jelly	Spirulina	Bilberry	Peppermint	Oats/Oatstraw
Licorice root	Bee pollen	Kirin ginseng root	Dong qual rt.	Ephedra	Garlic
Kelp & sea vegetables	Suma root	Barley grass	St. John's wort	Ginger root	Flax seed oil
Kola nut	Siberian ginseng	Echinacea root	Prince ginseng	Borage seed	Nettles
Chlorophyll-rich herbs	Panax ginseng	Chlorella	Hawthorn bry., lf., fl.	Dong qual	Nutritional yeast

❧ EXAMPLE FORMULAS OF REVITALIZING DEEP BODY ENERGY COMPOUNDS:

A RAINFOREST CNS ENERGY CAPSULE COMPOUND		(E - 3780)
Guarana seed	Suma root	Ginger root	Astragalus rt.
Kola nut	Bee pollen	Capsicum	

AN ADAPTOGENIC GINSENG ENERGY CAPSULE COMPOUND		(E - 2510)
Bee pollen	Gotu kola	Aralia root	Alfalfa
Siberian ginseng rt.	Fo-Ti root	Prince ginseng	Dong qual rt.
	Kirin ginseng root	Suma rt.	

SEE PAGE 1 FOR FORMULATING INSTRUCTIONS.

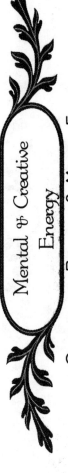

Mental & Creative Energy

OVERCOMING PHYSICAL & MENTAL FATIGUE

The brain controls the entire body, using over 20% of the body's energy supply. It takes 50% of our blood sugar and 20% of our inhaled oxygen. The brain is also the primary health maintenance organ and the seat of energy production. When it is functioning well, total body well-being is improved. Brain nutrients have a rapidly noticeable effect on increased brain performance. Consistent, neurotransmitter replenishing brain nourishment can straighten out even grave mental, emotional and coordination problems. The brain has a large appetite for blood sugars, oxygen, minerals, amino acids, vitamins and fatty acids. Antioxidants protect, nourish and fuel the brain. New tests are convincing many scientists that senile dementia and certain other brain nerve damage diseases have origins in free radical damage. Several herbs, like rosemary and ginkgo biloba have antioxidant properties to protect against free radical damage.

❧ ESSENTIAL CATEGORIES FOR MENTAL & CREATIVE ENERGY COMPOUNDS:

BRAIN NOURISHING HERBS	CIRCULATION SUPPORT	AMINO ACID SOURCES	ANTI-OXIDANT HERBS	CHOLINE & EFA SOURCES FOR MEMORY	POTASSIUM/IODINE SOURCES
Bee pollen/royal jelly	**Capsicum**	**Chlorella**	**Rosemary**	**Lecithin**	Kelp/sea vegetables
Damiana	**Ginger root**	**Spirulina**	**Kelp/sea vegetables**	**Brewer's yeast**	Irish moss
Hawthorn bry., lf., fl.	Bilberry	**Kelp/sea vegetables**	**Ginseng - all types**	**Borage seed**	**Spirulina**
Prickly ash bk.	**Ginkgo biloba**	**Brewer's yeast**	**Capsicum**	**Barley grass**	Burdock root
Fo-ti root	Cloves/Cinnamon	Panax ginseng	White pine bk.	**Panax ginseng**	Chlorella
Panax ginseng	Sarsaparilla root	Ephedra	**Bee pollen/royal jelly**	Chlorella	Watercress
Siberian ginseng	Panax ginseng	**Yellow dock rt.**	Prickly ash	**Licorice root**	**Garlic**
Gotu kola	**Siberian ginseng**	Alfalfa	Ginger root	**Evening primrose oil**	**Horsetail**
Rosemary	Cardamom	Fennel seed	Peppermint	**Flax seed**	Green tea

❧ ESSENTIAL HERBS FOR MENTAL & CREATIVE ENERGY COMPOUNDS:

PRIMARY HERBS		ASSISTING & COMPLEMENTARY HERBS		CATALYST & TRANSPORTING HERBS	
Ginkgo biloba	Burdock root	Ashwagandha rt.	Rosemary	Anise seed	St. John's wort
Bilberry	Fo-Ti root	Dong quai rt.	Alfalfa	Cardamom	Lecithin
Ginseng - all types	Kava kava root	Garlic	Kirin ginseng rt.	Cloves/Cinnamon	Watercress
Sarsaparilla root	Gotu kola	Nettles	Tienchi ginseng	Capsicum	Sage
Damiana	Royal jelly	Spirulina	Borage seed	Peppermint	Prickly ash bk.
Licorice root	Hawthorn bry., lf., fl.	Astragalus	Schizandra bry.	Brewer's yeast	Fennel seed
Kelp & sea vegetables	Suma root	Barley grass	Irish moss	Ginger root	Flax seed
White pine bk.	Siberian ginseng	Evening primrose oil	Prince ginseng rt.	Green tea	Lobelia
Chlorella	Panax ginseng	Bee pollen	Yellow dock rt.	Chamomile	Horsetail

❧ EXAMPLE FORMULAS OF MENTAL & CREATIVE ENERGY COMPOUNDS:

A MENTAL INNER ENERGY EXTRACT COMPOUNDS			(ε - 4440)	A MENTAL CLARITY CAPSULE COMPOUND			(ε - 3250)
Kava kava root	Dong quai rt.	Gotu kola	Prince ginseng rt.	Panax ginseng rt.	Kelp	Rosemary	Capsicum
Kirin ginseng rt.	Suma rt.	Kola nut	Ashwagandha rt.	Gotu kola	Ginkgo biloba	Schizandra bry.	Spirulina
Panax ginseng	Fo-Ti rt.	Ginkgo biloba		Fo-Ti rt.	Siberian ginseng rt.	Prickly ash bk.	
Siberian ginseng rt.							

SEE PAGE 1 FOR FORMULATING INSTRUCTIONS.

Sugar Imbalances & Adrenal Exhaustion

The inability to properly process glucose, the body's number one energy source, affects millions. At last count, more than twenty-five million Americans suffer from diabetes (high blood sugar) or hypoglycemia (low blood sugar). While seeming to be opposite problems, these two conditions really stem from the same cause - an imbalance between glucose and oxygen that puts the body under stress and leads to gland exhaustion. Poor nutrition is a common cause of both disorders, and both can be improved with a high mineral, high fiber diet, adequate usable protein, small frequent meals, and regular exercise.

HYPOGLYCEMIA is one of the most widespread disorders in modern industrial nations today. It is a direct effect of our excess intake of refined sweets, low fiber foods, and other processed carbohydrates. The pancreas reacts to this overload by producing too much insulin to reduce the blood sugar, and hypoglycemia results. Typical hypoglycemic symptoms include extreme irritability, fatigue, manic/depressive states, hunger and great cravings, over-eating, restlessness and insomnia, and mental confusion. After many years of this type of diet and pancreatic reaction, the whole endocrine system, especially the adrenals, reacts to hyper-insulinism, sometimes causing hypoglycemia to become a precursor of diabetes.

DIABETES is also a disease of the modern diet, in which people regularly eat too much sugar, refined carbohydrates and caffeine, and drink too much alcohol. When excess carbohydrates are not used correctly, blood sugar stays too high because too little balancing insulin is produced. The pancreas becomes exhausted, and glucose cannot enter the cells to provide body energy. Instead it accumulates in the blood, resulting in various symptoms from mental confusion to coma. Typical diabetic symptoms include excessive thirst and urination, failing vision, dry, itchy skin, poor circulation, lack of energy and kidney malfunction. Type 1, or juvenile onset diabetes is the more severe. Little or no insulin is produced, and insulin injections must be taken to sustain life. Type 2, or adult diabetes accounts for 90% of all cases. Pancreatic secretions which control the enzyme activity for digestion and food assimilation are inhibited, so obesity almost always results from diabetes. Enzymes relating to immune health also stem from the pancreas, so diabetics easily fall prey to other degenerative conditions as well.

ADRENAL EXHAUSTION reduces immune response, too, so you may lose the ability to fight off illness. The continual necessity to react and fight exhausts the adrenals to a point where they cannot recover naturally. Symptoms of poor adrenal function include low blood pressure, low energy, chronic constipation, brittle nails, dry skin, puffy ankles and eyelids, PMS, low metabolism and the inability to lose weight, brown spots on the skin, frail nerves, mental spaciness, and sparse body hair. Nutrient absorption is affected because the adrenals help to synthesize cholesterol, and influence metabolism of carbohydrates and sugars.

Balancing your blood sugar can change your life - literally. Erratic gland function, and the sugar-balancing hormones they secrete, cause havoc with your personality, moods, and outlook on life. Most people in our stressful, over-extended, high carbohydrate, increasingly polluted environment have experienced blood sugar problems at one time or another. Herbs are concentrated nutrients that your body identifies and absorbs readily. They can work faster in the bloodstream than raw glandulars or isolated vitamin/mineral tablets - without upsetting your system. Without question, there must be diet and lifestyle change for there to be permanent improvement, but herbal support is a safe, natural way to start off on the right foot. When sugar imbalances are under control, there is a feeling of well-being. You are aware that the herbs are working and helping while you concentrate on diet improvement.

✤FORMULAS FOR BALANCING BLOOD SUGAR FUNCTIONS HELP IN THE FOLLOWING CONDITIONS:
•Mood & Personality Swings   •Drug & Alcohol Addiction & Withdrawal   •Gum Disease & Gingivitis   •Diabetic Retinopathy   •Hyperactivity   •Epileptic Incidences   •Schizophrenia   •Cataracts & Glaucoma   •Adrenal Exhaustion   •Weight Control

✤COMPOUNDS FOR FORMULATION SHOULD INCLUDE:
•Controlling hypoglycemia reactions
•Overcoming diabetes
•Revitalizing exhausted adrenal glands

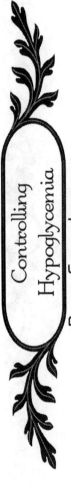

Controlling Hypoglycemia

BLOOD SUGAR IMBALANCES

Hypoglycemia (low blood sugar) is a result of too much dietary sugar and refined carbohydrates, foods that quickly raise blood glucose levels, causing the pancreas to over-compensate and produce too much insulin, which then lowers body glucose levels too far and too fast. It's been called a "sugar epidemic" in America, and is particularly harmful to the brain, the most sensitive organ to blood sugar levels, which requires glucose energy to think clearly. Small fluctuations disturb one's feeling of well-being. Large fluctuations cause feelings of depression, anxiety, mood swings, fatigue and aggressive behavior. Sugar balance is also needed for muscle contractions, the digestive system and nerve health. A low glycemic, high fiber, vegetable protein diet, along with potassium and chromium-rich herbal compounds can help prevent sudden sugar fluctuations. Small, frequent meals with plenty of fresh foods also promote stable blood sugar levels.

❧ ESSENTIAL CATEGORIES FOR HYPOGLYCEMIA CONTROLLING COMPOUNDS:

BLOOD SUGAR BALANCERS	PROTEIN STABILIZING HERBS	CHLOROPHYLL-RICH HERBS	PANCREAS SUPPORT HERBS	ADRENAL GLAND SUPPORT HERBS	NERVE SUPPORT TONIC HERBS
Licorice root	**Bee pollen**	**Barley grass**	Dandelion root	**Kelp/sea vegetables**	**Gotu kola**
Barley grass	Royal Jelly	Spirulina	Bilberry	**Sarsaparilla rt.**	**St. John's wort**
Spirulina	Kelp/sea vegetables	**Alfalfa**	**Licorice root**	**Astragalus**	**Rosemary**
Gotu kola	Alfalfa	Nettles	**Saw palmetto bry.**	Dandelion root	**Kava kava**
Wild yam rt.	Brewer's yeast	Kelp/sea vegetables	Goldenseal root	Uva ursi	Passionflower
Suma rt	Miso powder	Parsley leaf	**Siberian ginseng**	**Licorice root**	Ashwagandha
Sarsaparilla root	Spirulina	Chlorella	**Panax ginseng**	Capsicum/Ginger root	Red raspberry
Panax ginseng	Barley grass	Comfrey leaf	Capsicum	**Ginkgo biloba**	Scullcap
Cedar berry	Rice protein pwr.	Peppermint	Pau d' arco bark	Schizandra bry.	**Nutritional yeast pwr.**

❧ ESSENTIAL HERBS FOR HYPOGLYCEMIA CONTROLLING COMPOUNDS:

PRIMARY HERBS		ASSISTING & COMPLEMENTARY HERBS		CATALYST & TRANSPORTING HERBS	
Bee pollen	Pau d'arco bark	Dandelion root	Ginger root	Capsicum	Red raspberry
Kelp/sea vegetables	Sarsaparilla root	Goldenseal root	Saw palmetto bry.	Horseradish rt.	Nutritional yeast pwr.
Ginkgo biloba	Ashwagandha	Bilberry	Prince ginseng rt.	St. John's wort	Parsley rt & lf.
Siberian ginseng	Brewer's yeast	Kava kava rt.	Scullcap	Ginkgo biloba	Comfrey leaf
Licorice root	Astragalus	Peppermint	Passionflower	Rosemary	Uva ursi
Barley grass	Panax ginseng	Cedar berry	Nettles	Red clover	Rice protein pwr.
Fo-Ti root	Gotu kola	Wild yam rt.	Black cohosh	Guar gum	Juniper bry.
Suma rt	Spirulina	Burdock root	Royal Jelly	Watercress	Evening primrose oil
Ginseng - all types	Chlorella	Alfalfa	Schizandra bry.	Miso broth powder	Anise seed

❧ EXAMPLE FORMULAS OF HYPOGLYCEMIA CONTROLLING COMPOUNDS:

A LOW BLOOD SUGAR CAPSULE COMPOUND			(p - 2800)	A LOW BLOOD SUGAR TEA COMPOUND		(p - 5660)
Licorice rt.	Alfalfa	Spirulina	Horseradish rt.	Licorice rt.	Gotu kola	Bee pollen
Dandelion root	Wild yam rt.	Barley grass	Suma root	Dandelion root	Prince ginseng rt.	Anise seed
Cedar berry	Gotu kola	Panax ginseng	Guar gum	Alfalfa	Peppermint	
					Nettles	

SEE PAGE 1 FOR FORMULATING INSTRUCTIONS.

102

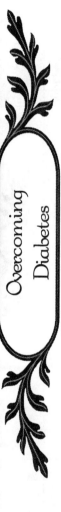

Overcoming Diabetes

BLOOD SUGAR IMBALANCES

Adult-onset diabetes mellitus, is a chronic degenerative disorder in which the body's ability to use carbohydrates is impaired by disturbances in normal insulin mechanisms. It is usually brought on by dietary habits that include too many sugary foods and alcohol, and refined carbohydrates. Pancreatic activity and other vital organs become damaged, the body loses the ability to produce enough insulin, and high blood sugar results. As less and less insulin is produced, refined, simple carbohydrates and sugars, which require large insulin secretions for metabolism, accumulate in the body and are stored as fat. A correcting diet should have a low-glycemic index, with slow-burning, complex carbohydrate fuels that do not need much insulin for metabolism. Meals should be small, frequent, largely vegetarian, and low in fats of all kinds, with protein from soy foods and whole grains that are rich in lecithin and chromium. Herbs can supply sugar-balancing, mineral-rich support.

❧ ESSENTIAL CATEGORIES FOR DIABETES MANAGEMENT COMPOUNDS:

BLOOD SUGAR BALANCING HERBS	PANCREATIC SUPPORT	CIRCULATION TONIC HERBS	MILD, BODY-FLUSHING HERBS	ADRENAL SUPPORT SOURCES	FIBER-RICH, LOW GLYCEMIC HERBS
Ginkgo biloba	Dandelion root	**Capsicum**	**Dandelion leaf**	**Royal jelly**	**Aloe vera**
Bilberry	Bilberry	**Ginger root**	**Cornsilk**	**Bee pollen**	**Guar gum**
Spirulina	**Licorice root**	**Gotu kola**	Parsley root & lf.	**Kelp/sea vegetables**	Slippery elm
Dandelion root	**Saw palmetto bry.**	Bilberry	**Uva ursi**	**Borage seed**	Oats/Oatstraw
Gymnema sylvestre	Goldenseal root	Hawthorn bry., lf., fl.	**Oatstraw**	**Panax ginseng**	Kelp/sea vegetables
Panax ginseng	**Siberian ginseng**	Horseradish rt.	Cleavers	**Sarsaparilla root**	**Flax seed**
Nettles	**Panax ginseng**	**Spirulina**	Fennel seed	**Licorice root**	**Fenugreek seed**
Licorice root	Capsicum	**Siberian ginseng rt.**	Watercress	**Evening primrose oil**	**Psyllium husk**
Wild yam root	Pau d' arco bark	**Ginkgo biloba**	**Green tea**	Hawthorn bry., lf., fl.	**Burdock root**

❧ ESSENTIAL HERBS FOR DIABETES MANAGEMENT COMPOUNDS:

PRIMARY HERBS		ASSISTING & COMPLEMENTARY HERBS		CATALYST & TRANSPORTING HERBS	
Gotu kola	Aloe vera	Parsley root & lf.	Evening primrose oil	Horseradish rt.	Horsetail
Dandelion rt.	St. John's wort	Alfalfa	Goldenseal root	Guar gum	Rosemary
Ginseng - all types	Ginkgo biloba	Green tea	Elecampane rt.	Tienchi rt.	Watercress
Sarsaparilla root	Wild yam root	Pau d' arco bark	Mullein	Capsicum	Reishi mushroom
Astragalus root	Royal jelly	Spirulina	Bilberry	Peppermint	Oats/Oatstraw
Licorice root	Bee pollen	Kirin ginseng root	Uva ursi	Cornsilk	Fennel seed
Kelp & sea vegetables	Suma root	Barley grass	Saw palmetto bry.	Ginger root	Flax seed
Cedar berry	Siberian ginseng	Echinacea root	Prince ginseng	Borage seed	Cleavers
Chlorella	Panax ginseng	Yellow dock root	Hawthorn bry., lf., fl.	Gymnema sylvestre	Aralia rt.

❧ EXAMPLE FORMULAS OF DIABETES MANAGEMENT COMPOUNDS:

A HIGH BLOOD SUGAR CAPSULE COMPOUND			(D - 2850)
Cedar berry	Mullein	Kelp	Capsicum
Licorice rt.	Guar gum	Horseradish rt.	Ginger root
Dandelion rt.	Wild yam root	Bilberry	
Elecampane rt.	Uva ursi	Spirulina	

A SUGAR-LOWERING GINSENG SUPER TEA COMPOUND			(PD - 6830)
Prince ginseng rt.	Suma rt.	St. John's wort	Fennel seed
Siberian ginseng rt.	Pau d' arco bark	Panax ginseng	Tienchi rt.
Kirin ginseng rt.	Echinacea root	Guar gum	Ginger rt.
Aralia rt.			

See page 1 for formulating instructions.

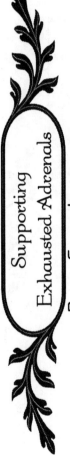

Supporting Exhausted Adrenals

BLOOD SUGAR IMBALANCES

Adrenal insufficiency is suffered by tens of millions of Americans. Its incidence is rising every year largely due to worsening nutritional deficiencies from an over-processed food diet and chronic mental and emotional strain. The adrenal glands are the primary organs for fighting stress. They are responsible for warding off the ill effects of every conceivable mental and/or physical stressor. Emotional strain, especially anger, causes significant, even profound disruption of adrenal function. Adrenal failure is associated with hypoglycemia and blood sugar imbalance, because the adrenals exert potent control over blood sugar status. Their job is to prevent blood sugar levels from dropping suddenly as a result of stress. Herbs can help strengthen and nourish weakened adrenal glands for those who suffer from the symptoms of blood sugar imbalance syndromes like diabetes and hypoglycemia.

❧ ESSENTIAL CATEGORIES FOR EXHAUSTED ADRENAL SUPPORT COMPOUNDS:

ADRENAL CORTEX STIMULANTS	IODINE/POTASSIUM SUPPORT	STRESS-REDUCING HERBS	ANTI-OXIDANT HERBS	ENZYME THERAPY HERBS	GLAND & HORMONE BALANCERS
Astragalus	**Kelp/sea vegetables**	**Scullcap**	**Rosemary**	**Alfalfa**	**Licorice root**
Bee pollen/Royal Jelly	**Spirulina**	**Gotu kola**	**Kelp/sea vegetables**	**Dandelion root**	**Wild yam root**
Ginkgo biloba	Barley grass	Suma root	**Ginseng - all types**	**Chlorella**	**Sarsaparilla root**
Kelp/sea vegetables	Garlic	**Black cohosh**	**Capsicum**	Spirulina	**Burdock root**
Licorice root	**Alfalfa**	St. John's wort	**White pine bk.**	**Barley grass**	Bee pollen/royal jelly
Hawthorn lf., bry., fl.	Irish moss	Oatstraw	**Bee pollen/royal jelly**	**Fennel seed**	Kelp/sea vegetables
Borage seed	Horsetail	Kava kava root	Prickly ash	**Capsicum**	Evening primrose oil
Bayberry bark	Nettles	Uva ursi	Ginger root	**Ginger root**	Black cohosh
Sarsaparilla root	Watercress	Lobelia	Peppermint	**Green tea**	Flax seed

❧ ESSENTIAL HERBS FOR EXHAUSTED ADRENAL SUPPORT COMPOUNDS:

PRIMARY HERBS		ASSISTING & COMPLEMENTARY HERBS		CATALYST & TRANSPORTING HERBS	
Ginkgo biloba	Bee pollen	Ashwagandha rt.	Burdock root	Borage seed	St. John's wort
Bee pollen	Fo-Ti root	Black cohosh	Alfalfa	Vitamin C pwr.	Rosemary
Ginseng - all types	Kava kava root	Dandelion root	White pine bk.	Prickly ash	Watercress
Sarsaparilla root	Gotu kola	Nettles	Garlic	Capsicum	Irish Moss
Spirulina	Royal Jelly	Brewer's yeast	Bayberry bark	Peppermint	Carrot pwdr.
Licorice root	Hawthorn bry., lf., fl.	Astragalus	Goldenseal rt.	Uva ursi	Fennel seed
Kelp & sea vegetables	Suma root	Barley grass	Horsetail	Ginger root	Flax seed
White pine bk.	Siberian ginseng	Evening primrose oil	Red raspberry	Green tea	Lobelia
Chlorella	Panax ginseng	Wild yam root	Scullcap	Mullein	Oatstraw

❧ EXAMPLE FORMULAS OF EXHAUSTED ADRENAL SUPPORT COMPOUNDS:

AN ADRENAL ACTIVE EXTRACT COMPOUNDS		(E - 4638)	A BODY REBUILDING CAPSULE COMPOUND		(SA - 1450)
Licorice root	Bladderwrack	Irish Moss	Ginger root	Hawthorn bry., lf., fl.	Siberian ginseng	Wild cherry
Sarsaparilla root				Royal Jelly	Sarsaparilla root	Chlorella
				Barley grass	Red raspberry	Goldenseal rt.
				Carrot pwd.	Kelp	Mullein
				Spirulina		
				Bee pollen		
				Alfalfa		
				Vitamin C pwd.		

SEE PAGE 1 FOR FORMULATING INSTRUCTIONS.

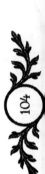

Digestive & Assimilation Problems

People today suffer from more digestive disorders than any other health problems. Digestive ailments are usually chronic, long standing, and deep seated. Bad breath, body odor, constipation, diarrhea, heartburn, bloating and flatulence are all signs of inadequate digestion. Poor digestion is also at the root of many serious diseases, like arthritis, anemia, candida albicans yeast overgrowth, hiatal hernia, liver and gallbladder disease, diverticulitis, Crohn's disease, colitis, ulcers, hypothyroidism, and even some kinds of cancer. The causes of digestive problems are almost as varied as the individuals who have them; food allergies and intolerances (especially to chemical food additives), poor food combining, stress, lack of minerals, long illness with prolonged use of drugs, pregnancy imbalances, over-use of antacids, overeating, eating too many fried, refined and acid-producing foods all contribute to poor digestion and nutrient absorption.

1) Refined foods with chemical additives are clearly the most prevalent cause of digestive problems, from gas to allergies to hiatal hernias to ulcers.
2) Too much red meat and too little soluble fiber in the diet results in food that stays too long in the stomach, depletes enzyme capacity, and favors constipation.
3) Unmetabolized fats and proteins are stored as body fat and cellulite resulting in obesity.
4) Lack of stomach HCl and bile affects digestion of acids and proteins, resulting in an over acid system, fermentation, and auto-toxemia.
5) Poor food combining causes food to be only partially digested, so that it just "sits there" in the stomach, partially fermented, causing gas and bloating.
6) Eating under stress brings on a vicious cycle. Enzyme production slows down to meet the metabolic demands of stress, and a heavy meal puts even more stress on the digestive systems. Meals eaten under stress are usually poorly chewed, further adding to enzyme depletion.

Good enzyme activity is important not only for digestion, but for total health. Most nutrient deficiencies result from the body's inability to absorb them, not from the lack of the nutrients themselves. Enzyme rich foods assure us adequate amounts of antioxidants to fight free radicals, and nutrients to keep our immune systems strong. Enzymes are the single most important factor that powers our bodies, the workhorses that drive metabolism which puts to use the nutrients we take in. The refining of food and fast-heat cooking methods have rendered the modern diet enzyme-deficient. Eating food devoid of enzymes means the pancreas and the liver have to use their enzyme stores. As a result, reserve enzymes for metabolic processes are pulled from their normal work, to digest food. But even this substitute measure does not make up for the missing enzymes that should be in our food, because without food enzymes the body can't break the food down correctly to deliver nutrients to the blood. So we end up with undigested food in the blood. White blood cell immune defenses are pulled from their jobs to take care of all the undigested food, so the immune system takes a dive. Eating enzyme rich foods or taking plant-based enzyme supplements takes care of this unhealthy cascade of reactions before it ever starts. Any enzymes left over after the digestion process go on to be used by the body as metabolic enzymes, which run our bodies and contribute to healing. **I believe Nature intended us to eat a largely plant-based diet, rich in fresh foods for the best digestion.** It is not necessary to always eat raw, live foods. But it is important to have a large percentage of the overall diet be enzyme rich. If you don't feel you get enough fresh foods, or you need extra enzyme concentration for healing through enzyme therapy, plant based, herbal enzyme supplements are the next best choice.

The natural approach for improving digestion is simple, successful, and free of substances that cause dependency. Enhance and maintain a high quality diet. Add plant enzymes from herbs or supplements to your daily nutritional intake. Restore and improve the beneficial bacteria in the colon and intestinal tract. Consciously try to reduce the stress in your life, especially when you eat.

❋ FORMULAS FOR NUTRIENT ABSORPTION AND ENZYME THERAPY HELP IN THE FOLLOWING:
• Gastritis & Gastro-enteritis • Food Intolerances & Sensitivities • Bad Breath & Body Odor • Gas, Bloating & Flatulence • Gum Disease & Gingivitis • Heartburn • Hemorrhoids • Chronic Constipation • Liver Malfunction • Colitis • Crohn's Disease • Diverticulitis • Stomach & Duodenal Ulcers

❋ COMPOUNDS FOR FORMULATION SHOULD INCLUDE:
• Controlling food allergies and sensitivities
• Healing stomach and duodenal ulcers
• Boosting enzyme activity for healing and nutrient absorption

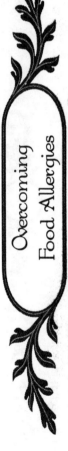

Overcoming Food Allergies

DIGESTIVE & NUTRIENT ASSIMILATION PROBLEMS

A food allergy is an antibody response to a certain food. **A food intolerance** is an enzyme deficiency to digest a certain food. This type of sensitivity is the fastest growing allergy group as people are more exposed to chemically altered, enzyme-depleted, processed foods. Without enzyme active foods, our bodies must assume all digestive responsibilities. This capacity eventually weakens, total food assimilation does not occur, and large amounts of undigested fats and proteins are left that the immune system treats as potentially toxic. It releases prostaglandins, leukotrienes, and histamines into the bloodstream to counteract the perceived threat, and allergy reactions occur. Common allergy foods include wheat, dairy products, fruits, sugar, yeast, mushrooms, eggs, soy, coffee, corn and greens. Although some of these foods are healthy in themselves, they are often heavily sprayed or treated, and in the case of animal products, may be affected by antibiotics and hormones.

❧ ESSENTIAL CATEGORIES FOR OVERCOMING FOOD ALLERGIES & SENSITIVITIES:

HISTAMINE-BALANCING HERBS	HERBS TO REDUCE ALLERGIC REACTIONS	DIGESTIVE TRACT CLEANSING HERBS	HERBS FOR NUTRIENT ASSIMILATION	CHLOROPHYLL-RICH IMMUNE BOOSTERS	ENZYME SUPPORT HERBS
Marshmallow root	**Bee pollen/Royal Jelly**	Aloe vera	**Garlic**	**Alfalfa**	**Chlorella/barley grass**
Vitamin C powder	Reishi mushroom	**Goldenseal root**	**Acidophilus pwdr.**	Chlorella	**Papaya**
Lobelia	**Kelp/sea vegetables**	Senna leaf	Bee pollen	Spirulina	**Fennel seed**
Gotu kola	Alfalfa	**Flax seed**	**Barley grass**	Barley grass	**Ginger root**
Parsley rt.	**Panax ginseng**	**Peppermint**	Pau d' arco bark	Nettles	Peppermint
Rosemary	**Miso powder**	Kelp/sea vegetables	Alfalfa	**Kelp/sea vegetables**	Cardamom
White pine bk.	Burdock root	Slippery elm	**Licorice root**	Parsley lf.	Dandelion root
Bee pollen	**Ginger root**	Lemon peel	**Dandelion root**	**Watercress**	Oregon grape rt.
Goldenseal root	**Wild cherry bk.**	Gentian root	**Ginger root**	Aloe vera	**Catnip**

❧ ESSENTIAL HERBS FOR OVERCOMING FOOD ALLERGIES & SENSITIVITIES:

PRIMARY HERBS		ASSISTING & COMPLEMENTARY HERBS		CATALYST & TRANSPORTING HERBS	
Bee pollen	Pau d'arco bark	Reishi mushroom	Wild cherry bk.	Capsicum	Red raspberry
Kelp/sea vegetables	Sarsaparilla root	Marshmallow root	Saw palmetto bry.	Cardamom	Acidophilus pwr.
Ginkgo biloba	Chlorella	Goldenseal root	Lobelia	Vitamin C powder	Parsley rt & lf.
Siberian ginseng	Pau d' arco bark	Aloe vera	Flax seed	Ginkgo biloba	Spearmint
Licorice root	Fennel seed	Peppermint	Papaya	Rosemary	Orange peel
Barley grass	Panax ginseng	Oregon grape rt.	Nettles	Senna leaf	Lemon peel
Fo-Ti root	Gotu kola	Garlic	White pine bk.	Gentian root	Slippery elm
Suma rt	Spirulina	Burdock root	Royal jelly	Watercress	Hibiscus
Dandelion root	Ginger root	Alfalfa	Slippery elm	Miso broth powder	Anise seed

❧ EXAMPLE FORMULAS OF COMPOUNDS FOR FOOD ALLERGIES & SENSITIVITIES:

A DIGESTIVE CLEANSING EXTRACT COMPOUND (CD - 4710)			A DIGESTIVE CLEANSING EXTRACT COMPOUND	AN ENZYME-ENCOURAGING EXTRACT COMPOUND (CO - 4650)		
Oregon grape rt.	Cardamom	Senna leaf	Peppermint	Peppermint	Orange peel	Papaya	Hibiscus
Gentian root	Lemon peel	Dandelion root	Honey	Spearmint	Lemon peel	Licorice root	

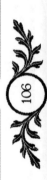

106

SEE "COOKING FOR HEALTHY HEALING" BY LINDA RECTOR PAGE FOR
A COMPLETE DIET PROGRAM TO OVERCOME FOOD ALLERGIES.

SEE PAGE 1 FOR FORMULATING INSTRUCTIONS.

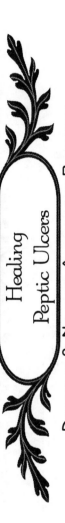

Healing Peptic Ulcers

DIGESTIVE & NUTRIENT ASSIMILATION PROBLEMS

A peptic ulcer is an open sore, an erosion of the lining in either the stomach or the duodenum (the first part of the small intestine). Most ulcers are caused by H. pylori, a common stomach bacterium which liberate copious amounts of damaging ammonia and carbon dioxide when the body's intestinal protective devices fail. While a stressful life-style and over-acidity play a role in ulcers, it is increasingly obvious that poor nutrition and refined foods are the primary culprits. Gastric ulcers are also often the result of alcohol abuse, or non-steroid anti-inflammatory drugs. Tagamet and Zantac drugs for ulcers, currently over a billion dollars in sales yearly, suppress HCL formation, cause eventual liver damage, and create dependency if discontinued. Herbal therapy focuses on gastric mucosal support and re-establishing intestinal balance. Rather than suppressing acid release into the stomach as drugs do, herbal combinations stimulate normal immune defenses that prevent ulcer formation.

❧ ESSENTIAL CATEGORIES FOR ULCER HEALING COMPOUNDS:

RELAXING, SOOTHING Herbs	H. PYLORI FIGHTING Herbs	ENZYME-PRODUCING Herbs	LIVER TONING Herbs	ANTI-SPASMODIC Herbs	ANTI-INFLAMMATORY Herbs
Slippery elm	**Licorice root**	**Licorice root**	**Dandelion leaf & rt.**	**St. John's wort**	Myrrh
Marshmallow root	Bilberry	**Chlorophyll-rich herbs**	**Goldenseal root**	**Valerian root**	**Garlic**
Irish moss	**Garlic**	Garlic	**Oregon grape root**	**Passionflower**	**Goldenseal root**
Aloe vera	**Chlorella**	**Dandelion root**	**Barberry bark**	**Kava kava rt.**	**Echinacea root**
Comfrey root	Panax ginseng root	Alfalfa	Yellow dock root	**Lobelia**	Aloe vera
Calendula	**Acidophilus powder**	Kelp/sea vegetables	**Milk thistle seed**	**Cramp bark**	Calendula
Flax seed	**Goldenseal root**	Goldenseal rt.	Capsicum	Peppermint	Pau d' arco
Parsley root	**Echinacea root**	**Ginger root**	Turmeric	Red raspberry	**White willow bark**
Chamomile	Pau d' arco bark	**Papaya**	Watercress	Catnip	**St. John's wort**

❧ ESSENTIAL HERBS FOR ULCER HEALING COMPOUNDS:

PRIMARY HERBS	ASSISTING & COMPLEMENTARY HERBS	CATALYST & TRANSPORTING HERBS
Ginger rt.	St. John's wort	Parsley root & lf.	Cramp bark	Aloe vera	Spearmint
Dandelion rt.	Chlorophyll-rich herbs	Red raspberry	Alfalfa	Barberry bark	Rosemary
Ginseng - all types	Ginkgo biloba	Lobelia	Peppermint	Chamomile	Watercress
Myrrh	Wild yam root	Pau d' arco bark	Marshmallow root	Acidophilus powder	Reishi mushroom
Goldenseal rt.	Royal Jelly	Spirulina	Bilberry	Kava kava rt.	Irish moss
Licorice root	Bee pollen	Slippery elm	Milk thistle seed	Papaya	Valerian root
Kelp/sea vegetables	Oregon grape root	Barley grass	Turmeric	Flax seed	Passionflower
Capsicum	Siberian ginseng	Echinacea root	Catnip	Comfrey root	Nettles
Chlorella	Panax ginseng	Yellow dock root	Garlic	White willow bark	Calendula

❧ EXAMPLE FORMULAS OF ULCER HEALING COMPOUNDS:

AN ULCER HEALING CAPSULE COMPOUND	(CO - 4180)	A PRE-MEAL, ANTI-INFLAMMATORY COMPOUND	(CO - 4908)
Goldenseal rt.	Capsicum	Bilberry	Ginger rt.	Fennel seed	Cramp bark	Spearmint
Slippery elm	Calendula		Peppermint	Catnip	Turmeric	Papaya
Licorice root						
Myrrh						

SEE PAGE 1 FOR FORMULATING INSTRUCTIONS.

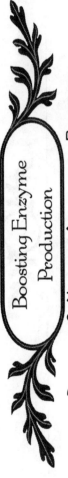

Boosting Enzyme Production

DIGESTIVE & NUTRIENT ASSIMILATION PROBLEMS

Enzyme production is at the heart of good digestion. Different foods require different enzymes for assimilation. Poor diet quality, poor food combining, and eating under stress often mean that the proper enzymes don't come into play at the right time for the right food. Herbal enzymes are in a natural unprocessed state, able to easily combine with digestive juices to enhance enzyme activity. They may be taken before meals, or as needed after distressful meals; and are effective even in cases where there is serious enzyme depletion, such as from over-use of drugs. There are three enzyme categories: metabolic enzymes, which run body processes, repair damage and heal; digestive enzymes, which assimilate carbohydrates, proteins and fats; and raw food enzymes, which start food digestion, and aid digestive enzymes. In fact, digestive enzymes are stronger than any of the body's other enzymes, and are more concentrated than any other enzyme combination found in nature.

✤ ESSENTIAL CATEGORIES FOR BOOSTING ENZYME PRODUCTION COMPOUNDS:

ENZYME PRODUCING HERBS	PANCREAS STIMULATING SUPPORT	BODY CHEMISTRY BALANCING HERBS	NUTRIENT ASSIMILATION SOURCES	LIVER & BILE STIMULANTS	CHLOROPHYLL SOURCES
Licorice root	Fenugreek seed	Chlorella/barley grass	Garlic	Parsley root & lf.	Alfalfa
Chlorophyll-rich herbs	Mullein	Papaya	Acidophilus pwr.	Senna lf.	Chlorella
Garlic	Saw palmetto bry.	Red raspberry	Bee pollen	Capsicum	Spirulina
Dandelion root	Burdock root	Ginger root	Barley grass	Oregon grape root	Barley grass
Alfalfa	Anise seed	Peppermint	Lemon/citrus peel	Cardamom seed	Nettles
Kelp/sea vegetables	Cascara bark	Catnip	Alfalfa	Goldenseal root	Kelp/sea vegetables
Chamomile	Barberry bark	Garlic	Miso powder	Milk thistle seed	Parsley lf.
Chickweed	Fennel seed	Fenugreek seed	Ginger root	Yellow dock root	Peppermint
Goldenseal root	Lemon peel	Brewer's yeast	Spirulina	Ginger root	Aloe vera

✤ ESSENTIAL HERBS FOR BOOSTING ENZYME PRODUCTION COMPOUNDS:

PRIMARY HERBS		ASSISTING & COMPLEMENTARY HERBS		CATALYST & TRANSPORTING HERBS	
Nettles	Ginseng - all types	Yellow dock root	Chlorophyll-rich herbs	Barberry bark	Acidophilus pwdr.
Goldenseal rt.	Bee pollen	Milk thistle seed	Alfalfa	Papaya	Chickweed
Oregon grape root	Ginkgo biloba	Dandelion root & lf.	Senna lf.	Chamomile	Watercress
Sarsaparilla root	Gotu kola	Cardamom seed	Garlic	Capsicum	Irish Moss
Spirulina	Royal jelly	Goldenseal root	Catnip	Peppermint	Cascara bark
Licorice root	Hawthorn bry., lf., fl.	Saw palmetto bry.	Miso powder.	Anise seed	Fennel seed
Kelp & sea vegetables	Burdock root	Barley grass	Aloe vera	Ginger root	Brewer's yeast
Parsley root & lf.	Siberian ginseng	Fenugreek seed	Red raspberry	Lemon peel	Lobelia
Chlorella	Panax ginseng	Wild yam root	Mullein	Apple pectin	Dulse

✤ EXAMPLE FORMULAS OF ENZYME PRODUCTION BOOSTING COMPOUNDS:

A GREEN ENZYME DRINK COMPOUND		A (SA - 8150)		A MINERAL SPECTRUM ENZYME COMPOUND		(SA - 3200)	
Barley grass	Acerola cherry	Dandelion lf.	Oatstraw	Nettles	Alfalfa	Barley grass	Borage seed
Alfalfa	Sarsaparilla root	Gotu kola	Lemon peel	Irish moss	Yellow Dock rt.	Kelp	Dulse
Bee pollen	Chlorella	Licorice root	Rice protein pwr	Watercress	Dandelion root	Parsley rt. & lf.	
Siberian ginseng	Dulse	Dandelion rt.	Apple pectin				

SEE PAGE 1 FOR FORMULATING INSTRUCTIONS.

108

Herbal Compounds For Elimination Problems

Much pain and disease that we endure extends from deficient drainage. One of the greatest factors in improving health is removing toxic waste from the system. Problems start with back-up and fermentation in the colon, like a walking pressure cooker, and end with the body actually re-absorbing unreleased waste material, which settles in weak tissues that are unable to "clean house." Continuing accumulation of this toxic build-up results in sluggish organ and glandular functions, poor digestion and assimilation, lowered immunity, faulty circulation, tissue degeneration and disease.

ELEMENTS CAUSING CONSTIPATION AND COLON TOXICITY COME FROM THREE BASIC AREAS:

1) Chemical-laced foods, and pollutants in the environment, ranging from relatively harmless to very dangerous. The body can tolerate a certain level of contamination, but when that individual level is reached, and immune defenses are low, toxic overload causes illness. A strong system can metabolize and excrete many of these toxins, but when the body is weak or constipated, they are stored as unusable substances. As more and different chemicals enter and build up in the body they tend to interreact with those that are already there, forming mutant, second generation chemicals far more harmful than the originals. Evidence in recent years has shown that most bowel cancer is caused by environmental agents.

2) Over-accumulation of body wastes and metabolic byproducts that are not excreted properly. These wastes can also become a breeding ground for parasite infestation. A nationwide survey reveals that one in every six people studied had one or more parasites living somewhere in their bodies! An astounding figure.

3) Slowed elimination time, allowing waste materials to ferment, become rancid, and then recirculate through the body tissues as toxic substances.

The key to avoiding elimination back-up is almost always nutritional. A fiber-rich diet along with appropriate herbal combinations is important for both normalization and prevention. Diet improvement can also correct the diseases waste elimination problems cause. Even a gentle and gradual improvement from low fiber, low residue foods helps almost immediately. In fact, graduated change is often better than a sudden, drastic about-face, especially when the colon, bowel or bladder are painful and inflamed. A complete change, over several months, to unrefined, whole foods with all their nutrients intact, is much better for therapeutic results than continuing with refined foods, and just adding a fiber supplement or a few fiber foods to the diet.

The protective level of fiber in your diet can be easily measured. The following GOOD PROTECTION TEST can help you monitor your support-system health on a regular basis. Essentially it is a dietary fiber check; enough dietary fiber to make the stool float is the protective level against poor waste elimination diseases.

- Bowel movements should be regular daily, and almost effortless.
- The stool should be almost odorless (signalling faster transit time in the bowel with no fermentation) .
- There should be very little gas or flatulence.
- The stool should float rather than sink.

Herbs can improve waste elimination problems both for long and short term results, but it takes from 3 to 6 months to rebuild the bowel and colon to adequate tone and elasticity with good systol/diastol action. There is no instant, easy route, but the rewards of a regular, healthy, energetic life are worth it.

✴ FORMULAS FOR WASTE MANAGEMENT ARE EFFECTIVE FOR THE FOLLOWING CONDITIONS:

•Chronic Constipation & Diarrhea •Irritable Bowel Syndrome (IBS) •Colitis •Crohn's Disease •Diverticulosis •Gas, Bloating & Flatulence •Badder Infections & Cystitis •Hemorrhoids •Kidney Malfunction •Bladder Incontinence •Low Energy & Immune Response •Varicose Veins •Internal Parasites & Worms

✴ COMPOUNDS FOR FORMULATION SHOULD INCLUDE:

- •Herbs to overcome constipation and normalize colon and bowel activity
- •Herbs to overcome chronic bladder infections
- •Herbs to help deal with kidney inflammation and kidney stones
- •Herbs to help get rid of intestinal parasites

109

SEE ALSO DETOXIFICATION & CLEANSING SECTION IN THIS BOOK FOR MORE INFORMATION.

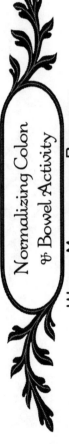

Normalizing Colon & Bowel Activity

WASTE MANAGEMENT PROBLEMS

The colon and bowel are the depository for all waste material after food nutrients have been extracted and processed to the bloodstream. It is hardly any wonder that up to 90% of all diseases generate from an unclean colon. Decaying food ferments, forms gases, as well as 2nd and 3rd generation toxins, and the colon becomes a breeding ground for putrefactive bacteria, viruses, parasites, yeasts, molds, etc. Ideally, one should eliminate as often as a meal is taken in. Constipation is normally a chronic problem, and while body cleansing progress can be felt fairly quickly with a diet change, it takes from three to six months to rebuild bowel and colon elasticity with good systolic/diastolic action. Bowel transit time should be approximately 12 hours. To promote healthy bowel function, include plenty of fiber and liquids in your diet, add helpful herbal combinations when you need them, exercise regularly and establish a regular daily time for elimination.

ESSENTIAL CATEGORIES FOR COLON & BOWEL NORMALIZING COMPOUNDS:

COLON & BOWEL CLEANSING HERBS	ANTISPASMODIC, SOOTHING HERBS	BODY CHEMISTRY BALANCERS	MINERAL-RICH HERBS	ANTI-INFLAMMATORY HERBS	FIBER-RICH HERBS
Cascara bark	Slippery elm	Lemon balm	**Kelp/sea vegetables**	**St. John's wort**	**Flax seed**
Butternut bark	Peppermint	Peppermint	**Horsetail**	**Chamomile**	**Aloe vera**
Rhubarb root	**Marshmallow root**	**Burdock root**	**Yellow dock root**	Gotu kola	**Psyllium husks**
Psyllium husk	**Wild yam root**	Aloe vera	**Pau d' arco bark**	**White willow bark**	Marshmallow root
Senna leaf	**Lobelia**	Parsley lf. & rt.	Alfalfa	**Marshmallow root**	Slippery elm
Aloe vera	Irish moss	**Chlorella/Barley grass**	**Dandelion root**	**Yarrow**	Pau d' arco bark
Licorice root	Scullcap	Milk thistle seed	Spirulina	**Calendula**	**Kelp/sea vegetables**
Ginger root	Red raspberry	**Hawthorn lf. flr. & bry.**	**Nettles**	Plantain	**Guar gum**
Irish moss	**Chamomile**	Calendula	**Oatstraw**	**Aloe vera**	**Irish moss**

ESSENTIAL HERBS FOR COLON & BOWEL NORMALIZING COMPOUNDS:

PRIMARY HERBS		ASSISTING & COMPLEMENTARY HERBS		CATALYST & TRANSPORTING HERBS	
Sarsaparilla root	Chlorella	Alfalfa	Chamomile	Capsicum	Horsetail
Licorice root	Barley Grass	Marshmallow root	Turkey rhubarb	Lobelia	Rosemary
Goldenseal root	Irish moss	Flax seed	Oatstraw	Irish moss	Garlic
Dandelion rt. & lf.	Senna leaf	Yellow dock root	Red raspberry	Ginger root	Red raspberry
Buckthorn bark	Nettles	Slippery elm	Lemon balm	Fennel seed	Parsley rt. & lf.
Burdock root	Spirulina	Wild yam root	Peppermint	Guar gum	Plantain
Pau d'arco bark	Kelp & ocean plants	St. John's wort	Yarrow	Milk thistle seed	Comfrey root
Aloe vera	Butternut bark	Scullcap	Barberry	Gotu Kola	Calendula
Cascara	Psyllium husks	Lobelia	Pau d' arco bark	Ginkgo Biloba	White willow bark

EXAMPLE FORMULAS OF COLON & BOWEL NORMALIZING COMPOUNDS:

A FIBER & HERBS CLEANSING CAPSULE COMPOUND			(CD - 2350)
Butternut bark	Psyllium husks	Licorice root	Capsicum
Cascara	Barberry	Ginger root	Lobelia
Turkey rhubarb	Fennel seed	Irish moss	

A TONING, ANTI-INFLAMMATORY CAPSULE COMPOUND			(CD - 1560)
Peppermint	Slippery elm	Pau d' arco bark	Lobelia
Aloe vera	Marshmallow root	Wild Yam root	Ginger root

SEE PAGE 1 FOR FORMULATING INSTRUCTIONS.

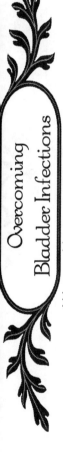

Overcoming
Bladder Infections

WASTE MANAGEMENT PROBLEMS

If you have frequent, urgent, burning, painful urination, especially at night, chronic lower back and abdomen pain below the navel, unexplained chills, fever, turbid, foul-smelling urine, cloudy or bloody urine and unusual fluid retention, you may be feeling the symptoms of a bladder infection. Recurrent bladder infections are common in women; less common in men (theirs are mostly as a result of prostate problems). Bladder infections are the most frequent reason a woman seeks medical attention. and the pain can be severe during the acute stage. Over 75% of American women have at least one urinary tract infection in a ten year period, almost 30% have one once a year. About 15% of menopausal women experience bladder infections, usually during early menopause when body chemistry is rapidly changing. Diabetics are prone to cystitis. A gentle, herbal bladder/kidney cleanse can help keep you from getting a serious bladder infection.

❧ ESSENTIAL CATEGORIES FOR BLADDER INFECTION HEALING COMPOUNDS:

CHLOROPHYLL-RICH HERBS	ANTI-SPASMODIC HERBS	ALKALIZING, BALANCING HERBS	ANTI-BIOTIC HERBS	GENTLE DIURETIC HERBS	ANTI-INFLAMMATORY HERBS
Chlorella	Slippery elm	Marshmallow root	**Echinacea root**	**Corn silk**	**Echinacea root**
Spirulina	Scullcap	Stone root	**Goldenseal root**	**Oatstraw**	St. John's wort
Aloe vera	**Marshmallow root**	**Kelp/sea vegetables**	Myrrh	**Uva ursi**	Yarrow
Nettles	Dandelion rt. & lf.	Plantain leaf	Garlic	**Juniper berry**	**Marshmallow root**
Parsley	Wild yam root	**Alfalfa**	**Pau d' arco bark**	**Dandelion leaf**	**White willow bark**
Alfalfa	**Lobelia**	Parsley lf. & rt.	**Burdock root**	**Fennel seed**	Chamomile
Barley grass	Irish moss	**Chlorella/barley grass**	Usnea barbata	**Cleavers**	Kelp/sea vegetables
Kelp/sea vegetables	**Thyme**	Goldenseal root	Licorice root	Parsley root & lf.	**Aloe vera**
Comfrey leaf	**Red raspberry**	Ginger root	Capsicum	Green tea	**Turmeric**

❧ ESSENTIAL HERBS FOR BLADDER INFECTION HEALING COMPOUNDS:

PRIMARY HERBS		ASSISTING & COMPLEMENTARY HERBS		CATALYST & TRANSPORTING HERBS	
Echinacea root	Slippery elm	Garlic	Turmeric	Capsicum	White willow bark
Goldenseal rt.	Dandelion rt. & lf.	Parsley rt. & lf.	Wild yam root	Gotu kola	Red raspberry
Marshmallow root	Licorice root	Chlorella	Juniper berry	Rosemary	Lobelia
Mullein	Kelp/sea vegetables	Cleavers	Myrrh	Bee pollen	Plantain
Corn silk	Nettles	Fenugreek seed	Bee polle	Ginger root	Irish moss
Pau d' arco barky	Chaparral	Barley grass	Burdock root	Peppermint	Cloves
Chamomile	Spirulina	Alfalfa	Usnea barbata	Oatstraw	Calendula
Comfrey root & lf.	Uva Ursi	Scullcap	Aloe vera	Green tea	Fennel
Juniper berry	Yarrow	Stone root	St. John's wort	Thyme	Hydrangea rt.

❧ EXAMPLE FORMULAS OF BLADDER INFECTION HEALING COMPOUNDS:

A HEALING DIURETIC CAPSULE COMPOUND			(CD - 1410)
Echinacea root	Ginger rt.	Dandelion rt.	
Goldenseal rt.	Stone root	Hydrangea rt.	
Parsley rt.	Lobelia		
Marshmallow rt.			

A CLEANSING, STRENGTHENING BLADDER TEA FORMULA			(CD - 5020)
Uva ursi	Parsley lf.	Dandelion lf.	Cleavers
Juniper berry	Cornsilk	Plantain	Marshmallow rt.

A HEALING DIURETIC CAPSULE COMPOUND		
Juniper berry		
Uva Ursi		
Mullein		

SEE PAGE 1 FOR FORMULATING INSTRUCTIONS.

**If infections develop regularly after intercourse, rinse the vagina and labia with goldenseal/echinacea tea.

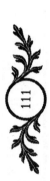

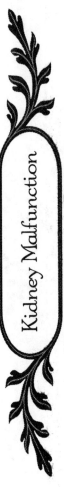

Kidney Malfunction

WASTE MANAGEMENT PROBLEMS

The kidneys are largely responsible for the elimination of waste products from protein breakdown. Concentrated protein wastes can cause chronic inflammation of the kidney filtering tissues, and can overload the bloodstream with toxins. Staph and strep infections also affect the kidneys - with an alarming number of cases resulting in kidney failure. If you have pain above the waist, it may be a kidney infection or kidney stones instead of a bladder infection. Kidney health is the reason most naturopaths recommend drinking 6 to 8 glasses of cleansing fluids every day, and limiting animal protein intake. A kidney cleanse is simple, and a good choice for herbal support. Eat plenty of fresh and cultured foods to alkalize the system. Avoid acid-forming foods, like caffeine, salty, sugary and fried foods, soft drinks, alcohol, and tomatoes. Also avoid mucous-forming foods, such as pasteurized dairy products, heavy grains, starches and fats to reduce sediment formation.

∼ ESSENTIAL CATEGORIES FOR KIDNEY MALFUNCTION COMPOUNDS:

CHLOROPHYLL SOURCE HERBS	MINERAL-RICH HERBS	KIDNEY TONE & DIURETIC ACTIVITY	ALKALIZING, BALANCING HERBS	BLOOD CLEANSING HERBS	ANTI-INFLAMMATORY HERBS
Chlorella	Kelp & sea vegetables	Uva ursi	Sarsaparilla root	Red clover	White willow bark
Spirulina	Horsetail	Hydrangea rt.	Parsley root & leaf	Goldenseal root	Marshmallow root
Nettles	Barley grass/chlorella	Parsley root & leaf	Marshmallow root	Burdock rt.	Coriander
Parsley	Marshmallow root	Plantain	Plantain	Licorice root	Alfalfa
Alfalfa	Yellow dock root	Corn silk	Aloe vera	Echinacea root	Aloe vera
Aloe vera	Dandelion root & lf.	Nettles	Chlorella & barley grass	Alfalfa	Yarrow
Barley grass	Nettles	Cranberry powder	Comfrey root & lf.	Capsicum	Turmeric
Kelp/sea vegetables	Oregon grape root	Kelp/sea vegetables	Miso powder	Dandelion root & leaf	Comfrey root
Comfrey leaf	Oatstraw	Juniper bry.	Fennel seed	Pau d' arco bark	St. John's wort

∼ ESSENTIAL HERBS FOR KIDNEY MALFUNCTION COMPOUNDS:

PRIMARY HERBS		ASSISTING & COMPLEMENTARY HERBS		CATALYST & TRANSPORTING HERBS	
Dandelion rt. & lf	Barley grass	St. John's wort	Pau d' arco	Capsicum	Black walnut hulls
Marshmallow root	Chlorella.	Alfalfa	Comfrey root & lf.	Oatstraw	Chamomile
Echinacea root	Licorice root	Plantain	Red clover	Miso	Wild yam root
Uva ursi	Cornsilk	Kava kava root	Turmeric	Peppermint	Yarrow
Kelp/sea vegetables	Nettles	Spirulina	Yellow dock root	Elecampane	Yarrow
Goldenseal root	Sarsaparilla root	Parsley rt. & lf.	Flax seed	Hydrangea rt.	Honey
Pau d' arco bark	Oregon grape root	Burdock root	Myrrh	Fennel seed	Irish moss
Aloe vera juice	Cranberry powder	Fenugreek seed	Horsetail	White willow bark	Calendula
Corn silk	Juniper bry.	Coriander	Ginger rt.	Fennel seed	Prickly ash bark

∼ EXAMPLE FORMULAS OF KIDNEY MALFUNCTION HEALING COMPOUNDS:

A KIDNEY CLEANSING EXTRACT COMPOUND			(CD - 4700)	A KIDNEY STRENGTHENING CAPSULE COMPOUND		(CO - 1420)
Cornsilk	Dandelion rt. & lf.	Goldenseal rt.	Parsley rt. & lf.	Cranberry powder	Coriander	Juniper bry.	Kava kava root
Juniper bry.	Marshmallow rt.	Ginger rt.	Honey	Echinacea root	Wild yam root	Uva ursi	Fenugreek sd.
Uva ursi					Dandelion rt. & lf.	Marshmallow rt.	

SEE PAGE 1 FOR FORMULATING INSTRUCTIONS.

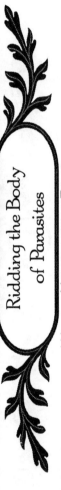

Ridding the Body of Parasites

WASTE MANAGEMENT PROBLEMS

Herbal combinations can help rid the body of some intestinal parasites, especially pinworms and threadworms. Worm and parasite infestations range from mild and hardly noticeable to serious and even life-threatening in a child. Other parasites move all over the body, including the brain, weakening the entire system. Common causes that allow parasite infestation are low immune strength, poor diet with too much sugar and refined carbohydrates (junk foods), too much red meat, poor hygiene, and fungal and yeast overgrowth conditions, infested, uncooked, poorly cooked, or spoiled meat. Herbal therapy, along with a short cleanse, a high resistance diet including onions and garlic, and restricted sugar intake, encourages parasites to release and pass from the body. Nutritional therapy is a good choice for thread and pin worms, but is very slow or ineffective in heavy infestations of hookworms, tape worms and blood flukes.

ESSENTIAL CATEGORIES FOR PARASITE ELIMINATION COMPOUNDS:

BOWEL & COLON CLEANSING HERBS	SOOTHING, ANTISPASMODIC HERBS	FRIENDLY FLORA SOURCES	IMMUNE STRENGTHENING HERBS	ANTI-INFLAMMATORY HERBS	VERMIFUGE, ANTI-FUNGAL HERBS
Cascara bark	**Valerian root**	**Aloe vera**	Bee pollen/Royal jelly	**Chamomile**	**Black walnut hulls**
Flax seed	**Slippery elm**	**Ginger root**	**Goldenseal root**	**Alfalfa**	**Wormwood**
Fennel seed	**Marshmallow root**	**Acidophilus powder**	**Astragalus**	Garlic	**Barberry bark**
Psyllium husk	Thyme	**Chlorella/barley grass**	**Pau d' arco bark**	**Turmeric**	**Tea tree oil**
Aloe vera	Irish moss/sea plants	Nettles	**Garlic**	**Calendula**	Garlic/Gentian root
Senna leaf	**Wild yam bk.**	Oregon grape rt.	Cardamom	Dandelion root & lf.	**Pumpkin seed**
Butternut bark	**Lobelia**	Parsley leaf	Myrrh	**White willow bk.**	**Aloe vera**
Rhubarb root	Hops	**Peppermint**	**Reishi mushroom**	**Yarrow**	Chaparral
Licorice root	Red raspberry	**Papaya**	Echinacea root	St. John's wort	**Mugwort**

ESSENTIAL HERBS FOR PARASITE ELIMINATION COMPOUNDS:

PRIMARY HERBS	ASSISTING & COMPLEMENTARY HERBS	CATALYST & TRANSPORTING HERBS
Black walnut hulls	Aloe vera	Valerian root	Wild yam root	Kelp/sea vegetables	Chamomile
Garlic	Dandelion root & lf.	Bee pollen/Royal jelly	Butternut Bark	False unicorn rt.	Irish moss
Slippery elm	Licorice root	Thyme	Mugwort	Ginger root	Turmeric
Marshmallow root	Chlorella/barley grass	Flax seed	Cascara bark	Chaparral	Hops
Barberry bark	Reishi mushroom	European mistletoe	Rhubarb root	Peppermint	Acidophilus powder
Psyllium husk	Astragalus	Lobelia	Fennel seed	White willow bk.	Myrrh
Pumpkin seed	Parsley rt. & lf.	Cardamom	Pau d' arco bark	Nettles	Papaya
Yarrow	Oregon grape rt.	Senna lf.	St. John's wort	Alfalfa	Reishi mushroom
Tea tree oil	Wormwood	Gentian root	Goldenseal root	Calendula	Echinacea root

EXAMPLE FORMULAS OF PARASITE ELIMINATION COMPOUNDS:

A VERMIFUGE CAPSULE FORMULA	(CD - 4200)	A BITTERS & LEMON EXTRACT FORMULA	(CD - 4710)
Black walnut	Cascara bark	Gentian	False unicorn rt.	Oregon grape rt.	Senna lf.	Cardamom	Peppermint
Garlic	Mugwort	Butternut Bark	Wormwood	Gentian root	Dandelion rt.	Lemon peel	Honey
Pumpkin seed	Slippery elm	Fennel seed					

SEE PAGE 1 FOR FORMULATING INSTRUCTIONS.

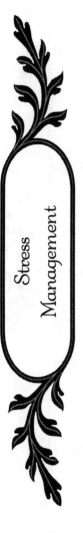

Stress Management

veryone is affected by varying degrees of stress. Stress is our physical and emotional response to the demands of life. The key to our health is how we respond to stress. Most Americans today are running harder and harder to stay in the same place. Financial obligations, job pressures, seeking work in an increasingly down-sized job market, family demands, health concerns, emotional problems, and lack of rest and leisure can overwhelm even the most stable, well-adjusted nature. Many people seem to be under stress most of the time. While facing challenges and difficulties helps us to grow and learn, (if we didn't have problems we would be bored silly). prolonged, chronic stress depletes energy reserves, and creates an imbalanced system that never allows for relaxation. We try to get as much done as we can in as short a time as possible. Sometimes we try to do as many things as possible at the same time!

Stress is a universal enemy affecting modern life. Everyone is affected by varying degrees of stress. It is experienced by people who work in polluted atmospheres, by people who are immobilized at control desks with machines demanding continual attention, by people who travel coast to coast constantly, by people with repetitive, boring jobs. At best, stress causes useless fatigue; at worst, it is dangerous to health. It is a major cause of headaches, hypoglycemia, arthritis, and some cancers. Indeed, most degenerative diseases are stress related. Stress irritates the body in the form of gastritis, ulcers and colitis. It irritates the mind in the form of moodiness, burn-out, overuse of drugs, depression and anxiety.

Stress is usually at the heart of heart disease. In fact, heart disease is a case where the failure to manage stress in your life can kill you. Stress directly depletes the adrenal glands. In prolonged stress, the adrenals cannot raise blood sugar when necessary and hypoglycemia results. Stress affects the reproductive organs, libido and sexual ability. It leads to irritable bladder, acne, eczema, psoriasis, nervous tics, muscle spasms, high cholesterol, and even to baldness. Profound emotional stress, such as that caused by job loss or the loss of a loved one can lead to serious depression. The inability to express our emotions, such as loneliness, or grief can be very damaging to health because immune response is reduced. Yet the human body is designed to handle stressful situations, if not indeed to thrive and be challenged by some of them. The goal should not be to avoid all stress, but to maintain a high degree of health to handle and survive stress well.

There are four levels of stress symptoms: 1) losing interest in enjoyable activities, eye-corner sagging, forehead creasing, becoming short-tempered, bored, nervous; 2) tiredness, anger, insomnia, paranoia, sadness; 3) chronic head and neck aches, high blood pressure, upset stomach, looking older; 4) skin disorders, kidney malfunction, susceptibility to frequent infections, asthma, heart disease, mental and nervous breakdown. Symptoms of fight or flight reactions are elevated heart rate, breathing changes, muscle tension, mental focus and fear or anger.

Herbs are wonderful therapeutics for overcoming stress naturally. They are rich in minerals, trace minerals, and enzymes. They provide inner strength with bio-active, stabilizing amino acids and electrolytes that help restore body and mind energy. They correct nutrient deficiencies with vitamin B complex, vitamin C and bioflavonoids that fortify you for inner calm when the going gets tough. Sometimes you can expect miracles. Effective herbal combinations help reduce stress and tension by repairing damaged nerve sheathing. Herbal nervines that calm and soothe the brain without the addictive side effects of valium compounds. Herbs support healthy nerve structure, and stabilize body balance during high stress times. Herbs help control acid-produced stress and emotional anxiety.

FORMULAS FOR MANAGING STRESS ALSO HELP IN THE FOLLOWING CONDITIONS:
●Mood & Personality Swings ●Anxiety & Depression ●Low Energy & Fatigue ●Hyperactivity ●Obsessive/Compulsive Disorders ●Schizophrenia ●Drug & Alcohol Addiction & Withdrawal ●Adrenal Exhaustion ●Epileptic Incidences ●Nerves & Nervous Tension ●Body Chemistry Imbalance

COMPOUNDS FOR FORMULATION INCLUDE:
●Dealing with stress and anxiety naturally
●Restoring a healthy nervous system
●Overcoming severe depression
●Herbal therapy for schizophrenia and psychosis

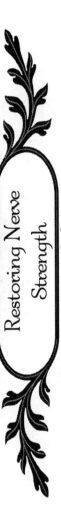

Restoring Nerve Strength

STRESS, ANXIETY & DEPRESSION

Along with the brain, the nervous system is the first to be affected by stress, tension and emotion. Poor nerve health can spawn a host of physical disorders, like Alzheimer's and Parkinson's disease, and inflammatory reactions like meningitis, or loss of muscular control, and coordination. The nervous system also affects mental balance - weak nerves result in neuroses, tension and anxiety. Over 25 million Americans will suffer from an anxiety disorder at some time during their lives. Anxiety is more than just tension before a stressful confrontation, a public speech or an airline flight. Anxiety and phobias (fear taken to extremes), are often due to long term, debilitating dread. Continued economic insecurity can generate this kind of fear, for instance. Anxiety and nerve stress are closely tied to high blood pressure, ulcer or colitis attacks, irritability, high blood pressure, TMJ, head and neck aches, loss of appetite, dizziness, heart spasms, even fatal heart disease.

❧ ESSENTIAL CATEGORIES FOR RESTORING NERVE STRENGTH COMPOUNDS:

ANXIETY-RELIEF NERVINES	STRESS-REDUCING ADAPTOGENS	MINERAL-RICH HERBS	LIVER SUPPORT HERBS	ADRENAL GLAND SUPPORT HERBS	NERVE SUPPORT TONIC HERBS
Rosemary	**Bee pollen/Royal Jelly**	**Barley grass/Spirulina**	**Dandelion root & lf.**	**Kelp/sea vegetables**	**Gotu kola**
Black haw bk.	**Panax ginseng**	**Alfalfa**	**Milk thistle seed**	**Sarsaparilla rt.**	Hawthorn lf. flr. & bry.
Gotu kola	**Kelp/sea vegetables**	**Dandelion rt. & lf.**	**Licorice root**	**Astragalus**	European mistletoe
St. John's wort.	**Alfalfa**	**Nettles**	**Wild yam root**	**Red raspberry**	Blessed thistle
Scullcap	White willow	**Kelp/sea vegetables**	Watercress	Lobelia	**Ashwagandha rt.**
Passionflower	Ginkgo biloba	**Parsley rt & lf.**	**Green tea**	**Licorice root**	**Chamomile**
Hops flwr.	**Spirulina/Barley grass**	**Yellow dock rt.**	**Oregon grape rt.**	Capsicum	Heartsease
Valerian rt.	Siberian ginseng	Pau d'arco bark	Bee pollen/royal jelly	Ginger root	Catnip
Kava kava rt.	**Black cohosh rt.**	**Oats/Oatstraw**	**Nutritional yeast pwr.**	Peppermint	**Wood betony**

❧ ESSENTIAL HERBS FOR RESTORING NERVE STRENGTH COMPOUNDS:

PRIMARY HERBS		ASSISTING & COMPLEMENTARY HERBS		CATALYST & TRANSPORTING HERBS	
Ashwagandha rt.	Pau d'arco bark	Dandelion rt. & lf.	Astragalus	Capsicum	Red raspberry
Black cohosh rt.	Sarsaparilla root	Chamomile	Yellow dock rt.	Oregon grape rt.	Nutritional yeast pdr.
Valerian rt.	Gotu kola	Milk thistle seed	Heartsease	Lobelia	Parsley rt & lf.
Siberian ginseng	Kelp/sea vegetables	Catnip	European mistletoe	Ginkgo biloba	Comfrey leaf
Licorice root	Hawthorn lf. flr. & bry.	Peppermint	Passionflower	Rosemary	Uva ursi
Barley grass	Panax ginseng	Black haw bk.	Nettles	Feverfew	Wood betony
St. John's wort	Kava Kava rt.	Wild yam rt.	Hops flwr.	Ginger root	Juniper bry.
Scullcap	Spirulina	Burdock root	White willow	Watercress	Evening primrose oil
Bee pollen/Royal jelly	Oats/Oatstraw	Alfalfa	Blessed thistle	Green tea	Anise seed

❧ EXAMPLE FORMULAS OF NERVE RESTORATION COMPOUNDS:

A RELAXING, NERVE REBUILDING CAPSULE COMPOUND		(RX - 3800)	A TEA COMPOUND FOR A STRESSED OUT FEELING		(RX - 6080)
Ashwagandha rt.	Valerian rt.	Lobelia	Rosemary	Peppermint	White willow
Black cohosh rt.	European mistletoe	Oatstraw	Chamomile	Heartsease	Feverfew
Scullcap	Wood betony		Catnip	Wood betony	Blessed thistle
					Gotu kola

SEE PAGE 1 FOR FORMULATING INSTRUCTIONS.

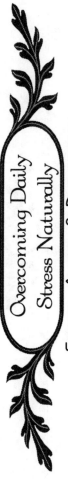

Overcoming Daily Stress Naturally

STRESS, ANXIETY & DEPRESSION

Herbs are wonderful medicinals for overcoming everyday stress and tension naturally. They are rich in replacement minerals, trace minerals, and plant enzymes. They provide inner strength with bio-active, stabilizing amino acids and electrolytes that help restore body and mind energy. They correct nutrient deficiencies with vitamin B complex, vitamin C and bioflavonoids that fortify you for inner calm when the going gets tough. Sometimes you can even expect miracles. Nervines like gotu kola, scullcap and Siberian ginseng reduce stress and tension by helping to repair damaged nerves. Herbs like passionflower and chamomile quiet and soothe without the addictive side effects of valium compounds. Herbs like hawthorn, ginkgo and St. John's wort support healthy nerve structure by balancing body chemistry, and provide a soothing influence on the brain. Herbal stress formulas work rapidly in many cases. Try a delicious, relaxing herbal "stress" tea the next time daily stress is getting you down.

❧ ESSENTIAL CATEGORIES FOR STRESS, TENSION & ANXIETY COMPOUNDS:

TONIC ADAPTOGEN HERBS	CALMING, NERVINE HERBS	BLOOD & CIRCULATION TONIC HERBS	BODY CHEMISTRY ALKALIZING HERBS	MENTAL, INNER ENERGY HERBS	B-VITAMIN SOURCE HERBS
Ginkgo biloba	**St. John's wort**	**Capsicum**	**Barley grass/Alfalfa**	**Ashwagandha rt.**	**Royal Jelly/Bee pollen**
Red clover	Catnip	Ginger root	**Lemongrass**	**Ginkgo biloba**	Dandelion rt. & lf.
Spirulina	**Kava kava rt.**	**Gotu kola**	**Aloe vera**	Fo-Ti root	**Black cohosh rt.**
Fo-Ti root	**Lemon balm**	Anise seed	Oats/Oatstraw	**Kava kava rt.**	**Red raspberry**
Siberian ginseng rt.	**Chamomile**	Hawthorn bry., lf., fl.	**White sage**	**Panax ginseng**	**Kelp/sea vegetables**
Panax ginseng	**Gotu kola**	Cinnamon	Spearmint	**Siberian ginseng**	Parsley root & lf.
Wild yam rt.	Horsetail	Sarsaparilla rt.	Pau d' arco bk.	**Licorice root**	**Fenugreek seed**
Licorice root	Passionflower	**Siberian ginseng rt.**	Spearmint	Suma root	Watercress
Hawthorn bry., lf., fl.	Scullcap	**Ginkgo biloba**	**Dandelion rt.**	Hawthorn bry., lf., fl.	**Burdock root**

❧ ESSENTIAL HERBS FOR STRESS, TENSION & ANXIETY COMPOUNDS:

PRIMARY HERBS		ASSISTING & COMPLEMENTARY HERBS		CATALYST & TRANSPORTING HERBS	
Gotu kola	St. John's wort	Parsley root & lf.	Evening primrose oil	Cinnamon	Stevia
Dandelion rt. & lf.	Fo-Ti root	Kava kava rt.	Alfalfa	Dulse	Rosemary
Ginseng - all types	Ginkgo biloba	Oats/Oatstraw	Passionflower	Orange peel	Watercress
Sarsaparilla root	Scullcap	Pau d' arco bark	Fenugreek seed	Capsicum	Anise seed
Bee pollen	Royal Jelly	Spirulina	Burdock rt.	Peppermint	Lobelia
Licorice root	Suma root	Lemongrass	Spearmint	Yerba santa	Fennel seed
Kelp & sea vegetables	Hawthorn bry., lf., fl.	Barley grass	Ashwagandha rt.	Ginger root	Flax seed
Red clover	Siberian ginseng	Red raspberry	White sage	Horsetail	Nettles
Lemon balm	Panax ginseng	Black cohosh rt.	Chamomile	Catnip	Rosebuds

❧ EXAMPLE FORMULAS OF STRESS, TENSION & ANXIETY COMPOUNDS:

AN ANTI-STRESS, RELAXING TEA COMPOUND		(RX - 5990)		A FEEL GREAT, TONIC TEA COMPOUND		(E - 5330)
Spearmint	Yerba santa	Passionflower		Red clover	Hawthorn bry., lf., fl.	Licorice rt.
Licorice root	Cinnamon	Rosebuds		Alfalfa	Spearmint	Stevia lf.
Orange peel	Rosemary	Anise seed		Siberian ginseng rt.	Dandelion rt.	Dulse
Lemon balm				Gotu kola		
Lemongrass						

SEE PAGE 1 FOR FORMULATING INSTRUCTIONS.

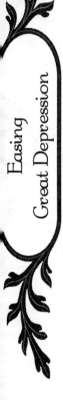

Easing
Great Depression

STRESS, ANXIETY & DEPRESSION

Depression is the most common adult psychiatric disorder, and it's on the rise worldwide. Mood disorders currently affect almost 16 million people, and up to 25% of us will experience an episode of great depression during our lives. Depression is both a mental and emotional state that stems from a wide range of causes, and affects women more than men. Depression is utterly individual and utterly personal, but certain common denominators include great loss, as of a spouse or child, and the inability to mourn or express grief; bottled-up anger and aggression turned inward; negative emotional behavior that controls a person's relationships; biochemical imbalances caused by nutrient deficiencies; or drug-induced depression. Many prescription drugs create nutrient deficiencies. New research, together with long standing empirical evidence may prove herbs to be viable alternatives for alleviating depression.

☙ ESSENTIAL CATEGORIES FOR SEVERE DEPRESSION COMPOUNDS:

NERVINE TONICS & BRAIN NOURISHERS	MUSCLE RELAXERS & ANTI-SPASMODIC HERBS	DIGESTIVE, ALKALIZING HERBS	ANTI-OXIDANT HERBS & FOODS	LIVER SUPPORT HERBS	GLAND & HORMONE BALANCERS
St. John's wort	Valerian root	Aloe vera	Rosemary	Pau d' arco bk.	Licorice root
Scullcap	Scullcap	Fennel seed	Kelp/sea vegetables	Dandelion root	Siberian ginseng root
Ginkgo biloba	Kava kava rt.	Ginger root	Ginseng - all types	Hawthorn bry., lf., fl.	Saw palmetto
Kelp/sea vegetables	Black haw	Pau d' arco bk.	Fo-ti root	Yellow dock rt.	Burdock root
Bee Pollen/Royal Jelly	Lobelia	Peppermint	White pine bk.	Watercress	Bee pollen/royal jelly
Gotu kola	Red raspberry	Slippery elm	Bee pollen/royal jelly	Parsley rt. & lf.	Ashwagandha
Panax ginseng rt.	Oatstraw	Red raspberry	Chlorella/Alfalfa	Red sage	Evening primrose oil
Black cohosh	Wild lettuce	Marshmallow rt.	Ginger root	Ginger root	Black cohosh
Wood betony	Chamomile	Catnip	Nutritional yeast	Milk thistle seed	Sarsaparilla rt.

☙ ESSENTIAL HERBS FOR SEVERE DEPRESSION COMPOUNDS:

PRIMARY HERBS		ASSISTING & COMPLEMENTARY HERBS		CATALYST & TRANSPORTING HERBS	
Ginkgo biloba	Pau d' arco bk.	Ashwagandha rt.	Red sage	Valerian root	Wild lettuce
Bee pollen/Royal Jelly	Fo-Ti root	Black cohosh	Alfalfa	Vitamin C pwr.	Rosemary
Ginseng - all types	Kava kava root	Dandelion root	Yellow dock rt.	Parsley rt. & lf.	Watercress
Sarsaparilla root	Gotu kola	Saw palmetto bry.	Chamomile	Capsicum	Nutritional yeast
Scullcap	Catnip	Burdock root	Wild cherry	Peppermint	Carrot pwdr.
Licorice root	Hawthorn bry., lf., fl.	Black haw	Goldenseal rt.	Aloe vera	Fennel seed
Kelp & sea vegetables	Spirulina	Chlorella/barley grass	Milk thistle seed	Ginger root	Marshmallow rt.
White pine bk.	Siberian ginseng	Oatstraw	Red raspberry	Slippery elm	Lobelia
St. John's wort	Panax ginseng	Evening primrose oil	Wood betony	Mullein	Miso powder

☙ EXAMPLE FORMULAS OF COMPOUNDS TO HELP SEVERE DEPRESSION:

A DEPRESSION-RELIEVING CAPSULE COMPOUND		(CO - 1985)	A BODY REBUILDING CAPSULE COMPOUND		(SA - 1450)
St. John's wort	Ashwagandha rt.	Fo-ti root	Spirulina	Hawthorn bry., lf., fl.	Wild cherry
Kava kava rt.	Gotu kola	Ginger root.	Bee pollen	Royal jelly	Chlorella
Panax ginseng rt.	Scullcap		Alfalfa	Barley grass	Goldenseal rt.
	Siberian ginseng		Vitamin C pwdr.	Carrot pwdr.	Kelp
	Rosemary			Siberian ginseng	Mullein
	Wood betony			Sarsaparilla root	
				Red raspberry	
				Kelp	

SEE PAGE 1 FOR FORMULATING INSTRUCTIONS.

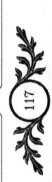

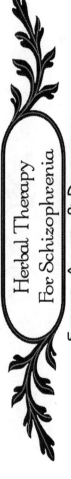

Herbal Therapy
For Schizophrenia

STRESS, ANXIETY & DEPRESSION

Schizophrenia is a form of psychosis with severe perception disorder characterized by hallucinations, delusions, extreme paranoia, and disturbed thought content. Personal relationships are abnormal, work is almost impossible, and the schizophrenic often withdraws emotionally and socially. Most researchers think that schizophrenia is linked to heavy metal and chemical toxicity and accompanied by nutritional deficiencies. Anti-psychotic (neuro-leptic) drugs may do more harm than good. Tardive dyskinesia is a side effect disorder, with slow, rhythmical, involuntary movements, caused exclusively by neuroleptic drugs used to treat schizophrenia and psychosis. It is bizarre in that the symptoms themselves are similar to a psychosis. Over 70% of the patients taking antipsychotic drugs develop this grim disorder which almost totally isolates them socially. Natural therapies have been successful in reversing TD.

❧ ESSENTIAL CATEGORIES FOR SCHIZOPHRENIA & PSYCHOSIS COMPOUNDS:

BODY CHEMISTRY BALANCING NERVINES	BRAIN NUTRIENTS & TONICS	EFA SOURCE HERBS	ANTI-OXIDANT, CIRCULATION HERBS	B VITAMIN SOURCE HERBS	IODINE, POTASSIUM & C SOURCES
Scullcap	**Kelp/sea vegetables**	**Evening primrose oil**	**Rosemary**	**Brewer's yeast**	**Aloe vera**
Black cohosh rt.	**Ginkgo biloba**	**Brewer's yeast**	**Kelp/sea vegetables**	**Royal jelly/Bee pollen**	**Kelp/sea vegetables**
St. John's wort	**Panax ginseng**	**Kelp & sea vegetables**	**Ginseng - all types**	**Parsley rt. & lf.**	Chlorella
Wood betony	**Siberian ginseng**	Chlorella	**Capsicum**	**Dong qual rt.**	Rosehips
European mistletoe	**Fo-Ti root**	Spirulina	**White pine bk.**	**Fenugreek seed**	**Bee pollen/royal jelly**
Kava kava root	**Gotu kola**	Black currant seed	**Bee pollen/royal jelly**	**Burdock rt.**	**Hawthorn bry., lf., fl.**
Ashwagandha rt	**Evening primrose oil**	Pumpkin seed	Prickly ash	**Kelp/sea vegetables**	Red clover
Black haw bark	**Schizandra berry**	Flax seed	Ginger root	**Dandelion root**	**Royal jelly**
Sarsaparilla root	**Rosemary**	Borage seed	Peppermint	**Alfalfa**	Capsicum

❧ ESSENTIAL HERBS FOR SCHIZOPHRENIA & PSYCHOSIS COMPOUNDS:

PRIMARY HERBS		ASSISTING & COMPLEMENTARY HERBS		CATALYST & TRANSPORTING HERBS	
Ginkgo biloba	Burdock rt.	Ashwagandha rt.	Valerian rt	Pumpkin seed	St. John's wort
Bee pollen	Fo-Ti root	European mistletoe	Alfalfa	Vitamin C pwdr.	Rosemary
Sarsaparilla root	Kava kava root	Dandelion root	Rosehips	Prickly ash	Borage seed
Spirulina	Gotu kola	Dong qual rt	Prince ginseng rt.	Capsicum	Oatstraw
Licorice root	White pine bk.	Aloe vera	Hops	Peppermint	Flax seed
Kelp & sea vegetables	Hawthorn bry., lf., fl.	White pine bk.	Black haw	Nutritional yeast	Black currant seed
Black cohosh rt.	Suma root	Barley grass	Horsetail	Ginger root	Flax seed
Chlorella	Siberian ginseng	Evening primrose oil	Fenugreek seed	Wood betony	Lobelia
Schizandra berry	Panax ginseng	Wild yam root	Scullcap	Lobelia	Kola nut

❧ EXAMPLE FORMULAS OF SCHIZOPHRENIA & PSYCHOSIS COMPOUNDS:

A MENTAL INNER ENERGY EXTRACT COMPOUND		(E - 4440)	A BODY RELAXING CAPSULE COMPOUND		(Rx - 3800)
Siberian ginseng	Fo-Ti root	Kola nut	Ashwagandha rt.	Valerian rt.	Lobelia
Prince ginseng rt.	Suma rt.	Gotu kola lf.	Black cohosh rt.	European mistletoe	Oatstraw
Dong qual rt.			Scullcap	Wood betony	

A MENTAL INNER ENERGY EXTRACT COMPOUND		
Kava kava root		
Kirin ginseng root		
Panax ginseng root		

SEE PAGE 1 FOR FORMULATING INSTRUCTIONS.

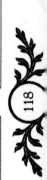

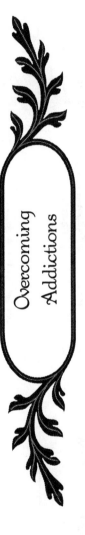

Overcoming Addictions

ddictions go hand in hand with chronic stress. Today, addictive abuse in one form or another has become a fact of modern life. American's high stress lifestyles deplete energy reserves, motivating us to want quick, "high voltage fixes" to overcome fatigue and relieve tension or boredom. Using drugs, sugar, alcohol, nicotine or caffeine as body fuel creates multiple nutritional deficiencies, and sets off chain reactions which result in more stress and noticeable cravings. The process repeats in a futile effort to satisfy increasing need, and addiction eventually occurs. For most people, this is just the beginning. Addictions reduce immune response, so conditions like hypothyroidism, fatigue syndromes, and auto-immune diseases can take hold. Even if serious disorders are avoided, the overwhelming majority of habitual addictive substance users suffer from nutrient and metabolic imbalances.

Nutritional support is essential to recovery from addictions. When the body is balanced, the need to get high by artificial means is sharply diminished. Herbs can establish a solid foundation for rebuilding a depleted system. Give yourself plenty of time for regeneration. It often takes up to a year to detoxify and clear drugs from the bloodstream.

Herbs can help overcome many kinds of addictions. A four stage program brings the most positive results:

1) **CLEANSE** addictive substance residues from your body as quickly as you can. Get a cleansing massage from a good massage therapist to help normalize your system. Take a hot sauna two or three times a week, or an herbal "sweating" bath with herbs like elder flowers, angelica root, thyme, jaborandi, pennyroyal and orange blossoms. Dry-brush your skin before the bath or sauna to remove residue toxins that come out on the skin. A liver flush herbal tea and lymph-clearing echinacea extract is indicated for all programs to overcome addictions.

2) **STRENGTHEN** your nervous system and adrenals with herbal formulas that increase energy without adding stimulants. Broad spectrum herbal nervines help control many of the problems faced during withdrawal from drugs or alcohol. Herbs can be a positive factor in "getting over the hump" of an addiction, reducing craving, relaxing nervous tension, boosting low energy, and, like gotu kola, helping to rebuild damaged nerve structure. Herbs like scullcap, kava kava, passionflower and valerian encourage restful sleep and soothe withdrawal headaches; herbs like Siberian ginseng and ginkgo biloba increase attention span and focus.

3) **BALANCE** your system with adaptogen herbs that normalize gland and hormone activity and restore body homeostasis. Look to herbs like panax, eleuthero, suma, gotu kola, ashwagandha, aralia and fo-ti from the ginseng family. Chinese herbs like astragalus, reishi and maitake mushrooms, and herbs like pau d' arco and St John's wort.

4) **ENERGIZE** your system so you won't fall back into old patterns and cravings. Most people recovering from addictions find their energy levels are very low as the body tries to carry on without its usual "high voltage fix". Herbs can help you through the energy crunch. They encourage better use of the body's own energy supply. Herbs like gotu kola, panax ginseng, kava kava, St. John's wort, damiana, red clover and peppermint make an excellent "weaning" tea for withdrawal fatigue. Don't forget regular exercise and deep breathing during this period, to help keep your mind clear, your head on straight, and your body cleansed of toxins.

❧ FORMULAS FOR OVERCOMING ADDICTIONS HELP IN THE FOLLOWING CONDITIONS:

•Drug Addiction & Withdrawal •Alcohol Addiction & Withdrawal •Caffeine & Nicotine Addiction & Withdrawal •Sugar Craving & Dependence •Hyperactive/Depressive Behavior •Unexplained Fatigue •Nervous Tension •Liver Malfunction •Mental Exhaustion •Compulsive/Obsessive Syndromes

❧ COMPOUNDS FOR FORMULATION TO HELP OVERCOME ADDICTIONS SHOULD INCLUDE:

•Formulas to address both prescription and recreational drug addictions
•Formulas to overcome alcohol abuse
•Formulas to help caffeine and nicotine addictions

119

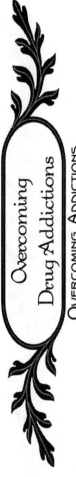

Overcoming Drug Addictions

OVERCOMING ADDICTIONS

So many people are taking drugs to alleviate boredom and fatigue, to relieve pain or to handle stress, that some believe that habitual use of both prescription and recreational drugs is the nation's number one health problem. Street drugs, like methamphetamines and crack cocaine are more powerful than ever, and more deadly to the user. Homicides and suicides are drug-related more than ever before. Accidental overdoses and poisonings due to the potency and toxicity of these substances are widespread. Yet, the most serious addictions are those to pharmaceutical drugs, especially those that alter mood like tranquilizers and antidepressants. All drugs deplete the body of nutrients and weaken immune response. Drug abusers are always either sick or coming down with something. As soon as one cold or bout of "flu," or bladder infection is treated, a new one takes its place. Work is impaired, job time is lost, and family and social life is greatly affected. It takes a year or more to detoxify the blood of drugs.

❧ ESSENTIAL CATEGORIES FOR OVERCOMING DRUG ADDICTIONS:

LIVER & BLOOD PURIFYING HERBS	DETOXIFICATION & CLEANSING HERBS	BLOOD SUGAR BALANCING HERBS	HERBS TO STRENGTHEN THE NERVES	HERBS FOR CRAVING & WITHDRAWAL	NORMALIZING & RESTORING HERBS
Nettles	Bee pollen/Royal Jelly	Gotu kola	Ginkgo biloba	Bee pollen	Chlorella/barley grass
Chlorella	Reishi mushroom	Sarsaparilla root	Scullcap	Kava Kava	Astragalus
Burdock root	Kelp/sea vegetables	Spirulina	St. John's wort	Scullcap	Suma root
Dandelion root	Alfalfa	Burdock root	Passionflower	Ginkgo biloba	Siberian ginseng root
Milk thistle seed	Panax ginseng	Aloe vera	Chamomile	St. John's wort	Pau d' arco bk.
Goldenseal root	Miso powder	Gymnema sylvestre	Rosemary	Kelp/sea vegetables	Fo-ti root
Chickweed	Burdock root	Wild yam root	Ashwagandha root	Wood betony	Garlic
Garlic	Ginger root	Yarrow	Panax ginseng root	Alfalfa	Schizandra
Yellow dock root	Echinacea root	Brewer's yeast	Gotu kola	Passionflower	Spirulina

❧ ESSENTIAL HERBS FOR OVERCOMING DRUG ADDICTIONS:

PRIMARY HERBS		ASSISTING & COMPLEMENTARY HERBS		CATALYST & TRANSPORTING HERBS	
Bee pollen/Royal Jelly	Pau d'arco bark	Reishi mushroom	Ashwagandha	Capsicum	Ginger root
Scullcap	Sarsaparilla root	Chamomile	Milk thistle seed	Lobelia	Acidophilus pwr.
Ginkgo biloba	Chlorella	Goldenseal root	Chamomile	Vitamin C powder	Dandelion root
Siberian ginseng	Kelp/sea vegetables	Wild yam root	Passionflower	Green tea leaf	Yellow dock root
Licorice root	Hawthorn lf. flr. & bry.	Astragalus	Oats/Oatstraw	Rosemary	Kola nut
Kava kava	Panax ginseng	Barley grass	Schizandra	Brewer's yeast	Echinacea root
Fo-Ti root	Gotu kola	Garlic	Nettles	Aloe vera	Yellow dock root
Suma rt	Spirulina	Burdock root	Wood betony	Chickweed	Yarrow
Valerian root	St. John's wort	Alfalfa	Prince ginseng	Miso broth powder	Wild lettuce

❧ EXAMPLE FORMULAS OF COMPOUNDS FOR OVERCOMING DRUG ADDICTIONS:

A GINSENG ENERGIZING CAPSULE COMPOUND (E - 2510)			A WITHDRAWAL SUPPORT CAPSULE COMPOUND (CO - 4330)		
Bee pollen	Fo-ti root	Prince ginseng	Alfalfa	Scullcap	St. John's wort	Licorice root
Siberian ginseng	Chinese ginseng	Suma root	Dong quai root	Siberian ginseng	Vitamin C powder	Capsicum
Gotu kola	Ashwagandha		Peppermint	Kava kava	Valerian root	Wood betony
				Gotu kola	Alfalfa	Ginkgo biloba

SEE PAGE 1 FOR FORMULATING INSTRUCTIONS.

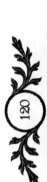

120

Overcoming Addictions

Alcohol abuse, the consumption of alcohol so that it interferes with performance of daily responsibility, destroys families and lives. Although usually treated as a character disorder, physiological factors, socio-psychological, and inherited factors all play a role. Seventy-six percent of alcoholics have a genetic disorder in metabolizing alcohol; up to thirty percent of all hospital admissions are alcohol related. Male alcoholics ultimately become impotent as the liver becomes so damaged through drinking that it is no longer able to control the estrogen levels in the blood. Alcoholics are often hypoglycemicsand usually mineral depleted. Symptoms include blackouts, dizziness, slurred speech, poor coordination, nervousness, irritability, tremors, heart disease, liver disease, increased cholesterol, and high blood pressure. The first step in treating alcoholism with herbal therapy is to cleanse and repair the damage done to the liver by excessive alcohol intake.

ESSENTIAL CATEGORIES FOR OVERCOMING ALCOHOL ABUSE COMPOUNDS:

Liver Repair & Support Herbs	Nervine, Relaxing Herbs	Herbal Energizers	Circulation/Elimination Stimulating Herbs	Herbs For Craving & Withdrawal	Adrenal Support Herbs
Nettles	Kava kava root	Suma root	Ginkgo biloba	Bee pollen	Gotu kola
Chlorella/Barley grass	Scullcap	Chlorophyll-rich herbs	Hawthorn lf., bry. & flr.	Kava kava root	Ashwagandha root
Bilberry	Black cohosh	Gotu kola	Oregon grape root	Scullcap	Licorice root
Dandelion root	Passionflower	Panax ginseng root	Prickly ash	Alfalfa	Kelp/sea vegetables
Milk thistle seed	Lobelia	Dong quai root	Spirulina	St. John's wort	Siberian ginseng root
Goldenseal root	Valerian root	Fo-ti root	Ginger root	Wood betony	Sarsaparilla root
Oregon grape root	Gotu kola	Prince ginseng rt.	Capsicum	Kudzu root	Schizandra bry.
Garlic	Panax ginseng root	Ashwagandha	Barberry bark	European mistletoe	Astragalus bark
Yellow dock root	European mistletoe	Damiana	Aloe vera	Passionflower	Wild yam root

ESSENTIAL HERBS FOR OVERCOMING ALCOHOL ABUSE COMPOUNDS:

Primary Herbs		Assisting & Complementary Herbs		Catalyst & Transporting Herbs	
Kava kava rt.	St. John's wort	Black cohosh	Astragalus bark	Aloe vera	Wood betony
Dandelion rt.	Kava kava root	Fo-ti root	Alfalfa	Barberry bark	Rosemary
Ginseng - all types	Ginkgo biloba	Hawthorn lf., bry. & flr.	Goldenseal root	Chamomile	Schizandra bry.
Ashwagandha	Suma root	Pau d' arco bark	Wild yam root	Capsicum	Reishi mushroom
Scullcap	Royal jelly/Bee pollen	Spirulina	Bilberry	Kudzu root	Irish mos
Licorice root	Gotu kola	Milk thistle seed	Passionflower	Oregon grape root	Valerian root
Kelp/sea vegetables	Siberian ginseng	Barley grass	European mistletoe	Ginger root	Garlic
Sarsaparilla root	Panax ginseng	Lobelia	Dong quai root	Damiana	Prickly ash
Chlorella	Nettles	Yellow dock root	Prince ginseng rt.	White willow bark	Angelica root

EXAMPLE FORMULAS OF OVERCOMING ALCOHOL ABUSE COMPOUNDS:

A MENTAL INNER ENERGY CAPSULE COMPOUND		(E - 2127)
Kava kava rt.	Fo-ti root	Ginkgo biloba
Chinese ginseng	Gotu kola	Ashwagandha
Panax ginseng	Prince ginseng rt.	
Siberian ginseng		
Dong quai root		
Suma root		

AN ADRENAL SUPPORT EXTRACT COMPOUND		(E - 4638)
Licorice root	Sarsaparilla root	Bladderwrack	Irish moss

See page 1 for formulating instructions.

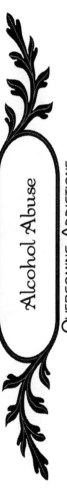

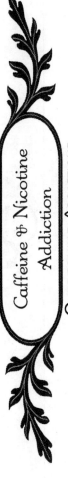

Caffeine & Nicotine Addiction

Overcoming Addictions

Caffeine and nicotine, although downplayed in our society as addictive substances, are the most widely used stimulants in the world. Caffeine is found in coffee, cocoa, chocolate and herbs such as kola nuts. It is a constituent of medicines like Excedrin, Anacin, Vanquish and Bromo-seltzer, and an ingredient of almost every appetite suppressant and many soft drinks. It is a quick energy pick-me-up and a memory stimulant, but excessive use of caffeine (over 4 cups of coffee a day) can lead to anxiety, sleeplessness, increased blood sugar levels, rapid heartbeat, exhausted adrenal and increased tolerance to its effects- all signs of addiction. Nicotine addiction is as powerful as heroin addiction. Cigarettes have over 4000 known poisons, any of which can kill in high enough doses. Secondhand or passive smoke, and chewing tobacco are just as dangerous, especially for women, increasing the instance of cervical, uterine and lung cancer, heart disease and osteoporosis.

❧ Essential Categories for Caffeine & Nicotine Addiction Compounds:

Withdrawal Support Herbs	Relaxing, Nervine Herbs	Blood Sugar Balancing Herbs	Natural Energy Sources	Normalizing, Antioxidant Herbs	Adrenal Support Sources
Bee pollen	**Kava kava root**	**Gotu kola**	**Suma root**	**Panax ginseng root**	**Gotu kola**
Kava kava root	**Scullcap**	**Sarsaparilla root**	**Bee pollen**	**Siberian ginseng**	**Ashwagandha root**
Scullcap	Hops	**Spirulina**	**Gotu kola**	**Rosemary**	**Licorice root**
Wood betony	**Passionflower**	**Licorice root**	**Panax ginseng root**	Ginkgo biloba	Kelp/sea vegetables
St. John's wort	Lobelia	**Siberian ginseng root**	Dong quai root	**Spirulina/Chlorella**	Siberian ginseng root
Oats/Oatstraw	Valerian root	**Miso powder**	Fo-ti root	**Gotu kola**	Sarsaparilla root
Chamomile	**Gotu kola**	Dandelion root	Ginkgo biloba	**Astragalus**	Brewer's yeast
Peppermint	**Oats/Oatstraw**	Wild yam root	**Ashwagandha**	**Bee pollen/Royal Jelly**	**Astragalus bark**
Passionflower	Black haw	Brewer's yeast	**Damiana**	**Hawthorn bry., lf., flr.**	Uva ursi

❧ Essential Herbs for Caffeine & Nicotine Addiction Compounds:

Primary Herbs	Assisting & Complementary Herbs	Catalyst & Transporting Herbs
Ginkgo biloba	Scullcap	Fo-ti root	Vitamin C powder	Acidophilus pwr.
Bee pollen	Kava kava root	Red clover	Rosehips	Dong quai root
Ginseng - all types	Dandelion root & lf.	Black haw	Spearmint	Stevia herb
Sarsaparilla root	Nettles	St. John's wort	Capsicum	Irish Moss
Spirulina	Alfalfa	Passionflower	Peppermint	Hops
Licorice root	Damiana	Miso powder	Prince ginseng rt.	Uva ursi
Kelp & sea vegetables	Barley grass	Aloe vera	Ginger root	Brewer's yeast
Astragalus	Wood betony	Oats/Oatstraw	Valerian root	Lobelia
Chlorella	Chamomile	Wild yam root	Rosemary	Dulse

❧ Example Formulas of Caffeine & Nicotine Addiction Compounds:

An adrenal support capsule compound		(e - 1000)	A natural energy capsule compound		(e - 3780)
Licorice root	Astragalus	Rose hips	Guarana seed	Astragalus	Capsicum
Sarsaparilla root	Capsicum	Vitamin C powder	Kola nut	Ginger root	
Bladderwrack	Uva ursi	Suma root			
	Irish moss	Bee pollen			
	Ginger root				

See page 1 for formulating instructions.

122

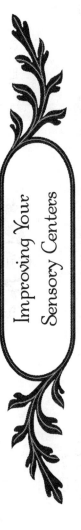

Improving Your Sensory Centers

e all know that air contaminates and impure drinking water aggravate chronic nasal, throat and sinus problems. Environmental and chemical pollutants are prime culprits for these allergy-type reactions. But we seldom realize how much our environment and lifestyle choices affect our senses. Optical, auditory, and olfactory problems are often the end result of toxins elsewhere in our bodies. Many can be addressed by correcting vitamin, mineral and other nutritional deficiencies, and boosting immune response at the body's deepest levels. A poorly functioning liver also opens the door for sensory center problems because of reduced immune response. Yet, we know the liver is remarkably adaptive, responding well to rich, green herbal nutrients, like those from sea vegetables and green grasses, and herbs with antioxidants and bioflavonoids to build immunity and improve poor circulation and capillary integrity.

Deteriorating vision is often directly related to both liver malfunction and environmental pollutants, as well as a diet with too much sugar and refined foods. No other sense is so susceptible to unhealthy lifestyle conditions. A good eyesight diet should have plenty of natural antioxidants and proteins from herbs, sea or soy foods, high mineral nutrients from leafy greens and green superfoods, and beta-carotene-rich foods like carrots, broccoli or sea vegetables. These nutrients not only build up immune response but also help keep the eyes protected from free radical damage and environmental pollutants. The most stressful eyesight situations are reading, using a computer for most of your workday, and a sedentary lifestyle. Take good care of your eyes!

Tinnitus, or ringing in the ears, may be blamed on exposure to excessively loud sounds from music or machinery. Today, noise pollution affects one out of every 10 people with some type of hearing impairment, (an astounding figure)! Hearing loss is the third most common health problem for people over 65. Eighty-five percent of these individuals suffer from tinnitus. Age-related hearing problems are also the result of arteriosclerosis, allergies, or sinus or chronic bronchial mastoid infections. Hypoglycemia, (low blood sugar) and inner ear imbalance are also implicated in tinnitus or ringing in the ears.

Meniere's syndrome mimics tinnitus. It is a recurrent, usually progressive group of symptoms that include both ringing and pressure in the ears, with some hearing loss and dizziness. Poor circulation and lack of oxygen to the brain is at the root of Meniere's. Supplementation with bioflavonoids or high flavonoid herbs like ginkgo biloba can increase capillary integrity, and improve hearing. Relaxation techniques and good daily nutrition are also keys to preventing attacks.

Sinusitis is an inflammation of the mucous membranes lining the sinuses, and regularly involving nasal polyps and scar tissue. It is often caused by a viral or bacterial infection triggered by an allergic conditions, environmentally based or otherwise. It is important to eliminate trigger foods in one's diet that may be implicated in sinus troubles and to try to stay away from the environmental conditions that aggravate them. Chronic sinusitis can result in taste or smell loss.

Taste and smell loss is often tied into mineral deficiencies, like zinc. A deviated septum, atrophied nerve endings, gland and hormone imbalances, even some over-the-counter and prescription drugs may all be involved. Highly absorbable minerals from herbs, along with herbal superfood greens like those in chlorella or spirulina can sometimes do wonders for people with this problem. In many cases, if total atrophy has not developed, at least partial tast and smell can be restored.

Drug therapy has been notably ineffective in improving problems of the sensory centers for two reasons: 1) the areas themselves are very subtle and delicately balanced in nature. They do not respond to the heavy hand of most drugs. 2) neither drug therapy, nor conventional medicine in general, address the cause of a problem, concentrating rather on its symptoms, yet sensory problems almost always stem from deep body imbalances and deficiencies. **Herbs can be effective "eye, ear, nose and throat specialists."** They support and strengthen these delicate areas, and are also capable of addressing specific problems. Herbs work with the body functions instead of outside them to remedy the cause of a problem at its source.

❧ FORMULAS FOR SENSORY CENTERS ARE ALSO EFFECTIVE FOR OTHER CONDITIONS:

•Deteriorating Vision & Night Blindness •Glaucoma •Conjunctivitis •Ear Infections •Chronic Low-Grade Throat & Sinus Infections •Post-Nasal Drip •Taste & Smell Loss •Ringing In The Ears •Deteriorating Hearing •Vertigo & Dizziness.

❧ COMPOUNDS FOR FORMULATION SHOULD INCLUDE:

•Herbal compounds for improving poor vision.
•Herbal compounds for arresting tinnitus and Meniere's syndrome.
•Herbal compounds for restoring taste and smell functions.

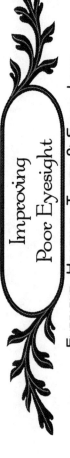

Improving
Poor Eyesight

EYESIGHT, HEARING, TASTE & SMELL LOSS

Ninety percent of what we learn during our lives we learn through sight. The eyes are not only the windows of the soul, but windows to body health as well. Your lifestyle profoundly affects your "eyestyle." You can often tell if your daily stress level is affecting your eyes if you see sparks or vivid colors when your eyes are closed. Eyes often reflect imbalances elsewhere in the system. As with so many other body systems, poor liver function is the most common cause of eye problems and the key to healthy eyes. The most stressful eyesight situations are reading, using a computer for most of your workday, (eyestrain will result in blurring vision as the day goes on), and a sedentary lifestyle. Natural treatment has been notably successful in improving poor vision, especially with herbs that support the liver, tone eye muscles and reduce eye fatigue. Take good care of your eyes!

❧ ESSENTIAL CATEGORIES FOR IMPROVING EYESIGHT COMPOUNDS:

EYESIGHT SUPPORT HERBS	BETA-CAROTENE-RICH HERBS	BIOFLAVONOID SOURCES	LIVER STIMULATION & SUPPORT HERBS	MINERAL-RICH HERBS	CIRCULATION TONERS & STIMULATORS
Ginkgo biloba	**Barley grass**	**Kelp & ocean plants**	**Dandelion root**	**Echinacea root**	**Hawthorn lf., flr., bry.**
Passionflower	Garlic	Cranberry powder	**Milk thistle seed**	**Spirulina**	**Ginger root**
Red raspberry	**Parsley**	**Bilberry berry**	Red sage	**Eyebright**	**Elder flower**
Parsley	**Alfalfa**	White pine bark	Parsley	Burdock root	**Ginkgo biloba**
Eyebright	**Nettles**	**Red raspberry**	**Oregon grape root**	Garlic	Capsicum
Capsicum	Black cohosh root	**Hawthorn berry**	**Hyssop**	**Alfalfa**	**Dong quai**
Goldenseal root	**Dandelion root & lf.**	Lemon peel	Bilberry	Bilberry	**Bilberry berry**
Rosemary	**Aloe vera**	Rosé hips	Fenugreek seeds	Barley grass	Angelica root
Fennel seed	**Watercress**	Hops	**Yellow dock root**	**Gotu kola**	Panax ginseng

❧ ESSENTIAL HERBS FOR IMPROVING EYESIGHT COMPOUNDS:

PRIMARY HERBS		ASSISTING & COMPLEMENTARY HERBS		CATALYST & TRANSPORTING HERBS	
Eyebright	Chlorella	Alfalfa	Astragalus	Capsicum	Aloe vera juice
Parsley	Barley Grass	Barberry bark	Angelica root	Elder flower	Rosemary
Ginkgo biloba	Sarsaparilla root	Oregon grape root	Hyssop	Ginger root	Green tea
Goldenseal root	Hawthorn lf. flr. & bry.	Yellow dock root	Myrrh	Fennel seed	Rosehips
Dandelion rt. & lf.	Nettles	Red sage	Plantain	Cinnamon	Wild cherry bk.
Licorice root	Bayberry bk.	Red Raspberry	Black cohosh root	Fenugreek seeds	Lemon peel
Burdock root	Kelp & ocean plants	Milk thistle seed	White pine bark	Hops	Cranberry powder
Bilberry bry.	Panax ginseng	Garlic	Gotu kola	Turmeric	Hibiscus
Pau d'arco bark	Passionflower	Echinacea root	Spirulina	Dong quai	Watercress

❧ EXAMPLE FORMULAS OF IMPROVING EYESIGHT COMPOUNDS:

AN EYESIGHT CAPSULE COMPOUND		(co - 4260)		AN EYESIGHT SUPPORT TEA COMPOUND		(co - 5300)	
Eyebright	Ginkgo biloba	Hawthorn lf., flr., bry.	Capsicum	Eyebright	Passionflower	Elder flower	Goldenseal root
Parsley	Goldenseal root	Red raspberry	Passionflower	Bilberry bry.	Plantain	Rosemary	Red Raspberry
Bilberry bry.	Bayberry bk.	Angelica					

SEE PAGE 1 FOR FORMULATING INSTRUCTIONS.

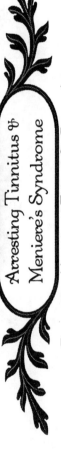

Arresting Tinnitus & Meniere's Syndrome

Eyesight, Hearing, Taste & Smell Loss

Many hearing loss problems, such as tinnitus and Meniere's syndrome may be addressed effectively with herbal and nutritional programs. In fact, rest, relaxation techniques and proper nutrition may be the keys to preventing ringing-in-the-ears attacks. Unfortunately, by the time most people figure out they have noise-induced tinnitus or hearing loss, hair cell damage to the inner ear is irreversible. (Internal bone fusions causing hearing loss need surgical attention.) The distress of hearing disorders can be helped by indicated herbal remedies, and avoidance of excessive use of nicotine, caffeine or alcohol which limit the flow of blood and nutrients to the brain. In addition, recreational drugs, such as cocaine, marijuana, LSD, and methamphetamines are balance-changing and likely to bring on aggressive attacks. Diet is very important. Reduce sugar, salt, and dairy along with a mild mucuos cleansing diet to keep passageways open and mucuos clog limited.

❧ ESSENTIAL CATEGORIES FOR ARRESTING TINNITUS PROBLEMS COMPOUNDS:

RESTORATIVE NERVINE HERBS	ANTIHISTAMINE SOURCE HERBS	B VITAMIN SOURCE HERBS	SILICA SOURCE HERBS	DISSOLVE CONGESTION, RELIEVE PAIN	CIRCULATION STIMULATING HERBS
Scullcap	**Ma huang (ephedra)**	**Bee pollen**	**Kelp/sea vegetables**	**Capsicum**	**Ginkgo biloba**
Black haw	Mullein	Royal Jelly	Echinacea root	Mullein	**Hawthorn bry., lf. flr.**
St. John's wort	**Marshmallow root**	**Kelp/sea vegetables**	**Burdock root**	**Marshmallow root**	**Capsicum**
Wood betony	**Goldenseal root**	**Dandelion root**	Horsetail	Echinacea root	**Ginger root**
Ashwagandha	**Burdock root**	Dong qual	Carrot powder	Goldenseal root	Bilberry bry.
Gotu kola	Parsley root	**Parsley root**	**Alfalfa**	Peppermint	Garlic
Lobelia	Acerola cherry	Red raspberry	**Oatstraw**	**Lobelia**	Cloves
European mistletoe	**Coltsfoot**	Burdock root	Ginger root	**Angelica root**	Astragalus
Black cohosh root	Bee pollen	Fenugreek seed	Orange peel	**Ginger root**	Peppermint

❧ ESSENTIAL HERBS FOR ARRESTING TINNITUS PROBLEMS COMPOUNDS:

PRIMARY HERBS		ASSISTING & COMPLEMENTARY HERBS		CATALYST & TRANSPORTING HERBS	
Ginkgo biloba	Slippery elm	Garlic	Alfalfa	Capsicum	Scullcap
Hawthorn bry., lf. flr.	Kelp/sea vegetables	Red raspberry	Black cohosh root	Wood betony	Black haw
Marshmallow root	Horsetail herb	Bilberry bry.	St. John's wort	Rosemary	Lobelia
Mullein	Coltsfooot	Burdock root	Myrrh	Dandelion root	European Mistletoe
Ma Huang	Nettles	Eucalyptus	Passionflower	Ginger root	Calendula
Elder flower & berry	Goldenseal root	Sage	Angelica root	Dong qual	Peppermint
Oatstraw	White pine bark	Echinacea root	Gotu kola	Lemon Peel	Orange peel
Bee pollen/Royal Jelly	Parsley root	Boneset	Astragalus	Rose hips	Anise seed
Fenugreek seed	Ashwagandha	Juniper berry	Acerola cherry	Carrot powder	Cloves

❧ EXAMPLE FORMULAS OF ARRESTING TINNITUS PROBLEMS COMPOUNDS:

AN ANTIHISTAMINE COMPOUND TO RELIEVE EAR PESSURE			(B - 1200)
Marshmallow root	Bee pollen	Burdock root	Rosemary
Fenugreek seed	White pine bark	Juniper berry	Mullein
Ma Huang	Goldenseal root	Parsley root	Capsicum
		Acerola cherry	Lobelia

A SILICA SOURCE COMPOUND FOR VASCULAR STRENGTH			(SA - 4950)
Horsetail herb	Oatstraw	Carrot powder	Orange peel

*Note: Ginkgo biloba extract is a specific for ringing in the ears and may be used in conjunction with any formula you choose to enhance your healing program.

SEE PAGE 1 FOR FORMULATING INSTRUCTIONS.

125

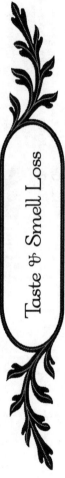

Taste & Smell Loss

EYESIGHT, HEARING, TASTE & SMELL LOSS

The decline or loss of the ability to smell odors or taste foods is a rising worry for many people, especially as they age. In times past a deviated septum (which must be corrected by surgery) was largely thought to be the cause. Yet, while the corrected deviation helped breathing, it often did not help taste senses. Today we see this disorder as a combination of modern lifestyle factors - from nutrient deficiencies, like zinc, to the effects of common colds and flu medicines, high blood pressure drugs, chemical diuretics or over use of antibiotics (which leach zinc from the body). In addition, nerve endings may be damaged from arthritis or osteoporosis (one of the reasons this problem afflicts older people more than younger people). The natural healing emphasis on overcoming nutritional deficiencies is often able to successfully address many of the root causes. In many cases, if total atrophy has not yet developed, at least partial taste and smell may be restored.

❧ ESSENTIAL CATEGORIES FOR TASTE & SMELL LOSS COMPOUNDS:

ELIMINATE LYMPH WASTE & CONGESTION	CIRCULATION STIMULATING HERBS	ADAPTOGENS HERBS FOR BODY CHEMISTRY	ZINC & MINERAL-RICH HERBS	B VITAMIN HERB SOURCES	BETA-CAROTENE HERB SOURCES
Echinacea root	**Capsicum**	**Ashwagandha**	**Kelp/sea vegetables**	**Bee pollen**	**Garlic**
Goldenseal root	**Hawthorn bry., lf., flr.**	Gotu kola	**Nettles**	**Dandelion root**	Nettles
Hawthorn bry., lf., flr.	**Ginkgo biloba**	**Schizandra berry**	**Alfalfa**	**Kelp/sea vegetables**	**Kelp/sea vegetables**
Panax ginseng	**Gotu kola**	Wild yam root	**Dandelion root**	**Parsley root & lf.**	**Parsley root & lf.**
Kelp/sea vegetables	St. John's wort	**Panax ginseng**	Spirulina/Barley grass	Red raspberry	Barley grass/Spirulina
Reishi mushroom	Burdock root	Suma root	**Horsetail**	**Burdock root**	**Peppermint**
Astragalus	Ginger root	Fo-Ti root	**Parsley rt. & lf.**	Fenugreek seed	Borage seed
Licorice root	**Siberian ginseng root**	**Black cohosh root**	Echinacea root	Royal jelly	Yellow dock root
Oregon grape root	Peppermint	**Siberian ginseng root**	Yellow dock root	Thyme	**Alfalfa**

❧ ESSENTIAL HERBS FOR TASTE & SMELL LOSS COMPOUNDS:

PRIMARY HERBS		ASSISTING & COMPLEMENTARY HERBS		CATALYST & TRANSPORTING HERBS	
Kelp/sea vegetables	Siberian ginseng root	Fo-Ti root root	Barley grass	Capsicum	Spearmint
Bee pollen	Dandelion root & leaf	St. John's wort	Alfalfa	Calendula	Lemon balm
Burdock root	Licorice root	Ashwagandha	Spirulina	Thyme	Parsley root
Hawthorn bry., lf., flr.	Wild Yam	Reishi mushroom	Myrrh	Peppermint	Borage seed
Panax ginseng	Nettles	Astragalus	Horsetail	Bilberry bry.	Turmeric
Echinacea root	Goldenseal root	Suma root	Black cohosh root	Lobelia	Propolis
Ginkgo biloba	Oregon grape root	Schizandra berry	Ginger root	Pau d' arco	Lemon peel
Gotu kola	Burdock root	Fenugreek seed	Yellow dock root	Dulse	Basil
Parsley root & lf.	Garlic	Royal Jelly	Red raspberry	Watercress	Cardamom

❧ EXAMPLE FORMULAS OF TASTE & SMELL LOSS COMPOUNDS:

A BROAD RANGE MINERAL SPECTRUM COMPOUND		(SA - 3200)
Nettles	Kelp	Borage seed
Irish miss	Parsley root	Dulse
Watercress		
Alfalfa		
Yellow dock rt.		
Barley grass		

A ZINC SOURCE EXTRACT COMPOUND		(SA - 4830)
Echinacea root	Peppermint	Propolis
Spirulina	Bilberry bry.	Spearmint
Gotu kola	Yellow dock rt.	
	Alfalfa	
	Barley grass	

SEE PAGE 1 FOR FORMULATING INSTRUCTIONS.

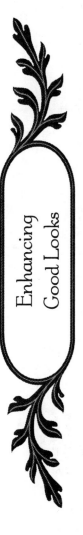

Enhancing Good Looks

We all want pleasing looks - to have sparkling eyes, radiant complexions, luxurious hair and healthy nails. There is no magic bullet for beauty, but there is truth in the maxim that good health means good looks, and many people who have embraced lifestyle changes, herbal therapy, and diet improvement have experienced remarkable success in enhancing both their health and their physical looks. Hormone imbalances, allergies to cosmetics and environmental pollutants, emotional stress, a low nutrient and EFA diet, and heredity are all factors that influence our cosmetic elements. A good diet is essential for good skin, healthy hair and strong nails. A diet with too much salt, lots of sweets, fatty, fried foods, and pasteurized dairy foods and red meats, shows up internally as a factor in chronic degenerative diseases like arthritis and circulatory problems, and externally in the health and beauty of our skin, hair and nails.

Diet improvement is a key. Reducing your intake of salt, sugar and caffeine and avoiding fatty, refined and preserved foods is a good start. Eliminating animal fats from the diet is a must. Focus on adding foods rich in silica and sulphur, like garlic, onions, sprouts, horseradish, green leafy veggies, carrots, bell peppers, eggs, apricots, cucumbers, rice and seeds to strengthen hair and nails and help to form collagen for skin beauty. Add soy foods for phyto-hormones, vegetable protein and vitamin E to help correct hormone imbalances that are at the root of some complexion and hair problems. Foods rich in iodine and potassium, such as sea vegetables and sea foods promote growth and thickness of the hair strengthen nails. Vitamin C, and bioflavonoid-rich foods like yellow and orange fruits and vegetables, and beta carotene foods like broccoli and sea vegetables help keep the body alkaline and skin, hair and nails nourished. A good looks diet should include six to eight glasses of water or healthy liquids a day to help the kidneys to flush out wastes, and filter out impurities that accumulate in the organs and bloodstream, and which ultimately show up on the skin, in the form of blemishes, rashes, etc. Remember that smoking is as bad for the your looks as it is for your health.

Herbs are uniquely suited to the care and nourishment of skin, hair and nails. Herbs are primary sources of organic minerals and trace minerals, the building blocks of our looks. They are rich in food source vitamins and concentrated food nutrients and are quickly capable of becoming part of the body to stimulate cleansing, encourage healthy cell growth and build tissue strength. As living remedies, herbs are uniquely effective for nourishing your hair skin and nails both from the inside out, and from the outside in, where drugs and commercial cosmetics are not.

Here are some watchwords for enhancing the appearance of your hair skin and nails:

• Beautiful skin, hair and nails need vitamin A, vitamin C, mineral-rich and high vegetable protein foods for collagen and interstitial tissue health. Herbs are high in collagen-producing elements such as organic silica and calcium.

• Glowing skin tone depends on a clear, hydrated system, flushed of toxic wastes and pH balanced. Herbs are cleansing, alkalizing agents that help purify the bloodstream, so that wastes are not dumped out through the skin. Many are high in soluble fiber to keep the system unclogged, and free of constipation.

• Vibrant hair needs vegetable protein for maximum growth and high carotenoids for health. Herbs are concentrated foods with easily absorbed protein nutrients.

• Stress is the primary cause of premature graying. Herbs help to relieve body stress; many are rich in B vitamins and amino acids that replenish hair deficiencies.

• Strong, hard nails need minerals for health. Herbs are concentrated forms of readily absorbable minerals and trace minerals.

• All the cosmetic elements need an oxygen-rich blood supply. Many herbs are high in antioxidant properties.

❧ FORMULAS FOR ENHANCING GOOD LOOKS HELP IN THE FOLLOWING CONDITIONS:

•Sallow complexion, Clogged Pores & Eczema •Adult Acne •Chronic Skin Infections & Dermatitis •Dry, Wrinkling Skin •Facial Blotching & Excess Pigmentation
•Easy Bruising •Split, Brittle Nails •Liver & Age Spots •Mental Exhaustion •Hair Loss & Alopecia •Dandruff & Seborrhea •Dry, Damaged Hair & Hair Color Loss

❧ COMPOUNDS FOR FORMULATION SHOULD INCLUDE:

•Formulas for boosting hair health and growth
•Formulas for complexion beauty and skin tone
•Formulas for dealing with adult acne
•Formulas for healing damaged skin
•Formulas for strengthening your nails

Boosting Hair Health & Growth

ENHANCING GOOD LOOKS

Nobody wants to lose their hair or go gray. Although heredity does play a role in male (and sometimes female) hair loss, so does poor nutrition. Disease, drugs and serious illness treatments, and hormonal imbalances may all manifest in a loss of hair or premature graying of the hair. Hair health depends on blood supply, circulation and nutrition. Hair consists of protein layers called keratin. In healthy hair, the cell walls of the hair cuticle lie flat like shingles, leaving hair soft and shiny. In damaged or dry hair, the cuticle shingles are often the first indication of nutritional deficiencies. Hair loss, alopecia and male pattern baldness affects 30 million men and 20 million women nationwide. Although androgenic alopecia is hereditary and not easily reversible, good nutrition and herbal hair care can indeed result in hair improvement, thickness and regrowth. Your therapy choice must be vigorously followed. Occasional therapy will have little or no effect. Two months is usually the minimum for really noticeable growth.

ESSENTIAL CATEGORIES FOR HAIR HEALTH & GROWTH COMPOUNDS:

HAIR STRENGTHENING HERBS	ESSENTIAL FATTY ACIDS (EFAs) FOR HAIR	MINERAL-RICH HERBS	SILICA SOURCE HERBS	CIRCULATION STIMULATING HERBS	B VITAMIN-RICH HERBS
Nettles	**Bee pollen/Royal Jelly**	**Alfalfa/Barley grass**	**Oatstraw**	Hawthorn lf. flr. & bry.	**Spirulina/barley grass**
Horsetail	**Evening primrose oil**	**Oatstraw**	Horsetail	Siberian ginseng	**Bee pollen/Royal Jelly**
Chamomile	**Flax seed**	**Yellow dock root**	**Kelp/sea vegetables**	Gotu kola	**Kelp/sea vegetables**
Burdock root	**Black currant seed**	**Watercress**	Eyebright	**Ginkgo biloba**	Red raspberry
Rosemary	Parsley root & lf.	**Nettles**	Echinacea root	Turmeric	**Fenugreek seed**
Oatstraw	Ginger root	Dandelion root & lf.	**Burdock root**	**Garlic**	Thyme
White sage	Burdock root	Pau d'arco bark	**Ginger root**	**Ginger root**	**Dandelion root**
Fo-Ti root	**Borage seed**	Kelp/sea vegetables	Spirulina	Capsicum	**Dong quai**
Yarrow	Pumpkin seed	Horsetail	**Orange peel**	Licorice root	Brewer's yeast

ESSENTIAL HERBS FOR HAIR HEALTH & GROWTH COMPOUNDS:

PRIMARY HERBS		ASSISTING & COMPLEMENTARY HERBS		CATALYST & TRANSPORTING HERBS	
Bee pollen/Royal jelly	Pau d'arco bark	Hyssop	Ginger root	Capsicum	Lemon balm
Evening primrose oil	Sarsaparilla root	Borage seed	Watercress	Turmeric	Thyme
Ginkgo biloba	Chlorella/Barley grass	Coltsfoot	Chamomile	Orange peel	White sage
Siberian ginseng	Kelp/sea vegetables	Oatstraw	Horsetail	Lemongrass	Peppermint
Licorice root	Hawthorn lf. flr. & bry.	Nettles	Dong quai root	Rosemary	Pumpkin seed
Saw palmetto bry.	Flax seed	Eyebright	Schizandra bry.	Brewer's yeast	Echinacea root
Fo-Ti root	Gotu kola	Garlic	Nettles	Stevia	Yellow dock root
Burdock root	Spirulina	Black currant seed	Fenugreek seed	Bilberry	Yarrow
Dandelion root/lf.	Parsley rt./lf.	Alfalfa	Red raspberry	Miso broth powder	Jojoba oil

EXAMPLE FORMULAS OF HAIR HEALTH & GROWTH COMPOUNDS:

AN IODINE & POTASSIUM HAIR STRENGTHENING COMPOUND			(SA - 4080)	A HEALTHY HAIR TEA COMPOUND			(BB - 5480)
Alfalfa	Licorice root	Horsetail	Schizandra bry.	Alfalfa	Horsetail	Parsley root/leaf
Oatstraw	Barley grass	Nettles	Rosemary	Lemongrass	Nettles	Peppermint
Dandelion lf.	Watercress	Fennel seed	Bilberry	Fenugreek seed	Rosemary	Stevia
Yellow dock rt	Pau d' arco bk.	Parsley rt./lf.	Spirulina			
Borage seed	Red raspberry	Siberian ginseng	Sea vegetables			

SEE PAGE 1 FOR FORMULATING INSTRUCTIONS.

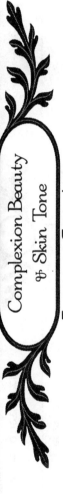

Complexion Beauty & Skin Tone

ENHANCING GOOD LOOKS

Beautiful skin is more than skin deep. Our skin is the essence of renewable nature... it sloughs off old, dying cells every day, and gives a chance for a new start. The skin is the body's largest organ of nourishment and elimination. The skin's protective acid mantle inhibits the growth of disease-causing bacteria for the whole body. Skin mirrors our emotional state and hormonal balance, too, and is a sure sign of poor nutrition. (Allergies show up first on the skin.) Skin problems reflect a stressed lifestyle almost immediately. Your complexion will benefit right away when you eliminate fried, fatty foods, red meats, caffeine and salty sugary foods. Relaxation, nourishment and improved nutrition show quickly in skin health and beauty. Herbs are great for skin - packed with absorbable minerals, anti-oxidants, EFAs and bioflavonoids, to cleanse, hydrate, heal, alkalize, and balance glands and hormones. Treat yourself to an herbal skin treatment at least once a week.

❧ ESSENTIAL CATEGORIES FOR BEAUTIFUL SKIN COMPOUNDS:

ANTIOXIDANT SUPPORT HERBS	STRESS RELIEVING NERVINE HERBS	BODY CHEMISTRY BALANCERS	MINERAL & PROTEIN RICH HERBS	SKIN CLEANSERS & DETOXIFIERS	GLAND & HORMONE BALANCING HERBS
Nettles	**Kava kava root**	**Suma root**	**Kelp & sea vegetables**	**Dandelion root & leaf**	**Black cohosh root**
Chlorella/Barley grass	**Scullcap**	**Chlorella-rich herbs**	**Royal Jelly/Bee pollen**	**Aloe vera**	**Ashwagandha root**
Alfalfa	**Black cohosh**	**Gotu kola**	Siberian ginseng	**Chickweed**	**Licorice root**
Dandelion root	**Passionflower**	**Panax ginseng root**	Dandelion root & leaf	**Alfalfa**	**Kelp/sea vegetables**
Ginger root	Lobelia	Dong qual root	**Spirulina**	Red raspberry	**Burdock root**
Rosemary	Valerian root	Fo-ti root	**Barley grass**	**Goldenseal root**	**Sarsaparilla root**
Kelp & sea vegetables	**Gotu kola**	Prince ginseng rt.	**Chlorella**	**Pau d' arco bark**	Schizandra bry.
Royal Jelly/Bee pollen	**Panax ginseng root**	**Ashwagandha**	**Nutritional yeast**	Echinacea root	**Dong qual root**
Suma root	Ashwagandha	**Alfalfa**	Soy powder	Buckthorn bark	**Wild yam root**

❧ ESSENTIAL HERBS FOR FOR BEAUTIFUL SKIN COMPOUNDS:

PRIMARY HERBS		ASSISTING & COMPLEMENTARY HERBS		CATALYST & TRANSPORTING HERBS	
Burdock rt.	St. John's wort	Parsley root & lf.	Kava kava	Aloe vera	Wood betony
Dandelion root & leaf	Kava kava root	Fo-ti root	Suma root	Nutritional yeast	Rosemary
Ginseng - all types	Ginkgo biloba	Hawthorn lf., bry. & flr.	Goldenseal root	Chamomile	Schizandra bry.
Ashwagandha	Suma root	Pau d' arco bark	Wild yam root	Capsicum	Reishi mushroom
Nettles	Royal jelly/Bee pollen	Spirulina	Red raspberry	Soy powder	Lobelia
Licorice root	Gotu kola	Chickweed	Scullcap	Red clover	Valerian root
Kelp/sea vegetables	Siberian ginseng	Barley grass	Rose hips	Ginger root	Passionflower
Sarsaparilla root	Panax ginseng	Buckthorn bark	Dong qual root	Damiana	Prickly ash
Chlorella	Yellow dock root	Echinacea root	Prince ginseng rt.	Bilberry	Irish moss

❧ EXAMPLE FORMULAS OF BEAUTIFUL SKIN COMPOUNDS:

A SKIN CLEANSING CAPSULE COMPOUND		(BB - 3950)	A SKIN NOURISHING, SOOTHING CAPSULE COMPOUND		(BB - 3960)
Dandelion rt.	Buckthorn bark	Red clover	Ginkgo biloba	Licorice root	Yellow dock root	White oak bark	Rose hips
Burdock root	Sarsaparilla root	Licorice root	Ashwagandha	Dandelion root	Alfalfa	Bilberry	Ginger root
Echinacea root				Burdock root	Sarsaparilla root	Wild yam root	
				Chickweed	Rosemary		

SEE PAGE 1 FOR FORMULATING INSTRUCTIONS.

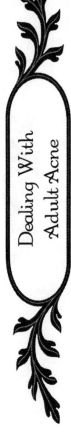

Dealing With Adult Acne

ENHANCING GOOD LOOKS

Acne is becoming more prevalent. In adults, acne is considered to be the result of poor diet (particularly a lack of green vegetables), a high stress lifestyle and environmental pollutants. Other causes of adult acne (as opposed to teen-age acne, which is mainly hormone-related, include poor digestion of fats, an EFA deficiency, poor liver function, and elimination/constipation problems. Herbal therapy incorporated with a healthy diet has shown clear improvement for adult acne, addressing blood purification, infections, oxidative stress, immune response and the nutritional needs of the body ... and herbs are effective without the side effects present in the commonly prescribed anti-biotics for acne. Herbs nourish and heal the skin, and the vital organs, glands and blood that support it. Adult acne doesn't have to ruin your life. Lower the fats in your diet, drink plenty of water, eat lots of fresh vegetables and use some of the healing herbs on this page.

❧ ESSENTIAL CATEGORIES FOR ADULT ACNE SKIN COMPOUNDS:

ANTIBACTERIAL, ANTIOXIDANT HERBS	BLOOD CLEANSING HERBS	MINERAL-RICH NUTRITIVE HERBS	ESSENTIAL FATTY ACID SOURCES	HORMONE & GLAND BALANCING HERBS	ANTI-INFLAMMATORY SOURCES
Echinacea root	**Dandelion root & lf.**	Kelp & sea vegetables	**Evening primrose oil**	**Black cohosh root**	**Yarrow**
Goldenseal root	**Burdock root**	**Echinacea root**	Bee pollen/Royal Jelly	Sarsaparilla root	Myrrh
Myrrh	**Sarsaparilla root**	**Dandelion root & lf.**	**Flax seed**	**Licorice root**	**Marshmallow root**
Pau d' arco	Kelp & sea vegetables	**Nettles**	Parsley root & lf	**Saw palmetto bry.**	Kelp/sea vegetables
Sarsaparilla root	**Licorice root**	**Chlorella/Barley grass**	Ginger root	**Burdock root**	**Turmeric**
Capsicum	Spirulina	Nettles	Lemongrass	**Panax ginseng root**	**Chamomile**
Kelp & sea vegetables	**Yellow dock root**	**Yellow dock root**	**Borage seed**	**Dong qual root**	**Lavender**
Rosemary	**Chickweed**	Oats/Oatstraw	White sage	**Ashwagandha**	**Aloe vera**
Aloe vera	Alfalfa	Brewer's yeast	Black currant seed	**Damiana**	Calendula

❧ ESSENTIAL HERBS FOR ADULT ACNE SKIN COMPOUNDS:

PRIMARY HERBS		ASSISTING & COMPLEMENTARY HERBS		CATALYST & TRANSPORTING HERBS	
Burdock root	Ashwagandha root	marshmallow root	Chickweed	Watercress	Acidophilus pwr.
Nettles	Goldenseal root	Aloe vera	Pau d' arco	Rose hips	Turmeric
Myrrh	Red raspberry	Dandelion root & lf.	Dong qual	Saw palmetto bry.	Stevia herb
Sarsaparilla root	Echinacea root	Black cohosh root	White sage	Capsicum	Lavender
Spirulina	Royal Jelly/Bee pollen	Oats/Oatstraw	Parsley root & lf.	Horsetail	Calendula
Licorice root	Hawthorn bry., lf., fl.	Damiana	Fennel seed	Lemongrass	Uva ursi
Kelp & sea vegetables	Suma root	Yellow dock root	Alfalfa	Ginger root	Nutritional yeast
Propolis	Siberian ginseng	Yarrow	Evening primrose oil	Bilberry	Lobelia
Chlorella/Barley grass	Panax ginseng	Chamomile	Wild yam root	Rosemary	Flax seed

❧ EXAMPLE FORMULAS OF ADULT ACNE SKIN COMPOUNDS:

AN ANTI-INFECTIVE CAPSULE COMPOUND		(PD - 1150)		A BEAUTIFUL SKIN TEA COMPOUND		(BB - 5000)	
Echinacea root	Capsicum	Marshmallow root	Turmeric	Licorice root	Rose hips	White sage	Chamomile
Goldenseal root	Myrrh	Echinacea root	Kelp	Burdock root	Sarsaparilla root	Thyme	Dandelion root
	Yarrow	Black walnut		Rosemary	Fennel seed	Parsley leaf	Stevia lf.
		Elecampane					

Note: Stevia extract drops have been shown to be a specific for adult acne. Follow directions carefully.

SEE PAGE 1 FOR FORMULATING INSTRUCTIONS.

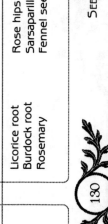

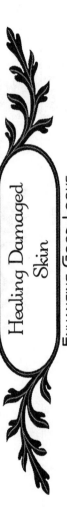

Healing Damaged Skin

ENHANCING GOOD LOOKS

For every sunburn you get that blisters, you double your risk of skin cancer. Even on a cloudy day, 80% of the sun's harmful UV rays come through. Sun damage is cumulative over a lifetime. Moderation is the key. Sunlight can help you avoid breast and prostate cancer. The newest research shows that a lack of protective vitamin D provided by sunlight may be involved). People who get almost no sun exposure are at higher risk for melanoma than those who get regular, moderate early morning sunshine. Practice good sun sense so that you dont fry now and pay later. Signs that your skin is damaged (beyond a simple cut or abrasion) include extraordinarily slow healing, loss of elasticity, blotchy, and reddened skin. If your tissues are loaded with carotene A, vitamin C, E and B complex, whether from food or food source supplements, your skin stands much less chance of being scarred or damaged, and will heal much quicker when it is damaged.

❧ ESSENTIAL CATEGORIES FOR HEALING DAMAGED SKIN COMPOUNDS:

ANTIOXIDANT, FREE RADICAL SCAVENGERS	VITAMIN C BIOFLAVONOID SOURCES	VITAMIN A, D & E NUTRITIVE HERBS	ESSENTIAL FATTY ACID SOURCES	SILICAL SOURCES FOR SCARRING	SKIN HEALING ANTI-INFLAMMATORIES
Siberian ginseng root	Rose hips	Kelp & sea vegetables	Evening primrose oil	Oatstraw	Yarrow
Ginkgo biloba	White pine bark	Dandelion root & lf.	Bee pollen/Royal Jelly	Horsetail	Myrrh
Nettles	Cranberry powder	Black cohosh root	Flax seed	Orange peel	Marshmallow root
Pau d' arco	Hawthorn bry., lf., fl.	Nettles	Parsley root & lf.	Kelp & sea vegetables	Kelp/sea vegetables
Sarsaparilla root	Peppermint	Burdock root	Ginger root	Spirulina/Chlorella	Turmeric
Licorice root	Red raspberry	Yellow dock root	Lemongrass	Burdock root	Chamomile
Kelp & sea vegetables	Chickweed	Saw palmetto berry	Borage seed	Ginger root	Lavender
Rosemary	Bee pollen	Aloe vera	White sage	Echinacea root	Aloe vera
Aloe vera	Bilberry berry	Watercress	Black currant seed	Eyebright	Calendula

❧ ESSENTIAL HERBS FOR HEALING DAMAGED SKIN COMPOUNDS:

PRIMARY HERBS	ASSISTING & COMPLEMENTARY HERBS	CATALYST & TRANSPORTING HERBS
Burdock root	Suma root	Marshmallow root	Pau d' arco bark	Ginkgo biloba	Eyebright
Nettles	Goldenseal root	Aloe vera	White pine bark	Saw palmetto	Calendula
Horsetail	Red raspberry	Dandelion root & lf.	White sage	Dulse	Stevia herb
Sarsaparilla root	Echinacea root	Black cohosh root	Chamomile	Capsicum	Lavender
Spirulina	Royal Jelly/Bee pollen	Oats/Oatstraw	Parsley root & lf.	Peppermint	Borage seed
Licorice root	Hawthorn bry., lf., fl.	Rose hips	Myrrh	Bilberry	Cranberry pwr.
Kelp & sea vegetables	Evening primrose	Barley grass	Orange peel	Ginger root	Nutritional yeast
Yellow dock root	Siberian ginseng	Yarrow	Grapefruit seed	Acidophilus pwr.	Black currant seed
Chlorella	Panax ginseng	Chickweed	Watercress	Rosemary	Flax seed

❧ EXAMPLE FORMULAS OF HEALING DAMAGED SKIN COMPOUNDS:

A BEAUTIFUL SKIN, HEALING CAPSULE COMPOUND				(BB - 1395)
Barley grass	Dulse	Goldenseal root	Dandelion root	
Horsetail	Rosemary	Cranberry pwr.	Nettles	
White sage	Echinacea root			

A TOPICAL SKIN, HEALING GEL COMPOUND				(BB - 7920)
Panax ginseng rt.	Suma root	Calendula	Aloe vera	
Kirin ginseng rt.	White pine bark	Rose hips	Lecithin	
		Chlorella	Grapefruit seed	
			Agar	

SEE PAGE 1 FOR FORMULATING INSTRUCTIONS.

131

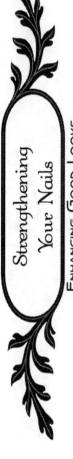

Strengthening Your Nails

ENHANCING GOOD LOOKS

Nails can be useful as an "early warning system" in evaluating health. If the eyes are the "windows to the soul," the nails are the "windows of the body." They are one of the last body areas to receive the nutrients carried by the blood, and show signs of trouble before better-nourished tissues do. Healthy nails are pink, smooth and shiny. Changes in their shape, color and texture signal the presence of disorder, deficiencies or disease in the body. When choosing nail products, keep in mind that commercial nail enamels and supplies carry some of the most toxic chemical pollutants. Fake nails and tips add weight to the nails, preventing them from thickening naturally; nail dyes penetrate the nail to the skin often causing allergic reactions. Simple beeswax spread on the nails and buffed to a shine will leave your nails naturally beautiful. Keep your diet rich in vegetable protein and calcium foods, like whole grains, sprouts, leafy greens, molasses and seafoods. Herbal programs for nails should be undertaken for at least 1 month.

❧ ESSENTIAL CATEGORIES FOR STRENGTHENING NAILS COMPOUNDS:

MINERAL-RICH HERBS	CIRCULATION STIMULATING HERBS	VITAMIN A, B & D NUTRITIVE HERBS	ESSENTIAL FATTY SOURCES	SILICA SOURCES FOR NAIL STRENGTH	ADRENAL SUPPORT SOURCES
Kelp & sea vegetables	**Hawthorn bry., lf., fl.**	Kelp & sea vegetables	**Evening primrose oil**	**Oatstraw**	**Gotu kola**
Dandelion root	Saw palmetto bry.	Dandelion root & lf.	**Bee pollen/Royal Jelly**	Horsetail	**Spirulina**
Black walnut hulls	Peppermint	**Gotu kola**	**Flax seed**	**Orange peel**	**Marshmallow root**
Nettles	**Ginkgo biloba**	**Burdock root**	Parsley root & lf.	Kelp & sea vegetables	Kelp/sea vegetables
Burdock root	Turmeric	**Siberian ginseng root**	Ginger root	Spirulina/Chlorella	**Echinacea root**
Spirulina	Ginger root	**Alfalfa/watercress**	Lemongrass	**Ginger root**	Sarsaparilla root
Horsetail	**Gotu kola**	Yellow dock root	**Borage seed**	**Burdock root**	Bilberry berry
Oats/Oatstraw	**Capsicum**	Red raspberry	White sage	**Spirulina**	**Alfalfa**
Yellow dock root	Watercress	Brewer's yeast	Black currant seed	**Eyebright**	Pau d' arco bark

❧ ESSENTIAL HERBS FOR STRENGTHENING NAILS COMPOUNDS:

PRIMARY HERBS		ASSISTING & COMPLEMENTARY HERBS		CATALYST & TRANSPORTING HERBS	
Alfalfa	Black walnut hulls	Ginkgo biloba	Fo-ti root	Evening primrose oil	Orange peel
Echinacea root	Horsetail	Saw palmetto bry.	Ashwagandha	Rose hips	Eyebright
Nettles	Burdock root	Dandelion root & lf.	Bilberry	Chamomile	Lemongrass
Sarsaparilla root	Gotu kola	Parsley rt. & lf.	Irish moss	Capsicum	Safflowers
Spirulina	Royal jelly/bee pollen	Yellow dock root	Passionflower	Peppermint	Lemon peel
Licorice root	Hawthorn bry., lf., fl.	Marshmallow root	White sage	Turmeric	Dulse
Kelp & sea vegetables	Suma root	Barley grass	Aloe vera	Ginger root	Nutritional yeast
Ginseng - all types	Siberian ginseng	Watercress	Oats/Oatstraw	Red raspberry	Borage seed
Chlorella	Panax ginseng	Chamomile	Flax seed	Rosemary	Garlic

❧ EXAMPLE FORMULAS OF STRENGTHENING NAILS COMPOUNDS:

A ZINC-RICH CAPSULE COMPOUND			(SA - 4390)	A MINERAL SPECTRUM CAPSULE COMPOUND			(SA - 3200)
Echinacea root	Gotu kola	Peppermint	Bilberry	Nettles	Dandelion root	Kelp	Garlic
Spirulina	Barley grass	Alfalfa	Yellow dock root	Irish moss	Parsley rt. & lf.	Dulse	Capsicum
				Watercress	Barley grass	Borage seed	
				Alfalfa	Yellow dock rt.		

SEE PAGE 1 FOR FORMULATING INSTRUCTIONS.

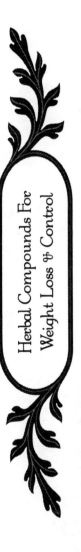

Herbal Compounds For Weight Loss & Control

eight loss is a national obsession in America. Yet 34 million American adults are obese. Another 45 million are overweight. (This doesn't count today's kids who are rapidly becoming an overweight generation.) At any given time, 25 million Americans are seriously dieting. As fried and fatty foods have increased in our diets, and the demand for physical labor has decreased, there has been a 500-800% increase in obesity in the 20th century. Wow! The answers to weight control aren't simple. Most serious dieters are able to lose about 10% of their body weight on a strict diet. Yet, typically, two-thirds of that weight is gained back within a year, and 90% is regained within five years. Even drastic diets don't make much of a difference in the long run. Most people who diet and fail, follow a "crash and burn" philosophy... crash dieting to burn calories fast, without any real change in lifestyle or eating habits. Crash diets, especially those that are almost totally fat-free, are impossible to stick with, intolerable for a normal lifestyle, and even dangerous to health because they are so unbalanced. In the end, crash dieters get burned by gaining the weight back.

Weight control is a strategy of prevention lifestyle - an attitude of keeping weight down. People today are more motivated for health reasons to control their weight. Even though Americans are always looking for the "miracle magic bullet" for slimness and body tone, everyone is slowly realizing that a good nutritional diet has to be front and center for permanent results. Weight control is a component of a sound nutritious eating plan, rather then a stab at the latest fad.

The Six Most Common Weight Control Problems

There are almost as many different weight loss problems as there are people who have them. Once you make the decision to be a thin person, analyze what your weight loss block really is. Identify your most prominent weight control problem, especially if there seems to be more than one. Best results are achieved by working on the worst problem first. As improvement is realized in the primary area, secondary problems are often overcome in the process. If lingering problems still exist, they may be addressed with additional supplementation after the first program is well underway and producing noticeable results.

After identifying, your personal difficulty, choose the weight loss products within that area that most appeal to you. Follow directions carefully. Since natural products work with the body to rebalance gland and hormone functions, product activity may be subtle and long-range for more permanent results. Overdosing is not productive, nor will it increase activity. Go slow, stick to it, improve your diet and your daily habits if necessary. Herbal therapy has shown success in treating each of the major weight loss problems. Don't weight.

Here are the six most common weight control problems. Does your weight loss difficulty fit in here?

1) **Lazy Metabolism & Thyroid Imbalance:** A poorly functioning thyroid invariably results in sluggish metabolism. Most people with underactive thyroids (hypothyroidism), have a weight problem. Factors that decrease thyroid activity and the rate at which the body burns calories, include certain nutrient deficiencies, thyroid exhaustion because of overstimulation by caffeine, sugar and other stimulants, and substances that inhibit thyroid function, like alcohol.

2) **Cellulite Deposits & Liver Malfunction:** Cellulite is a combination of fat, water and wastes. When circulation and elimination become impaired, connective tissue weakens, and unmetabolized fats and wastes become trapped just beneath the skin instead of just being eliminated by the body. Cellulite forms in areas of sluggish circulation, building up where normal cell exchange slows down.

3) **Overeating & Eating Too Much Fat:** Overeating on empty calories, like junk food, is the downfall of most dieters. Overeaters usually diet by eating one large meal a day and then try to eat nothing the rest of the time. Gnawing hunger for long periods makes the dieter irritable and miserable. This type of so-called diet taxes the willpower to the max and makes the dieter want a food binge.

4) **Poor Circulation & Low Body Energy:** For some dieters, initial weight loss is quite rapid, but then a plateau is reached and further weight loss becomes difficult, because restricted food intake slows down metabolism, helps convert stored fat to energy, and energizes circulation to help a dieter get over this plateau.

5) **Poor Elimination-Detoxing The Colon, Bowel, Kidney & Bladder:** Today, people make rich foods like red meats, rich cheeses, cream, butters and sweets, once reserved for festive occasions, a part of every meal. These foods are poor nutrition providers and difficult to eliminate. The environmental pollutants, pesticides, and chemical by-products in these foods also obstruct body processes. Clogged elimination systems especially impede the weight loss process.

6) **Sugar Craving & Body Sugar Imbalance:** Sugar provides a temporary "insulin rush," but is then followed by food cravings caused by low blood sugar levels. After a sugar binge, raised insulin levels mean more calories are transformed into fat. A low glycemic diet is a good answer for sugar cravers. It means fewer calories are turned into fat and more are burned for energy.

Weight Control After 40

There's no doubt about it. Weight loss gets more difficult after 40. Everybody goes through a change of life. The hormone changes of our middle years affect our body shapes, too .... for both men and women. One of the problems people face as they reach their late 40's and 50's is a disconcerting body thickening and a slow, upward rise in body weight. This seems to happen with everybody, even for people who have always been slender, who have a good diet, and who exercise moderately. Changes in estrogen levels for women and testosterone levels for men, mean that our body chemistry is in transition. Clearly, metabolic rates slow as we age, so it takes food longer to digest, and more of it goes into storage. People who could always lose weight when they were younger just by going on a crash diet for a weekend or a week whenever they gained a few pounds, find that strategy doesn't work anymore. Most of us also become less physically active as we age which leads to muscle loss, an important factor for a youthful body.

Weight control solutions have to be approached differently when your metabolism slows down. Just eating all the low fat or even no fat foods available today doesn't seem to make a difference. We tend to think we're getting a free ride, and eat too many of them, or we eat too much of something else to fill up the hunger hole left by not eating any fat. Even the free ride isn't free because most of the low fat foods have plenty of calories.

I have been working for several years to develop natural weight control techniques for people trying to maintain healthy body weight and tone after their metabolism changes. The program is showing promise and results. For success after 40, begin with two basic weight loss starting points: 1) Improve body chemistry at the gland and hormone level. 2) Re-establish better, long-lasting metabolic rates.

What about cellulite? Are there natural methods for overcoming this unsightly scourge?

The vast majority of Americans have cellulite. Many people don't need to lose weight as much as they need to lose cellulite. Eighty-six percent of U.S. women over the age of 20 have cellulite deposits on the hips and thighs. More than 50% of U.S. men over forty have cellulite deposits on their torso "love handles."

Cellulite is a combination of fat, water, and wastes. When the body's circulation and elimination become impaired, connective tissue loses its strength, and unmetabolized fats and wastes become trapped just beneath the skin instead of being expelled through body elimination. Over a period of time the wastes enlarge, harden and push through spaces in the connective fiber bands that anchor down skin. They cause bulges which appear as dimples, and form the puckering, distorted skin effect we know as cellulite. Definite skin undulations become apparent as cellulite layers build up. Unfortunately, this kind of fatty build up is not attached, so it is extremely difficult for the body to process through its elimination channels. Cellulite forms in areas of sluggish circulation, building up where normal cell exchange slows down. While fat is a generalized condition, cellulite deposits settle mainly on the hips, buttocks, thighs and knees. When regular fat is squeezed the skin appears smooth, but cellulite skin ripples like an orange peel, or has the texture of cottage cheese.

Herbs are good choices for improving cellulitic tissue tone, because they work at the cause of the problem, on body chemistry and metabolism, rather than on the external effect. The skin is a very complex organ. Regeneration of toned, elastic skin tissue works from the inside out. Man-made chemicals are rejected by the body's system functions, but plant-derived substances can pass through the powerful metabolic defenses of the skin's upper layers. Herbal sources of bioflavonoids and vitamin C help preserve vein and capillary integrity, encourage new collagen formation, and make it more difficult for cellulite to begin. Herbal support can help process fats through the system more normally, instead of being thrown off or stored as fatty "cottage cheese."

Weight loss is not easy in today's lifestyle. Reaching your ideal weight is a victory. Keeping it requires vigilance, especially in light of today's processed food products and fast lifestyles. Herbs can help your weight loss program be successful on a long-term basis, and without side effects.

✤FORMULAS FOR WEIGHT CONTROL PROBLEMS ALSO HELP IN THE FOLLOWING CONDITIONS:

•Weight Loss & Weight Control   •Adult Acne   •High Blood Pressure   •Boosting Energy   •Sluggish Thyroid & Poor Metabolism   •High Cholesterol   •Sluggish Circulation   •Cellulite   •Diabetic Obesity   •High Blood Pressure Obesity   •Bloating & Excess Fluid Retention   •Mental Exhaustion   •Liver Malfunction   •Constipation

✤COMPOUNDS FOR FORMULATION SHOULD INCLUDE:

• Formulas for addressing the six most common weight loss problems
• Formulas for controlling weight gain after metabolism change
• Formulas for controlling cellulite

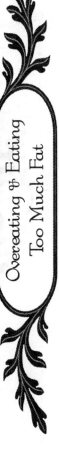

Overeating & Eating Too Much Fat

Weight Loss & Control

No matter what weight loss techniques or supplements you choose, the importance of cutting back on fat cannot be overstated. You can eat two to three times more volume of low-fat foods than high fat foods, and still lose weight. The average overweight person often has too high blood sugar and too low fat levels. This causes constant hunger - the delicate balance between fat storage and fat utilization is upset, and the body's ability to use fat for energy decreases. Overeating on empty calories like junk foods particularly aggravates this imbalance. Fat becomes non-moving energy, and fat cells become fat storage depots. Saturated fats are the hardest for the liver to metabolize. Stay away from them to control fat storage. Water can get you over weight loss plateaus. Drink it, and all liquids before eating to suppress appetite. Calorie burning, thermogenic herbs have a double-whammy for weight control; use enzyme therapy and thermogenic stimulants for calorie-burning.

❧ ESSENTIAL CATEGORIES FOR AN EFFECTIVE OVEREATING COMPOUND:

THERMOGENIC CALORIE BURNING HERBS	APPETITE SUPPRESSANT HERBS	HERBAL ENERGIZERS	BLOOD SUGAR STABILIZING HERBS	CIRCULATION STIMULATING HERBS	BODY CLEANSING HERBS
Kola nut	**Chickweed**	**Kola nut**	**Licorice root**	**Hawthorn lf. flr. & bry.**	Rhubarb root
Ephedra	**Barley grass/Spirulina**	**Bee pollen**	**Panax ginseng**	Safflowers	Irish moss
White willow bark	Fenugreek seed	**Gotu kola**	**Barley grass/Spirulina**	**Gotu kola**	**Cascara sagrada**
Kelp/sea vegetable	Oats/Oatstraw	**Sarsaparilla root**	Lecithin	**Ginkgo biloba**	Psyllium husks
Nettles	Kelp/sea vegetables	**Siberian ginseng root**	**Gotu kola**	Turmeric	**Butternut bark**
Parsley root & lf.	**Chlorella**	Hawthorn lf. flr. & bry.	Burdock root	Kelp	Apple pectin
Sarsaparilla root	**Fennel seed**	Barley grass	**Sarsaparilla root**	**Ginger root**	**Barberry**
Garcinia gambogia	**Alfalfa**	Suma root	Gymnema sylvestre	**Capsicum**	**Aloe vera**
Sida cordifolia	Flax seed	Guarana seed	Wild yam root	**Siberian ginseng root**	**Black walnut**

❧ ESSENTIAL HERBS FOR AN EFFECTIVE OVEREATING COMPOUND:

PRIMARY HERBS		ASSISTING & COMPLEMENTARY HERBS		CATALYST & TRANSPORTING HERBS	
Bee pollen	Nettles	Ginkgo biloba	Ephedra	Capsicum	Apple pectin
Royal Jelly	Dandelion root/lf.	Ginger root	Fo-Ti root	Turmeric	Psyllium husks
Barley grass	Chlorella	Watercress	Wild yam root	Orange peel	Rhubarb root
Gotu kola	Kelp/sea vegetables	Borage seed	Cascara sagrada	Lemongrass	Peppermint
Siberian ginseng root	Hawthorn lf. flr. & bry.	Chamomile	Guarana seed	Rosemary	White willow bark
Licorice root	Flax seed	Black walnut	Kola nut	Barberry	Lecithin
Sarsaparilla Rt.	Panax ginseng	Suma root	Fenugreek seed	Safflowers	Butternut bark
Spirulina	Chickweed	Oats/Oatstraw	Parsley lf., rt. & lf.	Acerola cherry	Irish moss
Burdock root	Alfalfa	Fennel seed	Aloe vera	Echinacea root	Gymnema sylvestre

❧ EXAMPLE FORMULAS OF OVEREATING WEIGHT LOSS COMPOUNDS:

AN ENERGY GREEN DRINK COMPOUND			(SA - 8150)	AN APPETITE CAPSULE COMPOUND			(D - 1310)
Barley grass	Chlorella	Gotu kola		Chickweed	Fennel seed	Lecithin	
Alfalfa	Dandelion root/lf.	Apple pectin		Gotu kola	Hawthorn lf. flr. & bry.	Ginger root	
Bee pollen	Dulse	Apple juice		Kelp	Safflowers	Spirulina	
Acerola cherry	Licorice root				Black walnut		

AN ENERGY GREEN DRINK COMPOUND			
Oats/Oatstraw			
Siberian ginseng root			
Sarsaparilla Rt.			
Spirulina			

SEE PAGE 1 FOR FORMULATING INSTRUCTIONS.

Lazy Metabolism & Thyroid Imbalance

WEIGHT LOSS & CONTROL

The thyroid gland produces hormones which profoundly influence the body's metabolic rate. A poorly functioning thyroid invariably results in sluggish metabolism Most people with underactive thyroids (hypothyroidism), have a weight problem. Factors that decrease thyroid activity and the rate at which the body burns calories, include certain nutrient deficiencies, thyroid exhaustion by overstimulation by caffeine, sugar and other stimulants, and substances that inhibit thyroid function, like alcohol. Herbal therapy may be helpful to jumpstart a healthy change for permanent weight control. Herbal supplements, like sea plants, rich in iodine and potassium, are a good choice to help metabolism and thyroid function. In addition to a mineral-rich oral combination, evening primrose oil boosts metabolism even more. A hot seaweed bath with thyroid stimulating ocean nutrients like kelp, kombu, bladderwrack, dulse and sea grasses is also effective.

❧ ESSENTIAL CATEGORIES FOR LAZY METABOLISM & THYROID IMBALANCE COMPOUNDS:

HERBAL METABOLIC STIMULATORS	IODINE & POTASSIUM SOURCE HERBS	ESSENTIAL FATTY ACID SOURCES	HERBAL ENERGIZERS FOR CALORIE BURNING	B VITAMIN & LIVER SUPPORT HERBS	ADRENAL SUPPORT HERBS
Nettles	**Spirulina**	**Bee pollen/Royal Jelly**	Kola nut	**Dandelion rt. & lf.**	**Astragalus**
Mullein	**Kelp/sea vegetables**	Evening primrose oil	Bee pollen	**Red raspberry**	Bee pollen
Watercress	**Parsley root & lf.**	Flax seed	Gotu kola	**Fenugreek seed**	Uva ursi
Parsley root & lf.	Alfalfa	**Black currant seed**	Ginsengs - all types	**Watercress**	**Kelp/sea vegetables**
Licorice root	Nettles	Parsley root & lf.	**Siberian ginseng root**	Lobelia	Irish moss
Cardamom	Chlorella	**Ginger root**	Guarana seed	Parsley root & lf.	**Sarsaparilla root**
Kelp/sea vegetables	**Barley grass**	Lemongrass	Barley grass	Dong quai	Saw palmetto bry.
Mustard seed	**Watercress**	**Borage seed**	Ginkgo biloba	**Royal Jelly/Bee pollen**	Fo-Ti root
Sarsaparilla root	Borage Seed	White Sage	Ginger root	**Burdock root**	**Siberian ginseng root**

❧ ESSENTIAL HERBS FOR LAZY METABOLISM & THYROID IMBALANCE COMPOUNDS:

PRIMARY HERBS		ASSISTING & COMPLEMENTARY HERBS		CATALYST & TRANSPORTING HERBS	
Burdock root	Royal Jelly/Bee pollen	Parsley root & lf.	Spirulina	Lemongrass	Lobelia
Echinacea root	Licorice root	Uva ursi	Uva ursi	Flax seed	Dong quai root
Dandelion ft. & lf.	Gotu kola	Astragalus	Astragalus	Ginkgo biloba	Carrot powder
Fo-Ti root	Kelp/sea vegetables	Suma root	Evening primrose oil	Thyme	White Sage
Gotu kola	Siberian ginseng	Hawthorn lf., bry. & flr.	Barley grass	Guarana seed	Black currant seed
Black cohosh root	Sarsaparilla root	Ginger root	Rose hips	Saw palmetto bry.	Borage seed
Irish moss	Panax ginseng	Fenugreek seed	Watercress	Capsicum	Mustard seed
Alfalfa	Chlorella	Red raspberry	Mullein	Vitamin C pwr.	Bilberry
Nettles	Ephedra leaf	Flax seed	Bladderwrack	Kola nut	Cardamom

❧ EXAMPLE FORMULAS OF LAZY METABOLISM & THYROID IMBALANCE COMPOUNDS:

A THYROID-STIMULATING CAPSULE COMPOUND			(D - 4150)
Parsley root & lf.	Mullein	Spirulina	
Watercress	Lobelia	Carrot powder	
Ginkgo biloba			

AN ADRENAL STIMULATING, STRENGTHENING COMPOUND			(B - 1000)
Licorice root	Uva ursi	Vitamin C pwr.	
Sarsaparilla root	Irish moss	Rose hips	Bee pollen
Bladderwrack	Ginger root	Astragalus	Mustard seed
		Capsicum	Cardamom

SEE PAGE 1 FOR FORMULATING INSTRUCTIONS.

136

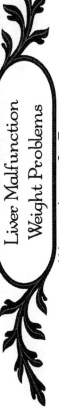

Liver Malfunction
Weight Problems

WEIGHT LOSS & CONTROL

Liver malfunction is directly connected to sugar metabolism as a cause of overweight. When the liver is working poorly, the blood becomes sugar-saturated, and stresses the pancreas, inviting diabetes (high blood sugar). Hypoglycemic (low blood sugar) attacks are due not only to improper insulin response, but also to a sluggish liver. Cellulite, a result of poorly metabolized fats, especially saturated fats, is a weight problem compounded by weak liver function. (See page 142 on cellulite problems in this section.) A liver cleansing formula with "bitters" herbs stimulates the liver to metabolize fats properly. I also recommend adding milk thistle seed extract for long term liver support, because it's gentle, and optimizes other liver cleansing choices. Other liver supports to help fat metabolism include bee pollen and royal jelly for amino acid and B vitamin support and bioflavonoid-rich herbs to help produce healthy collagen and tone skin tissue that's been affected by cellulite.

❧ ESSENTIAL CATEGORIES FOR EFFECTIVE LIVER MALFUNCTION COMPOUNDS:

LIVER CLEANSING & SUPPORT HERBS	FAT METABOLIZING LIVER HERBS	VITAMIN B/AMINO ACID SUPPORT HERBS	VITAMIN C/BIOFLAVONOID SUPPORT HERBS	WATER RETENTION BALANCERS	CIRCULATION STIMULANTS
Oregon grape root	Dandelion root & lf.	**Royal Jelly/Bee pollen**	**Bee pollen/Royal Jelly**	**Fenugreek seed**	**Ginger root**
Goldenseal root	**Fennel seed**	**Dandelion root**	**Red raspberry**	Kelp & sea vegetables	**Bilberry**
Dandelion root & lf.	**Fenugreek seed**	Thyme	**Hibiscus**	**Black cohosh root**	**Capsicum**
Licorice root	**Kelp & sea vegetables**	**Kelp & sea vegetables**	Hawthorn bry.,.lf., flr.	**Poria mushroom**	**Kelp/sea vegetables**
Milk thistle seed	**Licorice root**	**Parsley root & lf**	Lemon peel	**Cornsilk**	**Turmeric**
Red sage	Goldenseal root	**Spirulina**	**Bilberry bry.**	**Fennel seed**	Green tea
Aloe vera	**Chickweed**	Burdock root	Rose hips	Gotu kola	Peppermint
Cardamom	Poria mushroom	**Gotu kola**	**White pine bark**	Bilberry	**Kola nut**
Yellow dock root	Gotu kola	**Ginger root**	Ginkgo biloba lf.	Uva ursi	Ginkgo biloba

❧ ESSENTIAL HERBS FOR EFFECTIVE LIVER MALFUNCTION COMPOUNDS:

PRIMARY HERBS		ASSISTING & COMPLEMENTARY HERBS		CATALYST & TRANSPORTING HERBS	
Burdock root	Oregon grape rt.	Uva ursi	Corn silk	Fenugreek seed	Thyme
Nettles	Goldenseal root	Aloe vera	Green tea	Stevia	Bilberry bry.
Dandelion root & lf.	Wild yam root	Red sage	Milk thistle seed	Turmeric	Poria mushroom
Sarsaparilla root	Gotu kola	Black cohosh root	Cardamom pods	Green tea leaf	Ginger root
Spirulina	Royal jelly/Bee pollen	White pine bark	Red raspberry	Senna leaf	Hibiscus
Licorice root	Hawthorn bry., lf., flr.	Ginkgo biloba	Fennel seed	Barberry bark	White sage
Kelp & sea vegetables	Evening primrose oil	Yellow dock root	Alfalfa	Capsicum	Rose hips
Parsley root & lf.	Siberian ginseng	Kola nut	Flax seed oil	Peppermint	Wild cherry bk.
Chlorella/Barley grass	Ginkgo biloba lf.	Chickweed	Watercress	Lemon peel	Flax seed

❧ EXAMPLE FORMULAS OF EFFECTIVE LIVER MALFUNCTION COMPOUNDS:

A BITTERS & LEMON CLEANSE EXTRACT COMPOUND		(CD - 4710)	A LIVER CLEANSING & SUPPORT FLUSHING COMPOUND		(CD - 5780)
Oregon grape root	Senna leaf	Peppermint	Dandelion rt. & lf.	Pau d' arco bk.	Hibiscus
Gentian root	Dandelion root	Honey	Watercress	Hyssop	White sage
Cardamom pods			Yellow dock root	Parsley rt. & lf.	Stevia leaf
Lemon peel				Oregon grape rt.	
				Red sage	
				Licorice root	
				Milk thistle seed	

SEE PAGE 1 FOR FORMULATING INSTRUCTIONS.

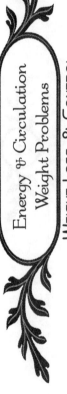

Energy & Circulation
Weight Problems

Weight Loss & Control

For some dieters, initial weight loss is quite rapid but then a plateau is reached and further weight loss becomes difficult because restricted food intake slows down metabolism. Sluggish circulation is also at the root of high blood pressure, varicose veins and blood sugar balance, things we know to be involved in weight control problems. Herbal stimulants, along with exercise, can help to reactivate metabolism, help convert stored fat to energy, and energize circulation to help a dieter get over this plateau. I also recommend a simple HAWTHORN BERRY, LEAF AND FLOWER EXTRACT as needed for circulation activation. Other energy and circulation supplements include: CoQ$_{10}$, about 60mg daily for antioxidant enzyme activity, the amino acids L-Glutamine and L-Carnitine for energy and body flow, bee pollen and royal jelly for B complex vitamins. Daily exercise and bodywork techniques that include alternating hot and cool showers provide noticeable benefits.

ESSENTIAL CATEGORIES FOR EXTRA ENERGY & CIRCULATION COMPOUNDS:

GENTLE HERBAL ENERGIZERS	MILD CIRCULATION STIMULATING HERBS	AMINO ACID & ANTIOXIDANT SOURCES	B VITAMIN & ENZYME SOURCES	BLOOD SUGAR STABILIZERS	ADRENAL SUPPORT HERBS
Schizandra berry	**Hawthorn lf. & bry.**	**Bee pollen/Royal jelly**	**Bee pollen/Royal Jelly**	**Panax ginseng**	**Sarsaparilla root**
Alfalfa/Spirulina	Ginger root	**Panax/Siber.ginseng**	**Fenugreek seed**	**Siberian ginseng rt.**	**Siberian ginseng**
Suma root	Kola nut	Miso	**Dandelion root**	**Fenugreek seed**	**Bee pollen/Royal Jelly**
Aralia root	Capsicum	**Ginger root**	Red raspberry	Pau d' arco bark	Bilberry
Guarana seed	Ginkgo biloba	**Barley grass/Alfalfa**	**Parsley root & lf.**	Burdock root	Kelp & sea plants
Fo-ti root	**Siberian ginseng**	Ginkgo biloba	Burdock root	**Licorice root**	**Licorice root**
Panax ginseng root	Butcher's broom	Chickweed	Thyme	Aloe vera juice	Alfalfa
Gotu kola	Cinnamon	**Gotu kola**	Dong quai	**Dandelion root & lf.**	**Gotu kola**
Astragalus	Yerba mate tea	**Suma root**	Watercress	**Gymnema sylvestre**	**Bladderwrack**

ESSENTIAL HERBS FOR EXTRA ENERGY & CIRCULATION COMPOUNDS:

PRIMARY HERBS		ASSISTING & COMPLEMENTARY HERBS		CATALYST & TRANSPORTING HERBS	
Siberian ginseng	Ginkgo biloba	Fo-ti root	Wild yam root	Bilberry	Aloe vera juice
Hawthorn lf. & bry.	Dandelion root & lf.	Royal jelly	Evening primrose oil	Green tea	Rosemary
Spirulina	Licorice root	Schizandra berry	Prince ginseng root	Ginger root	Parsley root & lf.
Bee pollen	Kelp & sea plants	Bladderwrack	Black cohosh	Capsicum	Cinnamon
Chlorella	Dong Quai	Burdock root	Red raspberry	Ephedra leaf	Fennel seed
Sarsaparilla root	Astragalus	Ashwagandha	Pau d' arco bark	Butcher's broom	Watercress
Gotu kola	Panax ginseng root	Chickweed	St. John's wort	Gymnema sylvestre	Thyme
Barley grass	Suma root	Fenugreek seed	Irish moss	Miso	Stevia leaf
Alfalfa	Guarana seed	Kola nut	Aralia root	Cinnamon	Yerba mate tea

EXAMPLE FORMULAS OF EXTRA ENERGY & CIRCULATION COMPOUNDS:

A RAINFOREST ENERGY SUPPORT FORMULA (E - 6470)			A GINSENG-BASED ENERGY & CIRCULATION FORMULA (E - 2510)		
Guarana seed	Suma root	Yerba mate tea	Stevia leaf	Bee pollen	Panax ginseng	Alfalfa
Kola nut		Cinnamon		Siberian ginseng root	Aralia root	Dong quai root
				Gotu kola	Suma root	Spirulina
				Fo-ti root		

138

SEE PAGE 1 FOR FORMULATING INSTRUCTIONS.

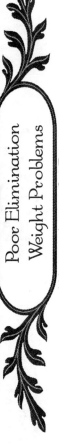

Poor Elimination
Weight Problems

WEIGHT LOSS & CONTROL

In times past, rich foods like red meats, rich cheeses, cream, butter, sugars and sweets were reserved for festive occasions. Today, people make them a part of every meal. The fat and sugar that makes these foods delicious, are both poor nutrition providers and difficult to eliminate. Environmental agents like pollutants, pesticides, and chemical by-products that appear in many dense foods also obstruct body processes. Nowhere are these factors more frustrating than when they impede the weight loss process. Herbal cleansing supplements can help reactivate normal elimination and body functions and aid in the weight loss process. In addition to the oral suggestions below, I recommend a **POUNDS OFF BATH** (with jaborandi, thyme, angelica root, elder flowers, pennyroyal and orange peel) that can begin a cleansing sweat in about 15 minutes. Take it once a week to enhance your ability to eliminate toxins easily.

❧ ESSENTIAL CATEGORIES FOR POOR ELIMINATION WEIGHT LOSS COMPOUNDS:

COLON & BOWEL FLUSHING HERBS	DIURETIC, FLUSHING HERBS	GREEN SUPERFOODS FOR ELIMINATION	FAT METABOLIZING HERBS	ESSENTIAL FATTY ACID SOURCE HERBS	GLAND ACTIVITY NORMALIZERS
Flax seed	**Fennel seed**	**Barley grass**	**Fenugreek seed**	**Evening primrose oil**	**Ginseng - all types**
Slippery elm	**Cleavers**	**Watercress**	**Gotu kola**	**Flax seed**	**Schizandra berry**
Senna leaf	**Parsley lf. & rt.**	**Kelp & sea vegetables**	Black cohosh	**Borage seed**	Suma root
Licorice root	Horsetail	**Spirulina**	**Chickweed**	**Black current seed**	Black cohosh root
Butternut bark	**Chickweed**	**Parsley lf.**	**Fennel seed**	Chlorella	Burdock root
Cascara	**Uva ursi**	Chlorella	**Red sage**	Spirulina	**Fo-Ti root**
Rhubarb root	**Kelp & sea vegetables**	Nettles	Goldenseal root	Pumpkin seed	**Gotu kola**
Barberry bark	**Juniper berries**	**Aloe vera**	Red sage	Safflower oil	Ashwagandha
Psyllium husks	Red clover	**Alfalfa**	Dandelion root & leaf	Kelp & sea vegetables	**Bee pollen**

❧ ESSENTIAL HERBS FOR POOR ELIMINATION WEIGHT LOSS COMPOUNDS:

PRIMARY HERBS		ASSISTING & COMPLEMENTARY HERBS		CATALYST & TRANSPORTING HERBS	
Flax seed	Spirulina	Ginseng - all types	Psyllium husks	Capsicum	Acidophilus
Fennel seed	Evening primrose oil	Rhubarb root	Gotu kola	Ginger root	Slippery elm
Fenugreek seed	Kelp & sea vegetables	Goldenseal root	Horsetail	Ashwagandha	Fo-Ti root
Dandelion root & leaf	Barley grass	Suma root	Cleavers	Miso	Pumpkin seed
	Uva ursi	Red clover		Bee pollen	Lemon peel
				Quassia chips	
		Panax ginseng		Borage seed	
		Schizandra berry		Irish moss	
		Watercress		Siberian ginseng	
		Black cohosh		Spearmint	
		Barberry bark		Black currant seed	
		Nettles		Safflower oil	
		Licorice root		Hibiscus	
		Red sage			
		Burdock root			

❧ EXAMPLE FORMULAS FOR POOR ELIMINATION WEIGHT LOSS COMPOUNDS:

A LEAN & CLEAN DIET SUPPORT CAPSULE FORMULA		(D - 6450)
Flax seed	Uva ursi	Hibiscus
Fennel seed	Parsley leaf & rt.	Burdock root
	Chickweed	Red clover
	Senna leaf	
	Lemon peel	
	Cleavers	

A FIBER & HERBS COLON CLEANSING FORMULA		(CD - 2350)
Butternut bark	Psyllium husks	Cayenne
Cascara	Barberry bark	Irish moss
Rhubarb root	Fennel seed	
	Ginger root	
	Licorice root	

SEE PAGE 1 FOR FORMULATING INSTRUCTIONS.

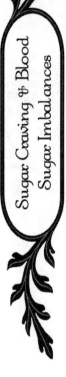

Sugar Craving & Blood Sugar Imbalances

Weight Loss & Control

Some dieters drastically lower fats, but then replace the fats with empty carbohydrates, like sugar and starches. Sugar binging is a common result of the overeating/non-eating diet pattern. Sugar provides a temporary "insulin rush," but then is followed by a powerful craving for more food, as blood sugar drops. (Sugar bingers routinely eat 60 to 70% more calories the following meal.) Few calories are burned after a sugar binge because raised insulin turns more calories into fat. Sugar dieters may even steadily gain weight, because the foods they do eat often contain more calories than 3 or 4 times that of healthy, whole foods they might normally consume. A low glycemic diet is a good answer for sugar cravers; it keeps insulin levels low so fewer calories are turned into fat and more are burned for energy. Low glycemic foods, exercise and certain herbal supplements can also optimize brain biochemistry, so the dieter feels more comfortable and can diet without binging.

❧ ESSENTIAL CATEGORIES FOR SUGAR CRAVING & IMBALANCE COMPOUNDS:

LOW BLOOD SUGAR BALANCING HERBS	HIGH BLOOD SUGAR BALANCING HERBS	METABOLISM STIMULATING HERBS	HIGH FIBER HERB SOURCES	BODY CHEMISTRY & LIVER SUPPORT	ADRENAL SUPPORT HERBS
Licorice root	**Cedar bry.**	**Bee pollen/Royal Jelly**	**Barley grass**	**Cedar berries**	**Sarsaparilla root**
Barley grass	**Dandelion root & lf.**	**Capsicum**	**Fennel seed**	**Gotu kola**	**Siberian ginseng**
Alfalfa	**Elecampane**	**Mustard seed**	**Oats/Oatstraw**	**Wild yam root**	**Bee pollen/Royal Jelly**
Cedar bry.	**Wild yam root**	**Ginger root**	**Flax seed**	Spirulina/Barley grass	Bilberry
Spirulina	**Mullein**	**Cinnamon**	Alfalfa	**Licorice root**	Irish moss
Ginseng - all types	Kelp & sea plants	Ginkgo biloba	Licorice root	Suma root	Licorice root
Gymnema sylvestre	**Licorice root**	Cloves	**Aloe vera**	**Dandelion root & lf.**	Alfalfa
Gotu kola	Bilberry	**Gotu kola**	**Guar gum**	**Milk thistle seed**	Gotu kola
Guar gum	**Gymnema sylvestre**	Horseradish rt.	**Psyllium seed**	Uva ursi	**Bladderwrack**

❧ ESSENTIAL HERBS FOR SUGAR CRAVING & IMBALANCE COMPOUNDS:

PRIMARY HERBS		ASSISTING & COMPLEMENTARY HERBS		CATALYST & TRANSPORTING HERBS	
Panax ginseng	Ginkgo biloba	Fo-ti root	Wild yam root	Mullein	Elecampame rot
Bee pollen/Royal Jelly	Dandelion root & lf.	Juniper berry	Slippery elm	Green tea	Red raspberry
Spirulina	Licorice root	Psyllium seed	Fennel seed	Ginger root	Parsley root & lf.
Chlorella	Kelp & sea plants	Bladderwrack	Mustard seed	Capsicum	Horseradish rt
Sarsaparilla root	Siberian ginseng root	Burdock root	Uva ursi	Milk thistle seed	Bilberry
Gotu kola	Elecampane	Garlic	Mullein	Aloe vera	Watercress
Barley grass	Pau d' arco	Chickweed	Oats/Oatstraw	Gymnema sylvestre	Cloves
Alfalfa	Suma root	Flax seed	Irish moss	Bayberry bark	Stevia leaf
Astragalus	Cedar berry	Guar gum	Cedar berry	Cinnamon	Yarrow

❧ EXAMPLE FORMULAS OF SUGAR CRAVING & IMBALANCE COMPOUNDS:

A SUGAR STABILIZING FORMULA FOR HIGH BLOOD SUGAR (b - 2850)		
Cedar berry	Licorice root	Wild yam root	Horseradish rt
Dandelion root	Mullein	Uva ursi	Bilberry
Elecampane	Guar gum	Kelp	Capsicum
Spirulina			

A SUGAR STABILIZING FORMULA FOR LOW BLOOD SUGAR (b - 2800)		
Licorice root	Spirulina	Barley grass	Horseradish rt.
Dandelion root	Gotu kola	Guar gum	Suma root
Alfalfa	Wild yam		
Cedar berry			

SEE PAGE 1 FOR FORMULATING INSTRUCTIONS.

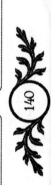

Note: All sugar cravers can use a panax ginseng and licorice root extract in water to balance blood sugar levels.

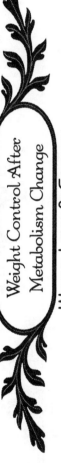

Weight Control After Metabolism Change

WEIGHT LOSS & CONTROL

As we age, our bodies go through major metabolism changes...for most of us that means a slowing of our metabolic rate. So it takes food longer to digest, and more of it goes into storage. But a lot of people don't realize that hormone changes during our middle years affect our body shapes, too... men as well as women. Changes in estrogen levels for women and testosterone levels for men change our body chemistry, so we need to make both diet and lifestyle changes if we're going to maintain slimness and body tone. Most of us also become less physically active as we age, which leads to muscle loss, and lean muscle tissue is very important to a youthful body. Clearly, we need to approach weight control differently than we have all our lives, but the good news is that we can do something about our weight, our body tone and our looks. Herbs offer good choices for keeping our bodies in the manner to which we are accustomed. Herbal weight loss combinations can help especially after forty.

✱ ESSENTIAL CATEGORIES FOR WEIGHT CONTROL AFTER FORTY COMPOUNDS:

THERMOGENESIS STIMULATING HERBS	LIVER SUPPORT HERBS	BODY CHEMISTRY BALANCERS	B VITAMIN & EFA SOURCES	CIRCULATION BOOSTERS & ENERGIZERS	APPETITE SUPPRESSANT HERBS
Green tea	**Oregon grape root**	**Bee pollen/Royal jelly**	**Evening primrose oil**	**Hawthorn lf. & bry.**	**Chickweed**
Spirulina	**Goldenseal root**	**Panax/Siber.ginseng**	**Flax seed**	**Ginger root**	**Licorice root**
Mustard seed	**Dandelion root & lf.**	Miso	**Borage seed**	Kola nut	**Fennel seed**
Ginger root	**Licorice root**	Ginger root	**Royal Jelly/Bee pollen**	**Capsicum**	Kola nut
Guarana seed	Milk thistle seed	**Barley grass/Alfalfa**	**Fenugreek seed**	**Ginkgo biloba**	Spirulina
green tea	Red sage	Ginkgo biloba	**Spirulina**	**Siberian ginseng**	**Guarana seed**
Ephedra or Sida cord.	Wild yam root	**Chickweed**	Burdock root	**Butcher's broom**	Ephedra leaf
Gotu kola	Cardamom	**Gotu kola**	Dandelion rt. & lf.	Cinnamon	**Gotu kola**
Kelp & sea plants	**Burdock root**	Suma root	Kelp & sea vegetables	Bilberry	**Kelp**

✱ ESSENTIAL HERBS FOR WEIGHT CONTROL AFTER FORTY COMPOUNDS:

PRIMARY HERBS		ASSISTING & COMPLEMENTARY HERBS		CATALYST & TRANSPORTING HERBS	
Siberian ginseng	Ginkgo biloba	Fo-ti root	Wild yam root	Bilberry	Butcher's broom
Hawthorn lf. & bry.	Dandelion root & lf.	Ephedra leaf/Sida cord.	Parsley lf. & rt.	Flax seed	Rosemary
Spirulina	Licorice root	Red sage	Senna lf.	Ginger root	Chickweed
Bee pollen/Royal jelly	Kelp & sea plants	Milk thistle seed	Black cohosh	Capsicum	Gymnema sylvestre
Chlorella	Ephedra leaf	Burdock root	Mustard seed	Dulse	Fennel seed
Sarsaparilla root	Guarana seed	Evening primrose oil	Oregon grape root	Borage seed	Lemon peel
Gotu kola	Panax ginseng root	Chickweed	Goldenseal root	Hibiscus	Cardamom
Barley grass	Kukicha twig/Green tea	Fenugreek seed	Suma root	Miso	Papaya powder
Alfalfa	Green tea	Kola nut	Red clover	Cinnamon	Lecithin

✱ EXAMPLE FORMULAS OF WEIGHT CONTROL AFTER FORTY COMPOUNDS:

A THERMOGENESIS STIMULATING EXTRACT FORMULA		(D - 4448)
Sida cordifolia	Spirulina	Ginger root
(or Ephedra leaf)	Bee pollen	Capsicum
Kukicha twig	Hibiscus	Ginkgo biloba
Green tea		

A THERMOGENESIS STIMULATING EXTRACT FORMULA	(D - 4448)
Sida cordifolia	Guarana seed
(or Ephedra leaf)	Panax ginseng
Kukicha twig	
Green tea	

A DIETING TEA TO RAISE & NORMALIZE METABOLISM		(D - 6450)
Flax seed	Senna lf.	Gymnema sylvestre.	Lemon peel
Fennel seed	Fenugreek seed	Burdock root	Hibiscus
Gotu kola	Parsley lf.	Red clover	Kelp
Uva ursi	Green tea lf.	Bladderwrack	Dulse

SEE PAGE 1 FOR FORMULATING INSTRUCTIONS.

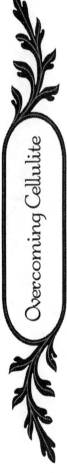

Overcoming Cellulite

WEIGHT LOSS & CONTROL

The vast majority of Americans have cellulite. Eighty-six percent of U.S. women have cellulite deposits on the hips and thighs. More than 50% of U.S. men over forty have cellulite deposits on their torso "love handles." Cellulite is a combination of fat, water, and wastes. When the body's circulation and elimination become impaired, connective tissue loses its strength, and unmetabolized fats and wastes become trapped beneath the skin instead of being expelled through body elimination. Hormones, mainly estrogen, play a part in forming cellulite. Men get less cellulite because of their lower estrogen levels, and differences in body structure. Women have more natural fatty areas for cellulite to accumulate, as on the hips, thighs and buttocks, and the outer layer of a woman's skin is thinner than a man's. Herbs are good choices for improving cellulitic tissue tone, because they work on body chemistry and metabolism, rather than on the external effect

❧ ESSENTIAL CATEGORIES FOR OVERCOMING CELLULITE COMPOUNDS:

LIVER SUPPORT & DETOXIFIERS	FAT METABOLIZING HERBS	SILICA SOURCES FOR CONNECTIVE TISSUE	CIRCULATION STIMULANT HERBS	VITAMIN C & BIOFLAVONOID SOURCES	WATER RETENTION BALANCERS
Fenugreek seed	**Green tea**	**Kelp/Sea vegetables**	**Ginger root**	**Bee pollen/Royal Jelly**	**Fenugreek seed**
Goldenseal root	Sarsaparilla root	Horsetail	**Juniper berry**	**Aloe vera**	Kelp/Sea vegetables
Dandelion root & lf.	**Peppermint**	Orange peel	**Capsicum**	**Chlorella**	**Black cohosh root**
Licorice root	Watercress	**Ginger root**	**Kelp/sea vegetables**	Hawthorn bry.,lf., flr.	**Poria mushroom**
Milk thistle seed	Mullein	**Spirulina/Barley grass**	**Dong qual**	Parsley root & lf.	Cornsilk
Red sage	Parsley root & lf.	Echinacea	Hawthorn lf. & bry.	**Billberry bry.**	**Fennel seed**
Bilberry	Lobelia	**Eyebright**	Peppermint	**Rose hips**	Gotu kola
Watercress	**Gotu kola**	**Burdock root**	**Kola nut**	**Red clover**	Bilberry
Turmeric	**Kelp & sea plants**	**Oatstraw**	Ginkgo biloba	Catnip	Uva ursi

❧ ESSENTIAL HERBS FOR OVERCOMING CELLULITE COMPOUNDS:

PRIMARY HERBS		ASSISTING & COMPLEMENTARY HERBS		CATALYST & TRANSPORTING HERBS	
Burdock root	Oregon grape rt.	Juniper berry	Bladderwrack	Orange peel	Red clover
Fenugreek seed	Goldenseal root	Aloe vera	Green tea	Eyebright	Grape seed oil.
Dandelion root & lf.	Garlic	Red sage	Milk thistle seed	Turmeric	Rosemary
Sarsaparilla root	Gotu kola	Black cohosh root	Kola nut	Quassia chips	Catnip
Spirulina	Royal Jelly/Bee pollen	Bilberry	Poria mushroom	Lobelia	Uva ursi
Licorice root	Hawthorn bry., lf., flr.	Guarana seed	Fennel seed	Horsetail	Lecithin
Kelp & sea vegetables	Evening primrose oil	Watercress	Dong qual	Capsicum	Rosehips
Parsley root & lf.	Siberian ginseng	Kola nut	Mullein	Peppermint	Horse chestnut
Chlorella/Barley grass	Ginkgo biloba lf.	Ginger root	Echinacea	Lemon peel	Cornsilk

❧ EXAMPLE FORMULAS FOR OVERCOMING CELLULITE COMPOUNDS:

A CELLULITE-RELEASING CAPSULE FORMULA		(D - 1760)	A SMOOTHING/TONING RUB-ON GEL FORMULA		(D - 7195)
Fenugreek seed	Red sage	Milk thistle seed	Bladderwrack	Guarana	Capsicum
Gotu kola	Goldenseal root	Kelp	Gotu kola	Rosemary	Horse chestnut
Black cohosh	Lecithin	Kola nut	Kola nut	Uva ursi	Eucalyptus
Quassia chips	Garlic		Green tea	Lemon peel	Horsetail
	Bilberry				Aloe vera gel
	Poria mushroom				Sea plants
	Fennel seed				Grape seed oil
	Turmeric				

SEE PAGE 1 FOR FORMULATING INSTRUCTIONS.

Note: A MILK THISTLE SEED EXTRACT may be used during all phases of celulite release for liver support.

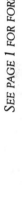

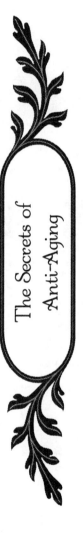

The Secrets of Anti-Aging

It's happening to everybody, most of the time faster than we'd like. But even though the hourglass tells us we're older, the passage of time isn't really what ages us. It's the process that reduces the number of healthy cells in the body. Whenever the gold and silver years begin for you, it's when the fun begins, when the hectic family life quiets down, financial strains ease, business retirement is here or not far off, and we can do the things we've always wanted to do but never had time for- travel, art, music, a craft, gardening, writing, quiet walks, picnics, more social life... doing what we want to do, not what we have to do. We all look forward to the treasure years of life and picture ourselves on that tennis court, bicycle path or cruise ship, healthy and enjoying ourselves. But, there's a catch - our freedom comes in the latter half of life, and many of us don't age gracefully in today's world.

There are so many interesting things to do and see in the world. We all want to extend our life spans with the best health possible. Fortunately, youth is not just a chronological age. It's good health and an optimistic spirit. The concept of anti-aging is gaining momentum as more people realize they can positively affect their own aging process. We can see this in today's elite athletes who perform at world class levels well into their thirties or even forties. Sparkling pockets throughout the world of healthy people living long life spans are proving that the downward spiral associated with aging need not happen.

The human life span is at least 20 to 30 years longer than most of us live today. It's astonishing to realize that we are living only two-thirds of the years our bodies are capable of! There is a paradox about aging: **Life expectancy lengthens as you age.** The average American child born in 1993 has a life expectancy of 75.4 years. But average life expectancy at 85 years is **six more years.** The longer you live, the longer your total expected life span becomes. **Age is not the enemy... Illness is.**

Our cells don't age; they're sloughed off as their efficiency diminishes to be replaced by new ones. When the body is given the right nutrients, cell restoration may continue for many years past current life expectancy. Environmental pollutants, a long standing diet of chemical laced, refined foods, vitamin and mineral deficiencies, overuse of prescription drugs and antibiotics, and high stress all prevent good cell restoration. Eighty percent of the population over 65 years old in industrial nations is chronically ill, usually with arthritis, heart disease, diabetes or high blood pressure.

Human lifespan can be increased. Youthfulness can be restored from the inside by strengthening lean body mass, metabolism, and immune response with good nutrition, regular exercise, fresh air, and a positive outlook. **A balanced life is the key to long life.** While cell life is largely genetically controlled, disease is usually the result of diet, lifestyle or environment. We can do something about these things. Slower aging means a better memory with no senility, better skin with fewer wrinkles, a strong heart, bones and immune response, flexible joints and muscles, a good metabolic rate and a healthy sex life, (organ and endocrine activity keeps your whole body youthful). Regular aerobic exercise like a brisk daily walk, prolongs fitness at any age. Exercise helps maintain stamina, strength, circulation and joint mobility. Stretching out every morning limbers the body, oxygenates the tissues, and helps clear it of the previous night's wastes and metabolic eliminations. Stretches at night before you retire help insure muscle relaxation and a better night's rest.

Don't worry. Be happy. Think positive to stay young. Clearly, the subtle energies of the mind effect the body. A pessimistic outlook on life depresses not only your personality, but your immune response. Even science is validating the "mind/body connection" in terms of the body's ability to heal. An optimistic, well-rounded, loving life needs friends and family. Regular contact is important for you and for them. Doing for, and giving to others at the stage of your life when there is finally enough time to do it graciously, makes a world of difference to your spirit.

The Fountain of Youth may have been available all along in the youth-extending nutrients of herbs and superfoods. Herbs have wide ranging properties, and far reaching possibilities as health restoratives. They can help with almost every aspect of human need as we age. The two main causes of aging are 1) cell and tissue damage caused by free radicals that aren't neutralized when the body lacks antioxidants; 2) reduced immune response that puts the body at risk for disease-causing stress and environmental toxic reactions. Herbal therapy is a premier agent for both of these aging actions. Antioxidant herbs quench and neutralize free radicals, energize and tone. Adaptogen herbs strengthen immunity, and equip the body to handle stress.

✳ COMPOUNDS FOR FORMULATION SHOULD INCLUDE:

•Boosting immunity against disease
•Averting cataracts and macular degeneration
•Counteracting Alzheimer's and age-related memory loss
•Slowing dry skin, wrinkling and gray hair

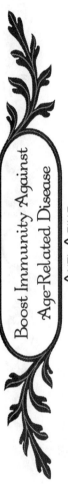

Boost Immunity Against Age-Related Disease

Anti-Aging

One of the main causes of aging is reduced immune response that puts the body at risk for disease-causing stress and environmental toxic reactions. The immune system is ever-vigilant, constantly searching for alien substances (antigens) that don't belong in our bodies. It can deal with a wide range of pathogens - viruses, funguses, bacteria and parasites. It can even recognize potential antigens, such as drugs, pollens, insect venoms and chemicals in foods, and malignant cells and foreign tissue, such as transplanted organs. Factors influencing reduced immune response are emotional stress, prolonged use of antibiotics and cortico-steroids drugs, glandular malfunction, usually the result of poor diet and nutrition, allergies, food and otherwise, staph infections, some immunization shots, environmental and heavy metal pollutants, and radiation. Building immune response with herbs and lifestyle therapy is a good preventative measure for those in their golden years to protect themselves against disease.

❧ ESSENTIAL CATEGORIES FOR BOOSTING IMMUNITY COMPOUNDS:

Anti-oxidant Herbs	Adaptogen Herbs For Resistance	Superfood Herbal Sources	Enzyme Therapy Herbs	Vitamin C & Bioflavonoid Sources	Mineral-Rich Herbs
Rosemary	**Bee pollen/Royal Jelly**	**Barley grass**	**Dandelion root & lf.**	**Kelp/sea vegetables**	**Gotu kola**
White pine bark	**Panax ginseng**	**Alfalfa**	**Milk thistle seed**	**Bilberry**	**Dandelion root & lf.**
Ginkgo biloba	**Pau d' arco bark**	**Royal Jelly/Propolis**	**Licorice root**	**Hawthorn lf. flr. & bry.**	Nettles
Reishi mushroom	**Alfalfa**	**Bee pollen**	**Nettles**	Aloe vera	**Alfalfa**
Maitake mushroom	Suma root	**Kelp/sea vegetables**	Goldenseal root	**Rosehips**	**Yellow dock rt.**
Astragalus	**Schizandra berry**	**Parsley rt & lf.**	**Green tea**	Cranberry powder	**Chamomile**
Alfalfa	**Siberian ginseng**	**Aloe vera**	**Oregon grape rt.**	Capsicum	Bee pollen
Hawthorn lf. flr. & bry.	**Ashwagandha**	Chlorella	Capsicum	Parsley leaf	Echinacea root
Ashwagandha rt.	Fo-Ti rt.	Spirulina	**Aloe vera**	Chlorella	**Burdock root**

❧ ESSENTIAL HERBS FOR BOOSTING IMMUNITY COMPOUNDS:

Primary Herbs		Assisting & Complementary Herbs	Catalyst & Transporting Herbs
Bee pollen/Royal Jelly	Pau d'arco bark	Dandelion rt. & lf.	Capsicum
Black cohosh rt.	Sarsaparilla root	Royal Jelly	Oregon grape rt.
Ginkgo biloba	Gotu kola	Fo-Ti root	Lobelia
Siberian ginseng	Kelp/sea vegetables	Bilberry	Milk thistle seed
Licorice root	Hawthorn lf. flr. & bry.	Peppermint	Rosemary
Barley grass	Spirulina	Goldenseal root	Propolis
Panax ginseng rt.	White pine bk.	Schizandra berry	Ginger root
Astragalus	Suma root	Burdock root	Watercress
Ashwagandha	Chlorella	Alfalfa	Green tea

Red raspberry, Nutritional yeast pwr., Parsley rt & lf., Chamomile, Echinacea root, Cranberry powder, Juniper bry., Evening primrose oil, Rose hips

Bee pollen, Yellow dock rt., Aloe vera, Panax ginseng, Dong quai rt, Nettles, Ashwagandha rt., Maitake mushroom, Reishi mushroom

❧ EXAMPLE FORMULAS OF BOOSTING IMMUNITY COMPOUNDS:

AN ANTI-AGING, ANTIOXIDANT CAPSULE COMPOUND   (SA - 1045)

Ginkgo biloba	Spirulina	Gotu kola
White pine bk.	Siberian ginseng	Reishi mushroom
Panax ginseng rt.	Suma root	Maitake mushroom
Wild yam rt.	Alfalfa	Astragalus
Hawthorn lf./flr./bry.	Bilberry	Sarsaparilla rt.

Dong quai rt, Licorice root, Ashwagandha, Damiana leaf, Royal Jelly

A FEEL GREAT, ADAPTOGEN CAPSULE COMPOUND   (E - 2250)

Bee pollen	Licorice root	Goldenseal root
Siberian ginseng	Suma root	Panax ginseng rt.
Gotu kola	Schizandra berry	Ginko biloba
Sarsaparilla root	Spirulina	Hawthorn lf./flr./bry.

Alfalfa, Wild cherry bk., Black cohosh rt., Kelp

SEE PAGE 1 FOR FORMULATING INSTRUCTIONS.

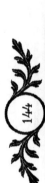

144

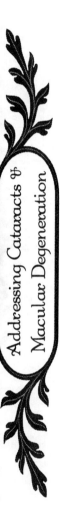

Addressing Cataracts & Macular Degeneration

Anti-Aging

Age-related macular degeneration (AMD), affects 9 million Americans and is the leading cause of blindness in the elderly. Lifestyle factors greatly influence vision as we age. Liver malfunction, environmental pollutants, or a poor diet can cause eye damage, especially free radical damage, so a diet rich in antioxidants makes a lot of sense. The carotenoids lutein and zeaxanthin, like spinach, kale, and collard greens, reduce the likelihood of getting (AMD) by up to 45%. **Cataracts** are the leading cause of impaired vision in America affecting over 4 million people. Even though cataract surgery is successful today, most operations have to be repeated in 2 to 5 years. Herbs are good choices for boosting your eye care because they can deliver highly absorbable carotenes, vitamin A, minerals and antioxidants very efficiently. Natural therapies can even arrest and reverse early cataracts. Reducing sugar intake, refined foods, pasteurized dairy, and red meats is also important as these foods slow metabolism and form crystallized clogs.

ESSENTIAL CATEGORIES FOR AGE-RELATED VISION PROBLEMS COMPOUNDS:

EYE SPECIFIC HERBS	ANTIOXIDANT SOURCE HERBS	LIVER CLEANSING & SUPPORT HERBS	VITAMIN C & BIOFLAVONOID HERBS	ALPHA & BETA CAROTENE SOURCES	SUGAR-REGULATING HERBS
Eyebright	**Ginkgo biloba**	**Goldenseal root**	**Parsley root & lf.**	**Spirulina**	**Royal jelly/Bee pollen**
Rosehips	Astragalus	**Beet root**	Hawthorn bry., lf., fl.	**Kelp & sea vegetables**	Dandelion rt. & lf.
Chamomile	Reishi mushroom	**Dandelion rt. & lf.**	**Aloe vera**	**Aloe vera**	**Mullein**
Bilberry berries	Maitake mushroom	**Oregon grape root**	Royal jelly	**Bilberry**	**Cedar berry**
Ginkgo biloba	**White pine bark**	**Milk thistle seed**	Rose hips	**Nettles**	**Elecampane**
Fennel seed	Siberian ginseng	Pau d' arco bk.	**Red raspberry**	Elder flowers	Parsley root & lf.
Aloe vera	Licorice root	Eyebright	Plantain	**Red raspberry**	**Licorice root**
Turmeric	Alfalfa	**Capsicum**	**Bilberry berries**	Bee pollen	Wild yam root
Kelp & sea vegetables	Rosemary	Echinacea root	Dandelion rt.	Garlic	**Gymnema sylvestre**

ESSENTIAL HERBS FOR AGE-RELATED VISION PROBLEMS COMPOUNDS:

PRIMARY HERBS		ASSISTING & COMPLEMENTARY HERBS		CATALYST & TRANSPORTING HERBS	
Eyebright	Parsley root & lf.	Elecampane	Red raspberry	Milk thistle seed	Reishi mushroom
Dandelion rt. & lf.	Chamomile	Goldenseal root	Alfalfa	Mullein	Goldeseal root
Ginseng - all types	Ginkgo biloba	Pau d' arco bk.	Red clover	Beet root	Turmeric
Bilberry	Aloe vera	Rose hips	Elder flowers	Capsicum	Oregon grape root
Bee pollen/Royal jelly	Rosemary	Spirulina	Licorice root.	Peppermint	Vitamin C powder
Gotu kola	Passionflower	Plantain	Garlic	Maitake mushroom	Fennel seed
Kelp & sea vegetables	Hawthorn bry., lf., fl.	Astragalus	Cedar berry	Ginger root	Lemon balm
Bayberry	Siberian ginseng	Wild yam root	Echinacea root	Horsetail	Nettles
White pine bark	White pine bark	Black cohosh rt'.	Calendula	Evening primrose oil	Gymnema sylvestre

EXAMPLE FORMULAS OF AGE-RELATED VISION PROBLEMS COMPOUNDS:

AN EYE NOURISHING ANTI-OXIDANT CAPSULE COMPOUND		(po - 3480)
White pine bark	Vitamin C powder	Licorice root	Garlic
Rosemary	Echinacea root	Astragalus	Bilberry
Siberian ginseng	Pau d' arco bk.	Capsicum	Hawthorn bry/lf.
Ginkgo biloba	Red clover	Lemon balm	Spirulina

AN EYEBRIGHT COMPLEX TEA AND EYEWASH COMPOUND		(co - 5300)
Eyebright	Plantain	Rosemary	Red raspberry
Bilberry	Elder flowers	Goldenseal root	
Passionflower			

SEE PAGE 1 FOR FORMULATING INSTRUCTIONS.

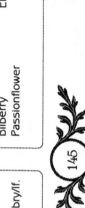

145

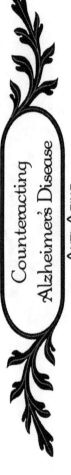

Counteracting Alzheimer's Disease

ANTI-AGING

Alzheimer's has become the most common form of senile dementia resulting in the loss of memory and almost every mental function. The brain develops "neuritic plaques" which consist of degenerating nerve terminals, and other brain material. There is hope for treating Alzheimer's disease nutritionally, especially with certain herbal remedies, that can help correct the deficiencies triggering memory loss, and can neutralize free radicals preventing further cell damage. Certain herbs, like ginkgo biloba, can be very beneficial for people with cerebral-vascular insufficiency. A vegetarian diet with fresh foods, high fiber, whole grains and cultured products is thought to prevent many forms of senile dementia (meat eaters are more likely to develop dementia than people who are vegetarians). Oxygen therapy and chelation therapy are very helpful in oxygenizing and detaching the plaque cells, showing marked improvements in the symptoms of dementia.

❧ ESSENTIAL CATEGORIES FOR ALZHEIMER'S DISEASE COMPOUNDS:

ANTIOXIDANT SOURCE HERBS	BRAIN NUTRIENTS & CHOLINE SOURCES	HERBAL AMINO ACID SOURCES	SILICA SOURCE, MINERAL-RICH HERBS	ESSENTIAL FATTY ACID BRAIN NUTRIENTS	CIRCULATION STIMULANTS
Ashwagandha	Gotu kola	Aloe vera	Horsetail	Evening primrose oil	Ginkgo biloba
Rosemary	Ginkgo biloba	Chlorella	Kelp/sea vegetables	Flax seed oil	Siberian ginseng root
Ginkgo biloba	Kava kava rt.	Garlic	Oatstraw	Borage seed	Cayenne/Goldenseal
Reishi mushroom	Bee pollen/Royal Jelly	Kelp & sea vegetables	Nettles	Chlorella	Ginger root
Licorice root	Schizandra bry.	Spirulina	Barley grass	Kelp/Dulse	Ginseng - all types
Garlic	Fo-Ti root	Royal Jelly/Bee pollen	Dandelion root & lf.	Spirulina/Barley grass	Hawthorn bry., lf., fl.
White pine bark	Wood betony	Barley grass	Carrot powder	Fennel seed	Bilberry
Grapeseed	Sarsaparilla root	Peppermint	Alfalfa	Burdock root	Suma root
Shiitake mushroom	Panax ginseng	Alfalfa	Irish moss	Dong quai	Prickly ash bk.

❧ ESSENTIAL HERBS FOR FOR ALZHEIMER'S DISEASE COMPOUNDS:

PRIMARY HERBS		ASSISTING & COMPLEMENTARY HERBS		CATALYST & TRANSPORTING HERBS	
Ginkgo biloba	Evening primrose oil	Rosemary	Prickly ash bk.	Peppermint	Aloe vera
Bee pollen/Royal Jelly	Fo-Ti root	Prickly ash bk.	Capsicum	Vitamin C pwr.	Rosemary
Ginseng - all types	Kava kava root	Dandelion root & lf.	Ginger root	Parsley rt. & lf.	Oatstraw
Sarsaparilla root	Gotu kola	Suma root.		Capsicum	Borage seed
Scullcap	Ashwagandha	Burdock root		Shepherd's purse	Irish moss
Licorice root	Hawthorn bry., lf., fl.	Bilberry		Aloe vera	Fennel seed
Kelp & sea vegetables	Spirulina	Barley grass		Ginger root	Black currant
White pine bk.	Siberian ginseng	Suma root		Shiitake mushroom	Dulse
Chlorella	Panax ginseng	Dong quai		Grapeseed	Carrot powder

❧ EXAMPLE FORMULAS OF ALZHEIMER'S DISEASE COMPOUNDS:

A MENTAL CLARITY CAPSULE COMPOUND		(E - 3520)	A COMPLEX GINSENG CAPSULE COMPOUND		(E - 2510)
Panax ginseng rt.	Kelp	Rosemary	Prickly ash bk.	Bee pollen	Fo-Ti root	Dong quai
Gotu kola	Ginkgo biloba	Schizandra bry.	Capsicum	Siberian ginseng	Panax ginseng rt.	Aralia root
Fo-Ti root	Siberian ginseng	Royal Jelly	Ginger root	Gotu kola	Prince ginseng	Alfalfa
Bee pollen						

SEE PAGE 1 FOR FORMULATING INSTRUCTIONS.

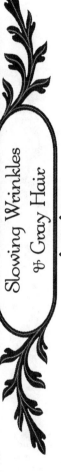

Slowing Wrinkles & Gray Hair
ANTI-AGING

Aging skin texture occurs when collagen becomes hard and cross-linked with neighboring collagen fibers, preventing it from holding water and maintaining elasticity. It collapses on itself, forming a kind of fish net below the surface of the skin, seen as wrinkles. The cause of cross-linking is free radical damage. Free radicals attack skin cell membranes, collagen and elastin proteins, resulting in dry skin and sagging skin contours. **Healthy hair** is a mirror of both good nutrition and common-sense, daily care. Hair consists of protein layers called keratin. In healthy hair, the cell walls of the hair cuticle lie flat like shingles, leaving hair soft and shiny. In damaged or dry hair, the cuticle shingles are broken and create gaps that make hair porous and dull. Skin and hair problems are often the first indication of nutritional deficiencies. Herbs have been used for centuries to maintain and improve the underlying vitality needs of healthy, youthful skin and hair.

✤ ESSENTIAL CATEGORIES FOR REVITALIZING SKIN & HAIR COMPOUNDS:

ANTIOXIDANTS FOR ANTI-WRINKLE EFFECTS	MINERAL-RICH HERBS	PHYTO-HORMONE SOURCE HERBS	ESSENTIAL FATTY ACID HERBS	B VITAMIN SOURCE HERBS	SILICA SOURCE HERBS
Sage	**Kelp/sea vegetables**	**Panax ginseng root**	**Evening primrose oil**	Brewer's yeast	**Horsetail**
Rosemary	Ginkgo biloba	Ashwagandha rt.	**Flax seed oil**	**Royal Jelly/Bee pollen**	**Kelp/sea vegetables**
Aloe vera	Spirulina/Chlorella	Damiana	Borage seed	Parsley rt. & lf.	**Oatstraw**
Reishi mushroom	Barley grass	**Sarsaparilla root**	**Fenugreek seed**	Dong qual rt.	**Nettles**
Evening primrose oil	**Dandelion rt. & lf.**	**Licorice root**	Kelp & sea vegetables	Thyme	**Barley grass.**
Wheat germ oil	Horsetail	**Wild yam root**	**Spirulina**	Burdock rt.	**Dandelion root & lf.**
White pine bark	Evening primrose oil	**Burdock root**	**Black currant seed**	**Kelp/sea vegetables**	Carrot powder
Grapeseed	Chickweed	**Black cohosh root**	Barley grass	Dandelion root	Alfalfa
Alfalfa	Chamomile	**Dong qual rt.**	**Safflowers**	Red raspberry	Irish moss

✤ ESSENTIAL HERBS FOR REVITALIZING SKIN & HAIR COMPOUNDS:

PRIMARY HERBS		ASSISTING & COMPLEMENTARY HERBS		CATALYST & TRANSPORTING HERBS	
Ginkgo biloba	Bee pollen/Royal Jelly	Ashwagandha rt.	Damiana	Chickweed	Carrot powder
Chamomile	Burdock rt	Yellow dock root	Alfalfa	Black currant	Wheat germ oil
Sarsaparilla root	Nettles	Dandelion root & lf.	Reishi mushroom	Coltsfoot	Oatstraw
Spirulina	Gotu kola	Dong qual rt.	Rosemary	Capsicum	Aloe vera
Licorice root	White pine bk.	White sage	Red raspberry	Thyme	Flax seed
Kelp & sea vegetables	Hawthorn bry., lf., fl.	Lemongrass	Watercress	Brewer's yeast	Peppermint
Black cohosh rt.	Suma root	Barley grass	Horsetail	Ginger root	Grapeseed
Chlorella	Siberian ginseng	Evening primrose oil	Parsley rt. & lf.	Safflowers	Fenugreek seed
Red Sage	Panax ginseng	Wild yam root	Irish moss	Squaw vine	Borage seed

✤ EXAMPLE FORMULAS OF REVITALIZING SKIN & HAIR COMPOUNDS:

A MINERAL SPECTRUM CAPSULE COMPOUND		(SA - 3200)	A PHYTO-HORMONE CONTAINING COMPOUND		(W -2150)
Nettles	Alfalfa	Yellow dock root	Dulse	Black cohosh rt.	Licorice root	Damiana	Wild yam rt.
Irish moss	Dandelion rt.	Borage seed	Bee pollen	Sarsaparilla rt.	Dong qual rt.	False unicorn	Blessed thistle
Watercress	Dandelion lf.	Barley grass	Parsley rt. & lf.			Squaw vine	

SEE PAGE 1 FOR FORMULATING INSTRUCTIONS.

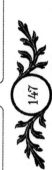

147

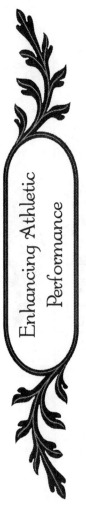

Enhancing Athletic Performance

Natural strength training supplements can be helpful for both the serious and casual athlete. They help build muscle tissue, maintain low body fat, and improve strength and endurance when the body is under the stress of a workout series. Supplements optimize recuperation time between workouts, are a proven adjunct to fitness and muscle growth, and speed healing from sports-related injuries. Antioxidants have become a byword for sports performance because they help maintain the body's defenses against exercise-induced free radicals to combat injury and speed muscle recovery. Mineral balance is critical for an athlete at any level. Macro and trace minerals are built into every biochemical reaction of athletic movement, from energy, to digestion, to utilization of vitamins and proteins, to nerve transmission, muscle contraction, the regulation of metabolism, cholesterol levels and blood sugar. Athletes regularly become deficient in minerals and can benefit greatly by replacing electrolytes (the ionized mineral salts found in the body fluids) lost after workouts.

Are Herbs A Good Choice For Athletes? Herbal supplements can be efficient partners in an exercise program, acting as concentrated food nutrients for body building, offering extra strength for energy and endurance. Herbs have been used by athletes since ancient times. Yarrow and other herbs were used by Roman gladiators to help heal wounds. Chinese and Japanese warriors and athletes have used herbs to increase endurance and strength from prehistory to the present. In Russia, Germany and Korea, herbs are extremely popular with sports enthusiasts and athletes. American athletes are just beginning to see the value of herbs for a winning body. Herb source minerals are highly absorbable, foundation nutrients that help the body build a good strength and stamina base. Proteins from plant superfoods like spirulina and barley grass provide strength and healing ability (you must have protein to heal) without the density or absorption problems

A Word About Steroids: As the standards of excellence rise in sports and competition, the use of steroids is increasing. Steroid enhancement has spread beyond the professional and Olympic arenas to dedicated weight lifters, body builders and team players at all levels. The dangers of synthetic steroids far outweigh any advantages. Steroid use leads to wholesale destruction of glandular tissue, stunted growth from bone closure in males, testicle shrinkage, low sperm counts with sterility noticeable after only a few months of use, enlargement and tenderness of the pectorals, weakening of connective tissue, jaundice from liver malfunction, circulation impairment, and adverse side effects of hostile personality behavior and facial changes.

Can Herbal Steroids Do The Sports Enhancement Job? Although there are no magic bullets for energy, endurance and healing of sports injuries, there are plant-derived steroids - phytosterols that have growth activity similar to that of free form amino acids and anabolic steroids. Amino acids from herbal sources and foods high in amino acids, can act as steroid alternatives to help build the body to competitive levels without chemical steroid consequences. These "natural steroids" help release growth hormone, promote ammonia and acid detoxification, stimulate immunity and liver regeneration. They maximize potential, promote fast recuperation, increase stamina and support peak performance. Testing still needs to be done on the herbs for anabolic effectiveness, especially on steroid strengths in normal herbal dosage form. Nevertheless, they may still be used with confidence in body building and endurance formulas. The most well-known of these herbs are: **damiana**, a mild aphrodisiac and nerve stimulant; **sarsaparilla root**, **Smilax**, coaxes the body to produce greater amounts of the anabolic hormones, testosterone and cortisone. A blood purifier for nitrogen-based waste products such as uric acid, sarsaparilla also speeds recovery time after workouts; **saw palmetto**, a urethral toning herb that increases blood flow to the sexual organs; **Siberian and panax ginsengs**, adaptogens for over-all body balance and energy; **wild yam**, an antispasmodic that prevents cramping; contains diosgenin, a phytoprogesterone; **yohimbe**, a testosterone precursor for body building, and potent aphrodisiac for both sexes.

Note: How you take training supplements is as important as what you take. Your program will be more productive if you balance supplements between workout days and rest days. Muscle growth occurs on "off" days as the body uses the workout you have been giving it. You can obtain increased enhancement by taking vitamins, minerals and glandulars on "off" days. Take proteins, amino acids, anabolics and herbs on "on" days, before the workout.

❖ COMPOUNDS FOR FORMULATION INCLUDE:

- •Increasing energy, stamina and endurance
- •Body building for competitive strength
- •Recovering from athletic injuries

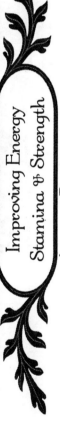

Improving Energy
Stamina & Strength

ATHLETIC PERFORMANCE

Stamina is the body's ability to withstand stress. Regular exercise is an integral part of building strength and endurance. A sedentary lifestyle has the same effect on heart disease risk as smoking a pack of cigarettes a day! We all know that exercise speeds results in weight loss and heart recovery. In reality, it strengthens the whole body - muscles, nerves, blood, glands, lungs, heart, brain, mind and mood. It increases metabolic rate, muscle mass, bone mass, tissue oxygen uptake, respiratory and circulatory vigor. Besides losing muscle mass, we also lose about 1% of bone mass every year if we don't exercise, beginning as early as age 35. Herbal stamina builders are a good choice for athletes wanting a strength and stamina edge to their performance. Herbs are full of minerals (you must have minerals to run). Many are rich in antioxidants, proteins and amino acids. Others help boost circulation and glandular activity.

❧ ESSENTIAL CATEGORIES FOR ENERGY, STAMINA & STRENGTH COMPOUNDS:

ENDURANCE & STAMINA ANTIOXIDANTS	ADRENAL TONIC HERBS	ENERGY SUPPORT HERBS	CIRCULATION STIMULATING HERBS	SUPERFOOD HERBS FOR STRENGTH & STRESS	METABOLIC ACTIVITY ENHANCING HERBS
Siberian ginseng	**Bladderwrack**	**Panax ginseng rt.**	**Ginkgo biloba**	**Spirulina**	**Royal Jelly/Bee pollen**
Schizandra berry	Alfalfa/Watercress	**Spirulina**	Hawthorn bry., lf., fl.	**Kelp & sea vegetables**	Panax ginseng
Panax ginseng rt.	**Suma root**	**Damiana**	**Ginger root**	**Barley grass**	**Fo-Ti root**
Chinese kirin ginseng	Sarsaparilla rt.	Kola nut	Bee pollen/Royal jelly	Bee pollen/Royal jelly	**White willow bk.**
Ginkgo biloba	Siberian ginseng	Capsicum	**Cayenne**	**Panax ginseng**	Evening primrose oil
Spirulina	**Gotu kola**	Suma root	Turmeric	Siberian ginseng rt.	Wild yam rt.
Sarsaparilla rt.	Kelp & sea vegetables	Saw palmetto	Yarrow	**Pau d' arco bk.**	**Licorice root**
Licorice root	Panax ginseng root	**Guarana seed**	**Bilberry berries**	Suma root	Yellow dock root
White pine bark	**Licorice root**	**Green tea**	**Siberian ginseng**	Schizandra berry	Dong quai root

❧ ESSENTIAL HERBS FOR ENERGY, STAMINA & STRENGTH COMPOUNDS:

PRIMARY HERBS		ASSISTING & COMPLEMENTARY HERBS		CATALYST & TRANSPORTING HERBS	
Spirulina	Sarsaparilla rt.	Royal jelly	Ginger root	White willow bk.	Reishi mushroom
Barley grass	Chamomile	Dandelion root	Capsicum	Mullein	Yarrow
Panax ginseng root	Ginkgo biloba	Pau d' arco bk.	Barley grass	Beet root	Turmeric
Bilberry	Aloe vera	Nutritional yeast		Capsicum	Yellow dock root
Bee pollen	Rosemary	Parsley rt. & lf.		Bladderwrack	Vitamin C powder
Gotu kola	Suma root	White willow bk.		Maitake mushroom	Irish moss
Kelp & sea vegetables	Hawthorn bry., lf., fl.	Astragalus		Ginger root	Watercress
Licorice root	Siberian ginseng	Wild yam root		Green tea	Nettles
White pine bark	Fo-Ti root	Dong quai root		Evening primrose oil	Ashwagandha

❧ EXAMPLE FORMULAS OF ENERGY, STAMINA & STRENGTH COMPOUNDS:

A HIGH PERFORMANCE CAPSULE COMPOUND		(ε - 2700)		AN ACTIVE, PHYSICAL ENERGY COMPOUND		(ε - 2125)
Siberian ginseng rt.	Gotu kola	Dandelion root	Ginger root	Am. Panax ginseng	Suma root	Sarsaparilla rt.
Bee pollen	Nutritional yeast	Yarrow	Capsicum	Chinese kirin ginseng	Fo-Ti root	Ginkgo biloba
Sarsaparilla rt.	Spirulina	Wild yam rt.	Barley grass	Siberian ginseng	Gotu kola	
Licorice root	Suma root	Alfalfa				

SEE PAGE 1 FOR FORMULATING INSTRUCTIONS.

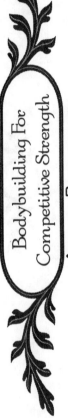

Bodybuilding For Competitive Strength

ATHLETIC PERFORMANCE

Whatever your personal bodybuilding regime, there are important bodywork watchwords to follow. **Cross train.** Besides your major sport or activity, supplement it with auxiliary exercise such as dancing, bicycling, jogging, walking, or swimming and aerobics. **Recuperation time is essential for optimum strength.** Muscles do not grow during exercise. They grow during rest periods. Alternate muscle workouts with rest days. Exercise different muscle sets on different days, resting each set in between. **Breathe deep.** Muscles and tissues must have enough oxygen for endurance and stamina. Vigorous exhaling is as important as inhaling for the athlete, to expel all carbon dioxide and increase lung capacity for oxygen. **Water is important.** Good hydration is necessary for high performance, cardiovascular activity and overheating. **Weight training is beneficial for both sexes.** Women do not get a bulky, masculine physique from lifting weights. They have low levels of testosterone, which influences their type of muscle development.

ESSENTIAL CATEGORIES FOR COMPETITIVE STRENGTH COMPOUNDS:

ANABOLIC ENHANCERS	MUSCLE RELAXERS & NERVE RESTORERS	METABOLIC ENHANCING HERBS	VITAMIN C & BIOFLAVONOID HERBS	STAMINA & ENDURANCE HERBS	PLANT PROTEIN SOURCES
Suma rt.	**Kava kava**	**Royal Jelly/Bee pollen**	**Bilberry**	**Siberian ginseng**	**Spirulina**
Sarsaparilla root	Ashwagandha rt.	Panax ginseng	Hawthorn bry., lf., fl.	Schizandra berry	**Wheat germ**
Siberian ginseng	Bee pollen/Royal Jelly	**Fo-Ti root**	**Rose hips**	**Panax ginseng rt.**	**Nutritional yeast**
Panax ginseng	**Gotu kola**	**Green tea**	Chlorella	Chinese kirin ginseng	**Whey protein**
Saw palmetto bry.	Oats/Oatstraw	Kola nut	Kelp & sea vegetables	Ginkgo biloba	**Barley grass**
Damiana	**Valerian**	Siberian ginseng rt.	**Spirulina**	**Spirulina**	**Chlorella**
Fo-Ti root	**Wood betony**	**Licorice root**	Royal Jelly	**Sarsaparilla rt.**	Bee pollen/Royal Jelly
Wild yam root	Scullcap	Sarsaparilla root	Aloe vera	**Licorice root**	Alfalfa
Yohimbe bark	**Black cohosh**	Ginger root	**Capsicum**	White pine bark	Soy & rice protein

ESSENTIAL HERBS FOR COMPETITIVE STRENGTH COMPOUNDS:

PRIMARY HERBS		ASSISTING & COMPLEMENTARY HERBS		CATALYST & TRANSPORTING HERBS	
Ginkgo biloba	Bee pollen	Ashwagandha rt.	Damiana	Goldenseal root	Wheat germ
Guarana seed	Burdock rt	Wild yam root	Alfalfa	Ephedra leaf	Soy & rice protein
Sarsaparilla root	Astragalus	Kava kava	Royal Jelly	Valerian	Dandelion root
Spirulina	Gotu kola	Dong quai rt	Evening primrose oil	Capsicum	Aloe vera
Licorice root	Kola nut	White pine bark	Scullcap	Rose hips	Bilberry
Kelp & sea vegetables	Hawthorn bry., lf., fl.	Fo-Ti root	Damiana	Nutritional yeast	Rosemary
Black cohosh rt.	Suma root	Barley grass	Horsetail	Ginger root	Soy & Rice protein
Chlorella	Siberian ginseng	Schizandra berry	Oats/Oatstraw	Chinese kirin ginseng	Wood betony
Saw palmetto bry.	Panax ginseng	Wild yam root	Green tea	Yohimbe bark	Orange peel

EXAMPLE FORMULAS OF COMPETITIVE STRENGTH COMPOUNDS:

A SUPER MAN'S ENERGY EXTRACT COMPOUND		(M - 4970)	A RAINFOREST ENERGY CAPSULE COMPOUND		(E -3780)
Sarsaparilla rt.	Siberian ginseng rt.	Capsicum	Guarana seed	Suma root	Astragalus
Saw palmetto bry.	Gotu kola	Orange peel	Kola nut	Bee pollen	Chlorella
Suma					

SEE PAGE 1 FOR FORMULATING INSTRUCTIONS.

150

Healing From Athletic Injuries

ATHLETIC PERFORMANCE

Although exercise is an integral part of good nutrition, and often times becomes a nutrient in itself, sports injuries are a pitfall of rigorous exercise and participation in different sports. **A strain** is any damage to tendons that anchor the muscle. **A sprain**, much harder to heal than a strain, is caused by a twisting motion that tears ligaments that bind up the joints. **Tendonitis** is the painful inflammation of a tendon, usually resulting from a strain. You can help yourself prevent sports injuries. Start your workout slowly; warm your body up at least 2 degrees before you start pushing yourself; end your workout with a cool down period to prevent lactic acid build-up. **Stretch out before and after a workout** to keep cramping down and muscles loose. Get some morning sunlight every day possible for optimal absorption of nutrient fuel. **No pain does not mean no gain.** Exercise doesn't have to hurt to be good for you. Once you work up to a good aerobic level, you don't need to push yourself ever harder to benefit.

ESSENTIAL CATEGORIES FOR ATHLETIC INJURY COMPOUNDS:

SILICA SOURCE HERBS	ANTI-INFLAMMATORY HERBS	NERVE-REBUILDING HERBS	ANTISPASMODIC HERBS	VITAMIN C & BIOFLAVONOID SOURCES	HERBS TO PREVENT LACTIC ACID BUILD-UP
Oats/Oatstraw	**White willow bk.**	**Oats/Oatstraw**	**Cramp bark**	**Bilberry**	**Sarsaparilla rt.**
Horsetail	**St. John's wort**	**Black cohosh rt.**	**Kava Kava**	**Hawthorn bry., lf., fl.**	**Siberian ginseng root**
Burdock rt.	**Devil's claw**	**Ashwagandha**	**Passionflower**	**Rose hips**	**Wild yam rt.**
Kelp & sea vegetables	**Yarrow**	**Scullcap**	**St. John's wort**	Chlorella	**Schizandra bry.**
Nettles	**Marshmallow rt.**	Gotu kola	**Wild yam root**	Kelp & sea vegetables	**Panax ginseng**
Garlic	Chamomile	**European mistletoe**	**Valerian root**	**Spirulina**	Spirulina
Echinacea rt.	Panax ginseng	**Parsley rt. & lf.**	Wild lettuce	Royal jelly	**Fo-Ti root**
Ginger root	**Turmeric**	Wood betony	Hops	Aloe vera	**White willow bark**
Eyebright	**Aloe vera**	White pine bk.	Lobella	**Capsicum**	**Barley grass**

ESSENTIAL HERBS FOR ATHLETIC INJURY COMPOUNDS:

PRIMARY HERBS		ASSISTING & COMPLEMENTARY HERBS		CATALYST & TRANSPORTING HERBS	
Yarrow	Eyebright	Aloe vera	Marshmallow rt.	Lobelia	Parsley rt. & lf.
Bee pollen	White willow bark	Red clover	Chamomile	Royal jelly	Rosemary
Horsetail	Kava kava root	Black cohosh rt.	Wild yam root	European mistletoe	Chaste tree berry
Sarsaparilla root	Gotu kola	Scullcap	Oatstraw	Capsicum	Wild lettuce
Schizandra bry.	Dandelion root	Burdock root	Nettles	Garlic	Rose hips
St. John's wort	Hawthorn bry., lf., fl.	Bilberry	Devil's claw	Black haw	Hops
Kelp & sea vegetables	Spirulina/Alfalfa	Barley grass	Echinacea Pur. rt.	Ginger root	Valerian
White pine bk.	Siberian ginseng	Chlorella	Echinacea Ang. rt.	Uva ursi	Red raspberry
Cramp bark	Panax ginseng/Fo-Ti	Passionflower	Wood betony	Turmeric	Ashwagandha

EXAMPLE FORMULAS OF ATHLETIC INJURY COMPOUNDS:

A POWERFUL ANTI-INFLAMMATORY CAPSULE COMPOUND		(co - 1180)		AN ANTISPASMODIC CAPSULE COMPOUND		(co - 1250)	
White willow bark	White pine bk.	Alfalfa	Chamomile	Cramp bark	Kava kava	Wild yam root	Kelp
St. John's wort	Gotu kola	Burdock root	Uva ursi	Black haw	Passionflower	St. John's wort	Lobella
Echinacea Ang. rt.	Red clover	Dandelion root	Ginger root	Rosemary	Red raspberry	Chaste tree berry	Valerian
Echinacea Pur. rt.	Devil's claw		Turmeric				

SEE PAGE 1 FOR FORMULATING INSTRUCTIONS.

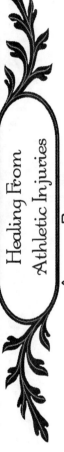

151

Optimizing Pregnancy & Childbearing

I n America today, one in six married couples of childbearing age has trouble conceiving and completing a successful pregnancy. Preconception planning has become important because neither our environment with its toxic pollutants, our diets full of fast foods, or our stressful lifestyles are conducive to successful child conception. Poor nutrition and stress are at the base of most fertility problems. Diet is an all-important key to successful conception: The body does not readily allow conception without adequate nutrition. Nature tries in every way possible to insure the survival and health of a baby. Gland and hormone health, the basis of reproductive health, is so primary and so potent that it must receive good nutrition for conception. Conscious attention needs to be made by both prospective parents to a healthy diet and lifestyle for at least six months before trying to conceive. (See also COOKING FOR HEALTHY HEALING by Linda Rector Page.)

Both men and women should avoid fatty, fried foods or reduce intake to between 5% and 10% of the diet. (This is good for your sex life, too.) Low-fat, fresh produce, whole grains, seafoods, turkey and chicken provide minerals, protein, fiber and complex carbohydrates to build gland function quickly, while avoiding cholesterol. Reduce or avoid full fat dairy foods, sugary foods, made from chemicals, and meats laced with nitrates and/or hormones.

Lifestyle habits are important, too. It is important to avoid or reduce consumption of tobacco, caffeine, and alcohol. (Moderate wine is okay until conception.) Get light exercise, and morning sunshine every day possible. Take alternating hot and cold showers to stimulate circulation and glandular secretions throughout the body. Apply alternating hot and cold compresses to the abdomen or scrotum to increase circulation to the reproductive areas.

Herbs and other nutritional supplements are valuable for both men and women trying to conceive a child.

Optimal Eating For Two During Pregnancy: A woman's body changes so dramatically during pregnancy and childbearing that her normal daily needs change. Promise yourself and your baby that at least during the months of pregnancy and nursing, your diet and lifestyle will be as healthy as you can make it. A largely vegetarian diet of whole foods provides optimum nutrition for pregnancy. Many staples of a lactovegetarian, seafood and poultry diet are nutritional powerhouses, such as whole grains, leafy greens, fish, turkey, eggs, legumes, nuts, seeds, green and yellow vegetables, nutritional yeast, bananas and citrus fruits. You can base your pregnancy diet on these foods with confidence that the baby will be getting the best possible nutrition.

Here are the keys:

• Protein is important. Most experts currently recommend 60 to 80 grams of protein daily during pregnancy, with a 10 gram increase every trimester. Eat a high vegetable protein diet, with whole grains, seeds and sprouts, with fish, seafood or turkey at least twice a week. Take a protein drink several times a week for optimal growth and energy. Even though protein requirements increase during pregnancy, it is the quality of the protein, not the quantity that prevents and cures toxemia.

• Have a fresh fruit or green salad every day. Eat plenty of soluble fiber foods like whole grains and vegetables for regularity. Eat complex carbohydrates foods like broccoli and brown rice for strength.

• Drink plenty of healthy fluids-pure water, mineral water, and juices throughout the day to keep the system free and flowing. Carrot juice at least twice a week is ideal. Include pineapple and apple juice frequently.

• Eat folacin rich foods, such as fresh spinach and asparagus for healthy cell growth.

• Eat carotene-rich foods, such as carrots, squashes, tomatoes, yams, and broccoli for disease.

• Eat zinc-rich foods, such as pumpkin and sesame seeds for good body formation.

• Eat vitamin C foods, such as broccoli, bell peppers and fruits for connective tissue. Eat bioflavonoid-rich foods like citrus and berries for capillary integrity.

• Eat alkalizing foods, such as miso soup and brown rice to combat and neutralize toxemia.

• Eat mineral-rich foods such as sea veggies, leafy greens, and whole grains for baby building blocks. Especially include silicon-rich foods for bone, cartilage and connective tissue growth, and for collagen and elastin formation; brown rice, oats, green grasses and green drinks.

• Eat small frequent meals instead of large ones.

❖ COMPOUNDS FOR FORMULATION INCLUDE:
• Herbs for prenatal health
• Herbs for pre-birth and labor ease
• Herbs for milk enrichment and nursing

Herbs For Prenatal Health

PREGNANCY & CHILDBEARING

Herbs have been used successfully for centuries to ease the hormone imbalances and discomforts of stretching, bloating, nausea and pain experienced during pregnancy, without impairing the development or health of the baby. Herbs are concentrated mineral-rich foods that are perfect for the extra growth requirements of pregnancy and childbirth. They are easily-absorbed and non-constipating. A developing child's body is very small and delicate. Ideal supplementation should be from food source complexes for best absorbability. Herbs are identified and accepted by the body's enzyme activity as whole food nutrients, lessening the risk of toxemia or overdose, yet providing gentle, easy nutrition for both mother and baby. Herbs are good and easy for you; good and gentle for the baby. Important Note: Early pregnancy and later pregnancy must be considered separately with herbal medicinals. If there is any question, always use the gentlest herbs.

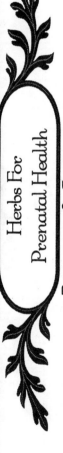

✍ ESSENTIAL CATEGORIES FOR PRENATAL HEALTH COMPOUNDS:

PREGNANCY SPECIFIC HERBS	ESSENTIAL FATTY ACID SOURCES	IODINE & POTASSIUM SOURCE HERBS	VITAMIN C & BIOFLAVONOID HERBS	MINERAL-RICH HERBS	HERBAL IRON SOURCES
Bilberry	**Flax seed oil**	Kelp & sea vegetables	**Bilberry**	**Yellow dock root**	**Beet root**
Chamomile	Alfalfa	Dandelion root & lf.	**Hawthorn bry., lf., fl.**	Kelp & sea vegetables	**Alfalfa**
Red raspberry	**Evening primrose oil**	Spirulina	**Rose hips**	**Watercress**	**Dandelion root & lf.**
Burdock root	**Spirulina**	**Barley grass**	**Parsley leaf**	Dandelion root & lf.	**Spirulina**
Nettles	**Chlorella**	**Capsicum**	Kelp & sea vegetables	**Parsley**	**Nettles**
Peppermint	Dulse	Nettles	**Spirulina**	**Spirulina**	**Yellow dock root**
Ginger root	Kelp & sea vegetables	Watercress	Royal jelly	Irish moss	**Parsley rt. & lf.**
Yellow dock root	Aloe vera	**Chlorella**	Red clover	**Barley grass**	Borage seed
Alfalfa	**Borage seed**	**Borage seed**	**Catnip**	Alfalfa	Kelp/sea vegetables

✍ ESSENTIAL HERBS FOR PRENATAL HEALTH COMPOUNDS:

PRIMARY HERBS		ASSISTING & COMPLEMENTARY HERBS		CATALYST & TRANSPORTING HERBS	
Red raspberry	Sarsaparilla rt.	Burdock root	Red clover	Dulse	Acerola cherry
Barley grass	Chamomile	Pau d' arco bk.	Catnip	Lemon peel	Yarrow
Alfalfa	Ginkgo biloba	Nutritional yeast	Damiana	Beet root	Hibiscus
Bilberry	Parsley leaf	Parsley root	Rose hips	Capsicum	Yellow dock root
Bee pollen	Rosemary	Ashwagandha	Borage seed	Bladderwrack	Chlorella
Gotu kola	Suma root	Astragalus	Flax seed oil	Orange peel	Irish moss
Kelp & sea vegetables	Hawthorn bry., lf., fl.	Wild yam root	Evening primrose oil	Ginger root	Apple pectin
Licorice root	Nettles	Peppermint	Schizandra berry	Green tea	Pear powder
Dandelion root & lf.	Royal jelly	Spirulina	Watercress	Aloe vera	Cranberry powder

✍ EXAMPLE FORMULAS OF PRENATAL HEALTH COMPOUNDS:

AN IODINE & POTASSIUM SOURCE CAPSULE COMPOUND		(SA - 2875)		A VITAMIN C & BIOFLAVONOID HERBAL COMPOUND		(PD - 8050)	
Alfalfa	Dulse	Nettles	Watercress	Pear powder	Acerola cherry	Hawthorn bry.	Hibiscus
Dandelion root	Spirulina	Borage seed	Bee pollen	Cranberry powder	Rose hips	Orange peel	Bilberry
Dandelion leaf	Barley grass	Kelp		Apple pectin	Lemon peel	Ginkgo biloba	Honey crystals

SEE PAGE 1 FOR FORMULATING INSTRUCTIONS.

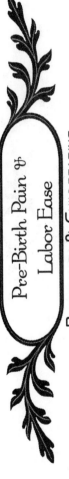

Pre-Birth Pain & Labor Ease

PREGNANCY & CHILDBEARING

Illness, body imbalance, even nutritional supplementation need to be handled differently during pregnancy, especially in the last trimester. A mother's body is very delicately tuned and sensitive at this time. Mega-doses of anything are not good for the baby's system. Dosage of all medication or supplementation should almost universally be about half of normal to allow for the infant's tiny systemic capacity. Ideal supplementation should be from food-source complexes for best absorbability. Herbs are an excellent choice for prenatal supplementation to ease pre-birth and contraction pain. During the last trimester: Rub vitamin E or wheat germ oil on the stomach and around the vaginal opening every night to make stretching easier and the skin more elastic. Begin to take extra minerals as labor approaches for an easier birth. During labor: Take natural vitamin E and calcium/magnesium to relieve pain and aid dilation. For afterbirth pain, herbal analgesic formulas help ease the lower back and spinal block area.

❦ ESSENTIAL CATEGORIES FOR PRE-BIRTH PAIN & LABOR EASE COMPOUNDS:

HERBAL CALCIUM & MAGNESIUM SOURCES	NERVINE HERBS FOR ANXIETY	LABOR-CONT. INDUCERS (USE VERY SMALL AMTS.)	LABOR PAIN EASING HERBS	HERBS TO HELP AGAINST HEMORRHAGING	HERBS FOR POST-PARTUM DEPRESSION
Oats/Oatstraw	**Chamomile**	False Unicorn	**Cramp bark**	**Cayenne**	**St. John's wort**
Catnip	**Passion flower**	Black cohosh rt.	**Kava Kava**	**Hawthorn bry., lf., fl.**	**Ginger root**
Ginger rt.	Scullcap	Blue cohosh rt.	**Wild lettuce**	Bilberry	Motherwort
Carrot powder	**Ashwagandha**	Mugwort	**St. John's wort**	**Nettles**	**Nettles**
Fennel seed	Lemon balm	Wild ginger	**Wild yam root**	**Red raspberry**	**False unicorn**
Alfalfa	Hops	European mistletoe	**Scullcap**	**Bayberry**	Dong quai
Wood betony	**Oats/Oatstraw**	Goldenseal	Ginger root	**False Unicorn**	**Black cohosh**
Parsley root & lf.	**Valerian**	Pennyroyal	White willow bk.	Squaw vine	**Kava kava**
Chamomile	**Catnip**	Wormwood	Lobelia	**Lobelia**	**Squaw vine**

❦ ESSENTIAL HERBS FOR PRE-BIRTH PAIN & LABOR EASE COMPOUNDS:

PRIMARY HERBS		ASSISTING & COMPLEMENTARY HERBS		CATALYST & TRANSPORTING HERBS	
Cramp bark	White willow bk.	Black cohosh rt.	Wild yam root	Orange peel	Motherwort
Kava kava	St. John's wort	Rosemary	Chamomile	Miso	Lemon peel
Black haw bark	Chamomile	Ginger rt.	Squaw vine	European mistletoe	Chaste tree berry
Wild lettuce	Alfalfa	Lemon balm	Nettles	Capsicum	Wild lettuce
Valerian rt.	False Unicorn	Burdock root	European mistletoe	Blue cohosh rt.	Wild ginger
Ashwagandha	Hawthorn bry., lf., fl.	Bilberry	Blue cohosh	Hops	Wormwood
Red raspberry	Catnip	Bayberry	Parsley root & lf.	Ginger root	Carrot powder
Scullcap	Oats/Oatstraw	Wood betony	Fennel seed	Mugwort	Pennyroyal
Passionflower	Lobelia	Passionflower	Wood betony	Dong quai	Goldenseal

❦ EXAMPLE FORMULAS OF PRE-BIRTH PAIN & LABOR EASE COMPOUNDS:

A LABOR-EASING EXTRACT COMPOUND		(co - 4740)	A LABOR-EASING CAPSULE COMPOUND		(co - 1380)
Black haw bark	Lobelia	Orange peel	Kava kava	St. John's wort	Capsicum
Cramp bark	Rosemary	Honey	Black haw bark	White willow bk.	
			Cramp bark	Wild lettuce	
				Valerian rt.	

SEE PAGE 1 FOR FORMULATING INSTRUCTIONS.

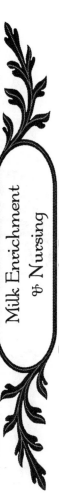

Milk Enrichment & Nursing

PREGNANCY & CHILDBEARING

Unless there is a major health or physical problem, mother's breast milk should be the only food for the baby during the first six months of life. Despite all the claims made for fortified formulas, nothing can take the place of breast milk for baby's health and ongoing well-being. Breast milk is a filtered food supply that prevents the baby from overdosing on higher potencies. The first thick, waxy colostrum is extremely high in protein, fats (needed for brain and nervous system development), and protective antibodies. A child's immune system is not fully established at birth, and the antibodies are critical, both for fighting early infections and in creating solid immune defenses that will prevent the development of allergies. The baby who is not breast-fed loses nature's "jump start" on immunity, and may face health disadvantages that can last a lifetime. Herbal supplements that were used during pregnancy may be continued during nursing.

❧ ESSENTIAL CATEGORIES FOR MILK ENRICHMENT COMPOUNDS:

PLANT PROTEIN SOURCES	SUPERFOOD SOURCES	CALCIUM & MAGNESIUM SOURCE HERBS	MILK PROMOTING HERBS	VITAMIN A & D SOURCE HERBS	ANTI-GAS & DIGESTIVE HERBS
Wheat grass	**Spirulina**	**Royal Jelly/Bee pollen**	**Marshmallow root**	**Alfalfa**	Vegetable acidophilus
Bee pollen/Royal Jelly	**Alfalfa lf. & sprouts**	Ginger root	**Red raspberry**	Kelp & sea vegetables	**Fennel seed**
Spirulina	Chlorella	**Parsley rt. & lf.**	**Fennel seed**	**Dandelion root**	**Catnip**
Alfalfa lf. & sprouts	**Barley grass**	**Spirulina**	**Dandelion rt. & lf.**	Cayenne	**Peppermint**
Chlorella	**Bee pollen**	**Alfalfa**	**Cumin seed**	**Spirulina**	**Thyme**
Barley grass	Kelp & sea vegetables	Sage	Vervain	**Red raspberry**	**Ginger rt.**
Wheat germ	**Royal Jelly**	**Chamomile**	Buckthorn	Bee pollen/Royal jelly	Papaya
Nutritional yeast	**Nutritional yeast**	**Fennel seed**	**Fenugreek seed**	**Licorice root**	Spearmint
Soy protein	Dulse	**Carrot powder**	**Blessed thistle**	Yellow dock rt.	Hibiscus

❧ ESSENTIAL HERBS FOR MILK ENRICHMENT COMPOUNDS:

PRIMARY HERBS		ASSISTING & COMPLEMENTARY HERBS		CATALYST & TRANSPORTING HERBS	
Red raspberry	Bee pollen/Royal jelly	Chamomile	Lemongrass	Thyme	Wheat germ
Fennel seed	Burdock rt	Wild yam root	Sage	Vegetable acidophilus	Wheat grass
Sarsaparilla root	Alfalfa lf. & sprouts	Kava kava	Vervain	Catnip	Anise seed
Spirulina	Gotu kola	Dong qual rt	Evening primrose oil	Capsicum	Peppermint
Licorice root	Nettles	Marshmallow rt.	Buckthorn	Papaya	Hibiscus
Kelp & sea vegetables	Hawthorn bry., lf., fl.	Yellow dock rt.	Blessed thistle	Nutritional yeast	Aloe vera
Black cohosh rt.	Fenugreek seed	Barley grass	Parsley rt. & lf.	Ginger root	Soy & Rice protein
Chlorella	Dandelion rt. & lf.	Spearmint	Oats/Oatstraw lf.	Carrot powder	Wood betony
Saw palmetto bry.	Panax ginseng	Dulse	Strawberry lf.	Cumin seed	Stevia lf.

❧ EXAMPLE FORMULAS OF MILK ENRICHMENT COMPOUNDS:

A MOTHERING TEA COMPOUND			(w - 5870)	A BREAST MILK PROMOTING TEA COMPOUND		
Red raspberry	Alfalfa	Lemongrass	Ginger rt.	Red raspberry	Red raspberry	Marshmallow rt.
Spearmint	Nettles	Fennel seed	Stevia lf.	Spearmint	Fennel seed	Alfalfa
	Horsetail	Strawberry lf.			Fenugreek seed	Anise seed
					Nettles	

SEE PAGE 1 FOR FORMULATING INSTRUCTIONS.

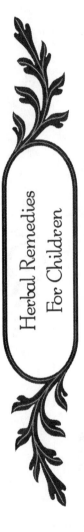

Herbal Remedies
For Children

nless unusually or chronically ill, children have well-developed, powerful immune systems. A child often needs only the subtle body-strengthening forces that nutritious foods, herbs or homeopathic remedies supply, rather than the highly focused medications of allopathic medicine which can have such drastic side effects on a small body. The undeniable ecological, sociological and diet deterioration in America during the last fifty years has had a marked effect on children's health. Declining educational performance, learning disabilities, mental disorders, drug and alcohol abuse, hypoglycemia, allergies, chronic illness, deliquency and violent behavior are all evidence of declining immunity and general health. You can get a lot of help from kids themselves in a natural health program. Kids don't want to be sick, they aren't stupid, they don't like going to the doctor any more than you do. They often recognize that natural foods and therapies are good for them.

Diet Help For Childhood Diseases: Diet is the most important way to keep a child's immunity and defense systems working. Pathogenic organisms and viruses are everywhere. But they aren't the major factor causing disease if the body environment is healthy. Well-nourished children are usually strong enough to deal with infection in a successful way. They either do not catch the "bugs" that are going around, or if they do, illness is short in duration, (childhood diseases are one of Nature's ways of building resistance), or, they get the problem over and done with quickly. A wholesome diet can easily restore a child's vitality. Even children who have eaten a junk food diet for years quickly respond to a diet of fresh fruits, vegetables, whole grains, low fats and sugars. I have noted great improvement in as little as a month's time. A child's hair and skin takes on new luster, they fill out if they are too skinny, and lose weight if they are too fat. They sleep more soundly and regularly. Their attention spans markedly increase, and many learning and behavior problems diminish or disappear.

Herbal Remedies For Healing Children: A child's body responds very well to herbal medicines. Herbal remedies are building, strengthening and non-traumatic to a child's system. I have found that children drink herbal teas, take herbal drops, syrups and homeopathic medicines much more readily than you might think. Most herbal remedies can be taken as needed, then reduced and discontinued as the problem improves. Take only one or two herbal combinations at the same time when working with a child's system. Choose the herbal remedy that addresses the worst problem first. One of the bonuses of a natural healing program is the frequent discovery that other conditions were really complications of the first problem, and often take care of themselves as the body comes into balance. In addition, rotating and alternating herbal combinations according to the changing health state of the child allows the body to remain most responsive to herbal effects. Reduce dosage as the problem improves - allowing the body to pick up its own work and bring its own vital forces into action. It's best to let herbs gently rebuild health. Even when a good healing program is working, and obvious improvement is being made, adding more of the remedy in an effort to speed healing can aggravate symptoms and worsen the condition. The way to use herbs is as important as the herbs you choose.

Herbal remedy effectiveness usually goes by body weight. Base dose decisions on weight for both adults and children. Child dosage is as follows:

$1/2$ dose for children 10-14 years.
$1/3$ dose for children 6-10 years.
$1/4$ dose for children 2-6 years.
$1/8$ dose for infants and babies.

Special Notes: •Do not use honey in teas for children less than one year old. Honey has been linked to infant botulism, which can be life threatening. •Do not use aspirin for a child's viral infection. Aspirin given during a viral infection has been linked to the development of Reye's syndrome, a dangerous liver disease in children. •Antibiotic drugs can be tough on a small child's system, especially over a long period of time. Question your doctor if an antibiotic prescription seems automatic, particularly if your child has a viral infection.

❧ COMPOUNDS FOR FORMULATION INCLUDE:

•Childhood allergies and sensitivities
•Dealing with acute childhood diseases
•Overcoming hyperactive attention deficit disorder
•Childhood epilepsy and seizures

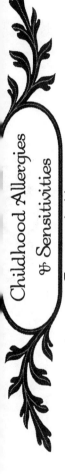

Childhood Allergies & Sensitivities

Children's Health

Children's allergies are on the rise, manifesting themselves not only as sneezing, headaches and rashes, but also as changes in personality and emotions. The greatest allergy increase in children is to foods, commonly to dairy, wheat, eggs, chocolate, nuts, seafood and citrus fruits. If your child is allergic, try eliminating one of these foods at a time for a few weeks and watch to see if there is improvement. Eliminate dairy foods and cooked fats and oils because they thicken and stimulate excess mucous. Give the child lots of water to thin secretions and ease expectoration. Essential fatty acids help regulate the inflammatory response. Use flaxseed oil for children, and mix into foods like salad dressings or in place of butter. In addition to the herbal remedies below, vitamin supplements for childhood allergies (in child amounts) might include: beta-carotene to help heal irritated mucous membranes, vitamin C with bioflavonoids as an anti-inflammatory, and calcium/magnesium for overreactive nerves.

Essential Categories for Childhood Allergy Compounds:

Expectorant Herbs	Demulcent, Soothing Herbs	Calcium/Magnesium Sources	Antihistamine, Anti-inflammatories	Vitamin C & Bioflavonoid Sources	Immune Boosters & Lymph Clearers
Wild cherry bark	**Licorice root**	**Barley grass**	**Ephedra leaf**	**Kelp/sea vegetables**	**Burdock root**
Anise seed	**Coltsfoot**	**Alfalfa**	**Marshmallow root**	**Bilberry**	**Dandelion root & lf.**
Fennel seed	Chickweed	**Catnip**	**Bee pollen**	**Hawthorn lf. flr. & bry.**	Licorice root
Elecampane	Burdock root	**Chamomile**	**Lobelia**	**Aloe vera**	Astragalus
Licorice root	Peppermint	**Fennel seed**	Pleurisy root	**Rose hips**	Yellow dock rt.
Plantain	**Flax seed**	**Parsley rt & lf.**	**Parsley**	Cranberry powder	Goldenseal root
Lobelia	**Irish moss**	**Carrot powder**	**Acerola cherry**	Red clover	**Bee pollen**
Mullein	**Marshmallow root**	**Wood betony**	Juniper berry	Parsley leaf	**Echinacea root**
Horehound	**Slippery elm**	**Ginger root**	**Ginger root**	Catnip	**Lobelia**

Essential Herbs for Childhood Allergy Compounds:

Primary Herbs		Assisting & Complementary Herbs		Catalyst & Transporting Herbs	
Bee pollen	Marshmallow rt.	Dandelion rt. & lf.	Parsley rt. & lf.	Wood betony	Red clover
Flax seed	Catnip	Fennel seed	Slippery elm	Anise seed	Rosebuds
Chamomile	Gotu kola	Ephedra leaf	Aloe vera	Carrot powder	Thyme
Acerola cherry	Kelp/sea vegetables	Echinacea root	Wild cherry bk.	Milk thistle seed	Chamomile
Licorice root	Hawthorn lf. flr. & bry.	Boneset	Rose hips	Irish moss	Calendula flower
Barley grass	Coltsfoot	Goldenseal root	Bilberry	Cloves	Cranberry powder
Lobelia	Mullein	Pleurisy root	Ginger rt.	Burdock rt.	Juniper bry.
Astragalus	Horehound	Elecampane	Peppermint	Stevia	Yellow dock rt.
Plantain	Chlorella	Alfalfa	Reishi mushroom	Green tea	Orange peel

Example Formulas of Childhood Allergy Compounds:

A Gentle Expectorant Tea Compound (B - 5930)

Licorice root	Mullein	Peppermint	Ginger rt.
Ephedra leaf	Rosehips	Fennel seed	Calendula flower
Pleurisy root	Marshmallow rt.	Boneset	Stevia

An Allergy, Antihistamine Tea Compound (B - 5960)

Horehound	Rose hips	Bee pollen	Orange peel
Peppermint	Ephedra leaf	Anise seed	Cloves
	Rosebuds	Ginger root	Burdock rt.

See page 1 for formulating instructions.

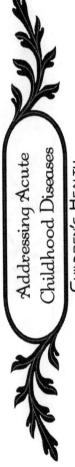

Addressing Acute Childhood Diseases

CHILDREN'S HEALTH

Keeping a child's resistance and immune response strong is the key to understanding and dealing appropriately with children's diseases. The current official government position on immunizations against a variety of childhood diseases has been to vaccinate early (and often several times). Yet, naturopaths are seeing that preventing children from ever getting ailments like chicken pox, measles or mumps, may be depriving them of a powerful childhood natural disease resistance process. Information is coming to light that adults who received all their childhood immunizations of the fifties and sixties did not get childhood diseases, but seem to be at far greater risk for disease as adults than their counterparts whose bodies were allowed to fight against a childhood disease and establish natural immunity. A fresh foods diet and herbal remedies as therapeutic complements to the natural body processes are a good choice for alleviating symptoms and making the child more comfortable.

❧ ESSENTIAL CATEGORIES FOR ACUTE CHILDHOOD DISEASE COMPOUNDS:

HERBS TO INCREASE PERSPIRATION	RELAXING NERVINE HERBS	EXPECTORANT HERBS	LYMPHATIC CLEANSING HERBS	HERB FOR UPSET STOMACHS	CIRCULATION STIMULATING HERBS
Yarrow	**Chamomile**	**Wild cherry bark**	**Burdock root**	**Catnip**	**Ginger root**
Hyssop	Lobelia	Anise seed	**Dandelion root & lf.**	Fennel	**Dandelion rt. & lf.**
Garlic	**Scullcap**	**Fennel seed**	Licorice root	**Peppermint**	**Hawthorn bry., lf., fl.**
Buchu	Passionflower	Elecampane	Astragalus	**Lemon Balm**	**Ginkgo biloba**
Boneset	Catnip	**Licorice root**	Goldenseal root	**Ginger root**	Bayberry
Elder flowers	**Oats/Oatstraw**	Plantain	**Myrrh**	**Chamomile**	Parsley root & lf.
Ginger root	Hops	**Lobelia**	**Acerola cherry**	**Spearmint**	**Bilberry**
Angelica root	Angelica root	**Mullein**	**Echinacea root**	Papaya leaf	Bee pollen/Royal jelly
Peppermint	Mullein	Horehound	**Lobelia**	Sage	**Cinnamon**

❧ ESSENTIAL HERBS FOR ACUTE CHILDHOOD DISEASE COMPOUNDS:

PRIMARY HERBS	ASSISTING & COMPLEMENTARY HERBS	CATALYST & TRANSPORTING HERBS
Catnip	Elecampane	Spearmint	Astragalus	Reishi mushroom
Dandelion rt. & lf.	Goldenseal root	Alfalfa	Mullein	Bayberry
Licorice root	Hyssop	Red clover	Nettles	Horehound
Bilberry	Rose hips	Elder flowers	Rosebuds	Sage
Acerola cherry	Scullcap	Oats/Oatstraw	Peppermint	Buchu
Chamomile	Plantain	Garlic	Papaya leaf	Burdock root
Ginger root	Yarrow	Parsley root & lf.	Hops	Wild cherry bk.
Bee pollen	Cinnamon	Echinacea root	Anise seed	Stevia leaf
Boneset	Fennel seed	Angelica root	Orange peel	Myrrh
Lobelia				
Bee pollen				
Ginkgo biloba				
Aloe vera				
Lemon balm				
Passionflower				
Hawthorn bry., lf., fl.				
Royal jelly				
White pine bark				

❧ EXAMPLE FORMULAS OF ACUTE CHILDHOOD DISEASE COMPOUNDS:

A RELAXING TEA COMPOUND			(RX – 5990)
Lemon balm	Spearmint	Yerba santa	Passionflower
Lemongrass	Licorice root	Cinnamon	Rosebuds
	Orange peel	Rosemary	Anise seed

A FIRST AID TEA FOR KIDS COMPOUND			(PD – 5320)
Chamomile	Lemon balm	Acerola cherry	Wild cherry bk.
Catnip	Fennel seed	Cinnamon	Stevia leaf

SEE PAGE 1 FOR FORMULATING INSTRUCTIONS.

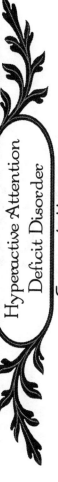

Hyperactive Attention Deficit Disorder

CHILDREN'S HEALTH

Hyperactive behavior and Attention Deficit Disorder have been serious problems for children since the nineteen-fifties. Hyperactivity seems to be the expression of either hypoglycemia or food allergies or both. Attention Deficit Disorder is slow learning caused by any or all of the learning disorders. Autism is almost a "mind-blind" condition, characterized by withdrawn behavior, lack of emotion and speech, and extreme sensitivity to sound and touch. Autistic children have a brain malfunction that creates a barrier between them and the rest of the world. Children at greatest risk are male, with a history of family diabetes or alcoholism. The current drugs of choice, such as Ritalin, have a history of unpleasant, even fearful side effects. Nutritional improvement and calming herbs are the cornerstones of successful treatment in overcoming hyperactivity.

❧ ESSENTIAL CATEGORIES FOR ATTENTION DEFICIT DISORDER COMPOUNDS:

CALMING, NERVINE HERBS	HERBS FOR INNER EAR BALANCE	B VITAMIN SOURCES	VITAMIN C & BIOFLAVONOID SOURCES	ESSENTIAL FATTY ACID BRAIN NUTRIENTS	CALCIUM/MAGNESIUM SOURCES
Chamomile	**Gotu kola**	Dandelion rt.	**Rose hips**	**Evening primrose oil**	**Chamomile**
Black haw	**Ginkgo biloba**	Bee pollen/Royal Jelly	**Kelp/sea vegetables**	**Flax seed oil**	**Fennel seed**
Scullcap	Kava kava rt.	**Thyme**	**Acerola cherry**	Borage seed	Sage
Passionflower	**Bee pollen/Royal Jelly**	**Kelp & sea vegetables**	**Aloe vera**	**Chlorella**	**Alfalfa**
Wood betony	**Ginger root**	**Red raspberry**	Hawthorn bry., lf., fl.	**Kelp**	**Catnip**
Oats/Oatstraw	Lobelia	Burdock rt.	**Dandelion root & lf.**	**Spirulina**	Ginger root
European mistletoe	St. John's wort	**Barley grass**	Red clover	**Black currant**	Parsley rt. & lf.
St. John's wort	Hawthorn bry., lf., fl.	Watercress	**Bilberry**	Barley grass	**Carrot powder**
Lobelia	**Peppermint**	Parsley rt. & lf.	Parsley rt. & lf.	**Dulse**	**Wood betony**

❧ ESSENTIAL HERBS FOR FOR ATTENTION DEFICIT DISORDER COMPOUNDS:

PRIMARY HERBS		ASSISTING & COMPLEMENTARY HERBS		CATALYST & TRANSPORTING HERBS	
Ginkgo biloba	Evening primrose oil	Rosemary	Thyme	Peppermint	Kelp
Bee pollen/Royal Jelly	Valerian rt.	Black cohosh root	Alfalfa	Aloe vera	Reishi mushroom
Acerola cherry	Kava kava root	Dandelion root & lf.	Horsetail	Rose hips	Watercress
Bilberry	Gotu kola	St. John's wort	Wood betony	Sage	Parsley rt. & lf.
Scullcap	Lobelia	Red raspberry	European mistletoe	Shepherd's purse	Red clover
Licorice root	Hawthorn bry., lf., fl.	Catnip	Burdock rt.	Borage seed	Fennel seed
Kelp & sea vegetables	Spirulina	Barley grass	Flax seed oil	Ginger root	Black currant
Flax seed oil	Ashwagandha	Oatstraw	Passionflower	Shiitake mushroom	Dulse
Chamomile	Wild lettuce	Black haw bark	Hops	Chlorella	Carrot powder

❧ EXAMPLE FORMULAS OF ATTENTION DEFICIT DISORDER COMPOUNDS:

A MENTAL CLARITY CAPSULE COMPOUND			(RX - 3800)	SINGLE HERB SPECIFICS
Ashwagandha	Kava kava rt.	European mistletoe	Lobelia	**Note:** EVENING PRIMROSE OIL (250 to 500mg for critical EFAs), WILD LETTUCE/VALERIAN extract (for calming), and GINKGO BILOBA extract (for inner ear balance) drops in water are specific herbs that may be used throughout treatment.
Black cohosh root	Black haw bark	Wood betony	Oatstraw	
Scullcap	Valerian rt.	Hops		

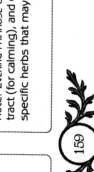

SEE PAGE 1 FOR FORMULATING INSTRUCTIONS.

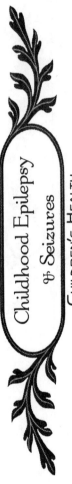

Childhood Epilepsy & Seizures

CHILDREN'S HEALTH

Epilepsy is a neurological disorder that involves recurrent electrical disturbances in the brain, causing seizures. 1) Petit mal involves short seizures with a blank stare and is the type most common in children; 2) Grand mal involves long seizures with falling, muscle twitching, incontinence, gasping, and ashen skin. 3) Partial seizures involve muscle jerking, and sensing things that do not exist. Most people have no memory of an attack. Many commonly used anticonvulsant drugs today are so strong and so habit forming (especially for children), that even non-epileptic people have bad reactions and seizures when cut off suddenly. Nutritional medicines can make drugs unnecessary. If you decide to use natural therapies, or try methods other than drugs, taper off gradually and always consult your physician. If seizures recur, return to the anti-convulsant drugs briefly to let the body adjust.

❧ ESSENTIAL CATEGORIES FOR CHILDHOOD EPILEPSY & SEIZURE COMPOUNDS:

ANTISPASMODIC HERBS	MINERAL-RICH HERBS	TONIC ADAPTOGEN HERBS	ESSENTIAL FATTY ACID HERBS	LIVER SUPPORT & B VITAMIN SOURCES	NERVE CALMING HERBS
Cramp bark	**Kelp/sea vegetables**	**Gotu kola**	**Evening primrose oil**	**Nutritional yeast**	**Chamomile**
Black cohosh	**Ginkgo biloba**	**Ashwagandha rt.**	**Flax seed oil**	**Royal Jelly/Bee pollen**	**Scullcap**
Kava kava	**Spirulina**	Suma root	Borage seed	Parsley rt. & lf.	**Oatstraw**
Black haw	**Barley grass**	**Schizandra berry**	**Chlorella**	**Milk thistle seed**	**European mistletoe**
Red raspberry	**Dandelion rt. & lf.**	**Licorice root**	Kelp & sea vegetables	**Watercress**	**Gotu kola**
Lemon balm	**Horsetail**	**Wild yam root**	**Spirulina**	**Pau d' arco**	**Valerian**
Wild yam root	**Yellow dock root**	**Burdock root**	**Black currant**	Kelp/sea vegetables	Catnip
Lobelia	**Chickweed**	**Black cohosh root**	Barley grass	**Dandelion root & lf.**	Rosemary
Scullcap	**Aloe vera**	**Dong qual rt.**	**Safflowers**	Yellow dock root	St. John's wort

❧ ESSENTIAL HERBS FOR CHILDHOOD EPILEPSY & SEIZURE COMPOUNDS:

PRIMARY HERBS		CATALYST & TRANSPORTING HERBS	
Ginkgo biloba	Bee pollen/Royal jelly	Chickweed	Anise seed
St. John's wort	Burdock rt	Soy protein	Hibiscus
Chamomile	Catnip	Safflowers	Oatstraw
Scullcap	Gotu kola	Dong qual rt.	European mistletoe
Licorice root	Black cohosh	Valerian	Flax seed
Kelp & sea vegetables	Hawthorn bry., lf., fl.	Nutritional yeast	Fennel seed
Cramp bark.	Kava kava	Ginger root	Miso
Suma root	Lobelia	Black currant	Milk thistle seed
Schizandra berry	Pau d' arco	Red sage	Borage seed

ASSISTING & COMPLEMENTARY HERBS	
Ashwagandha rt.	Red raspberry
Yellow dock root	Alfalfa
Dandelion root & lf.	Rosemary
Bilberry	Aloe vera
Spirulina/Chlorella	Lemon balm
Horsetail	Watercress
Barley grass	Milk thistle seed
Evening primrose oil	Parsley rt. & lf.
Wild yam root	Black haw

❧ EXAMPLE FORMULAS OF CHILDHOOD EPILEPSY & SEIZURE COMPOUNDS:

A SYSTEM STRENGTHENING DRINK MIX COMPOUND   (SA - 8230)

Alfalfa	Dandelion rt. & lf.	Fennel seed
Borage seed	Barley grass	Parsley rt. & lf.
Yellow dock root	Licorice root	Bilberry
Oatstraw	Watercress	Red raspberry	Schizandra berry
Miso	Soy protein	Rosemary	Sea vegetables

A LIVER SUPPORT TEA COMPOUND   (CD - 5780)

Dandelion rt.	Hyssop	Oregon grape rt.	Hibiscus
Watercress	Pau d' arco bk.	Red sage	White sage
Yellow dock rt.	Parsley lf.	Licorice rt.	Anise seed
Milk thistle seed			

SEE PAGE 1 FOR FORMULATING INSTRUCTIONS.

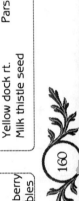

Herbal Remedies
For Pets

ur pets usually need more nutrition than is found in common commercial animal foods. Most pet foods are derived from low quality ingredients rejected for human consumption. Pet foods that are advertised as "Complete and Balanced" are regularly based on uncertain minimum nutrition requirements designed only for adequate health, not optimal health. We have come to accept canned and dried foods as being normal, but many vitamin and mineral nutrients are lost through "mixmaster" processing that relies heavily on chemical additives to make the food palatable and the shelf life long. Veterinarians today are seeing an abundance of premature and chronic health problems that seem to stem from substandard, low quality, processed foods.

Chemicals additives (many known to be toxic) can be legally included in animal foods. Some of the worst offenders, present in virtually every supermarket pet food include: sodium nitrite, red dye #40, BHA, BHT, MSG, sodium metabisulfite, artificial flavorings, propylene glycol, and ethoxyquin. Salt is used as a preservative in pet foods, which can irritate the intestines and contribute to high blood pressure and heart disease in pets. Sugar is a frequent additive, and causes animal problems like hypoglycemia, overweight, nervousness, cataracts, tooth decay, arthritis, and allergies, because sugar drains nutrients from the body. I recommend the chemical-free pet foods found in health food stores. Several veterinarians that use natural healing methods on pets and advise us for this book feel that many of today's pet ailments are a result of chemical laced foods and environmental pollutants... just like people.

Animals' bodies rely on enzymes even more than ours. It's the reason some animals, even some whole breeds, tend to eat waste excrement- for the enzymes. Besides being the driving force behind all life processes, enzymes are responsible for keeping internal systems working. A lack of sufficient enzymes promotes degenerative disease. Almost all pet food is cooked, pasteurized, canned or microwaved, which means most enzymes are destroyed. Uncooked, whole foods contain enzymes, as well as vitamins, minerals and chlorophyll, so it is important to add some fresh greens and vegetables to an animal's diet. (See Healthy Healing 10th Edition for complete diet information.)

Herbs and homeopathic medicines can help maintain pet health. Herbal remedies have proven very effective for animal illness, and are successful as gentle, non-toxic aids in maintaining animal health. Herbs are, of course, food source supplements and can be used efficiently and easily by an animal's system. Natural therapies create an environment in which the animal's body can support its own healing functions, especially with the aid of a good diet. Both dogs and cats are comfortable taking herbs internally as pills, powders, teas and tinctures. The trick is knowing how to give them quickly and with a minimum of fuss. Oftentimes they will lick and eat herbs as they do foods, or they will take them as "treats." Be careful that the base/solidifying/emulsifying ingredients that you use for ointments, salves and other topical applications are safe for ingestion since most animals will try to lick them off. (Sometimes this is a good way to get the herbs into their systems!)

How to give Tinctures, Extracts, Syrups and Liquids to Cats and Dogs:

Pry open mouth by firmly grasping the animal's upper jaw with one hand and inserting thumb and a finger in the gap between the teeth. Tilt the head back slightly. Most animals will relax their mouths slightly at this point so that you can pour the liquid with a spoon or dropper between the teeth, letting the liquid run down the throat. Stroke the throat to make the animal swallow. If there is resistance, wrap the animal in a towel, or get someone to hold it if it backs away. Teas and other therapeutic drinks, such as protein drinks or chlorophyll liquid in water, may be simply given in a bowl to be lapped up; both cats and dogs will usually drink enough of the mixture naturally throughout the day for therapeutic effectiveness. If there is resistance, spoon or eyedropper it into the mouth. Always be gentle and speak positively during the process so the animal doesn't feel frightened and anxious.

How to give Pills and Capsules to Cats and Dogs:

Open the mouth as described above for giving liquids. Hold the pill between the thumb and forefinger and keep the lower jaw pressed down with the other fingers. Quickly place the pill on the back of the tongue and push it as far back into the throat as you can. Hold the muzzle shut and stroke the throat so the animal will swallow.

**Remember that dosage for herbal and natural medications is by body weight, as it is for humans. Animals seventy pounds and over can usually take the same amount as an adult human, half doses for 30 to 65 pounds, quarter doses for 15 to 25 pounds, and eighth doses for babies and very small animals.

❧ COMPOUNDS FOR FORMULATION INCLUDE:

- Overcoming animal arthritis and displaysia
- Enhancing skin, coat and eyes
- Ridding your pet of parasites and worms

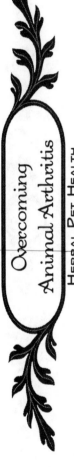

Overcoming Animal Arthritis

HERBAL PET HEALTH

Arthritis and other joint problems are more common in dogs than in cats. Most cases could be prevented if female dogs are fed properly during pregnancy (See HEALTHY HEALING: 10TH EDITION for a complete diet program for pets and more details.) Herbs can support body cleansing, detoxification and and improvement of body chemistry; they can dissolve and flush out inorganic mineral deposits, and help replace them with non-mucous forming nutrients. Where serious inflammation is evidence that the animal is not producing enough natural cortisone, herbs are particularly effective for adrenal gland nourishment. Many herbs are high in vitamin C and organic silica for the rebuilding of healthy collagen and tissue. Even in advanced and chronic cases of pain, inflammation and joint degeneration, with major digestive disorders and attendant toxic syndromes of depression and exhaustion, diet and herbs can effect improvement.

❧ ESSENTIAL CATEGORIES FOR ANIMAL ARTHRITIS COMPOUNDS:

HERBS TO COMBAT JOINT DEGENERATION	ANTI-INFLAMMATORY EFA HERBS	MINERAL RICH SOURCES	ACID/ALKALINE BALANCERS	VITAMIN C & BIOFLAVONOID SOURCES	ANTIOXIDANT HERBS
Kelp/sea vegetables	Devil's claw	Barley grass	Burdock rt.	Kelp/sea vegetables	Kelp/sea vegetables
Bilberry	Dandelion root & lf.	Alfalfa	Marshmallow root	Bilberry	Dandelion root & lf.
Parsley lf.	Comfrey root	Catnip	Aloe vera	Hawthorn lf. flr. & bry.	Ginkgo biloba
Royal jelly/Bee pollen	Aloe vera	Chamomile	Catnip	Aloe vera	Bilberry
Licorice root	Yarrow	Aloe vera	Chamomile	Rosehips	Mullein
Red clover	Flax seed	Parsley rt & lf.	Parsley	Cranberry powder	Wheat germ
Lobelia	Yucca	Oats/Oatstraw	Uva ursi	Papaya	Bee pollen
Ginger rt.	Turmeric	Yellow dock rt.	Alfalfa	Parsley leaf	Echinacea root
Spirulina	Slippery elm	Pau d' arco bark	Barley grass	Catnip	Garlic

❧ ESSENTIAL HERBS FOR ANIMAL ARTHRITIS COMPOUNDS:

PRIMARY HERBS	ASSISTING & COMPLEMENTARY HERBS	CATALYST & TRANSPORTING HERBS
Bee pollen	Marshmallow rt.	Dandelion rt. & lf.	Parsley rt & lf.	Nutritional yeast	Royal jelly
Flax seed	Catnip	Devil's claw rt.	Ginkgo biloba	Acidolphilus powder	Comfrey root
Yucca	Gotu kola	Oats	Aloe vera	Papaya leaf	Lobelia
Garlic	Kelp/sea vegetables	Bilberry	Pau d' arco bark	Sodium Ascorbate C	Chamomile
Licorice root	Hawthorn lf. flr. & bry.	Buckthorn	Burdock rt.	Wheat germ	Uva ursi
Barley grass	Spirulina	Black cohosh	Dulse	Irish moss	Cranberry powder
Sarsaparilla rt.	Yarrow	Slippery elm	Ginger rt.	Rice protein	Mullein
Red clover	Nutritional yeast	Yellow dock rt.	Siberian ginseng	Apple pectin	Rose hips
Alfalfa leaf/seed	Chlorella	Oatstraw	Turmeric	Acerola cherry	Echinacea root

❧ EXAMPLE FORMULAS OF ANIMAL ARTHRITIS COMPOUNDS:

AN ARTHRITIS-EASING COMPOUND			(A - 9050)
Nutritional yeast	Garlic	Bilberry	Licorice rt.
Alfalfa leaf/seed	Yucca	Black cohosh	Parsley lf. & rt.
Sodium Ascorbate	Turmeric	Buckthorn	Slippery elm
Vitamin C	Devil's claw rt..	Yarrow	Dandelion rt.

A CLOROPHYLL-RICH GREEN DRINK COMPOUND			(SA - 8150)
Barley grass	Acerola cherry	Dandelion lf.	Oats
Alfalfa	Sarsaparilla rt.	Gotu kola lf.	Rice protein
Bee pollen	Chlorella	Licorice rt.	Apple pectin
Siberian ginseng	Dulse	Dandelion rt.	

SEE PAGE 1 FOR FORMULATING INSTRUCTIONS.

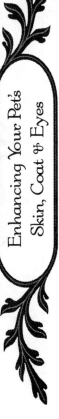

Enhancing Your Pet's Skin, Coat & Eyes

Herbal Pet Health

Unhealthy skin, coat and eye conditions are the most frequent problems of pets today, ranging from flea infestations to mange, eczema and dermatitis. Eye infections cause cloudy eyes, styes and itchy, mucous-clogged eyes. Many of these disorders are the result of a poor, unbalanced diet **with no fresh foods for critical enzymes,** contaminants from pest control sprays and pesticides, and environmental pollutants. A successful herbal skin formula should seek to address the cause of these problems by neutralizing acidity, improving digestion and elimination, adding hydrating elements, and healing damaged tissue.

Herbs are a good choice to help your pet in these areas. As concentrated foods, they work at the deepest levels of the body processes, where most skin, coat and eye problems occur and where they can be helped the most for the most permanent results.

ESSENTIAL CATEGORIES FOR ENHANCING YOUR PET'S BEAUTY COMPOUNDS:

HERBS TO HELP PURIFY THE BLOOD	ACID/ALKALINE BALANCERS	DIGESTION/ELIMINATION ENHANCERS	GREEN SUPERFOOD HERBS	HYDRATING, SOOTHING HERBS	ANTIBIOTIC, ANTIOXIDANT HERBS
Nutritional yeast	**Chamomile**	**Dandelion rt. & lf.**	**Spirulina**	**Catnip**	**Burdock root**
Kelp & sea vegetables	Aloe vera	**Catnip**	**Dandelion leaf**	**Slippery elm**	**Dandelion rt. & lf.**
Garlic	**Burdock root**	**Papaya leaf**	Nettles	Aloe vera	**Wheat germ**
Alfalfa	**Marshmallow root**	Peppermint	Alfalfa	**Marshmallow root**	**Echinacea**
St. John's wort	**Catnip**	Miso	Kelp & sea vegetables	**Yellow dock root**	Rosemary
Ginger root	**Dandelion rt. & lf.**	**Fenugreek seed**	**Aloe vera**	**Chamomile**	Parsley root & lf.
Parsley root & lf.	Bee pollen	Kelp & sea vegetables	**Barley grass**	**Thyme**	**Sage**
Yarrow	Barley grass	**Acidophilus**	**Chlorella**	Papaya leaf	Lecithin
Fennel seed	Alfalfa	Comfrey leaf	Parsley root & lf.	Peppermint	**Garlic**

ESSENTIAL HERBS FOR ENHANCING YOUR PET'S BEAUTY COMPOUNDS:

PRIMARY HERBS		ASSISTING & COMPLEMENTARY HERBS		CATALYST & TRANSPORTING HERBS	
Alfalfa	Garlic	Licorice root	Oatstraw	Miso	Rosemary
Dandelion rt. & lf.	Catnip	Pau d' arco	Yellow dock root	Acidophilus	Red raspberry
Lecithin	Dulse leaf	Horsetail	Red clover	Nutritional yeast	Slippery elm
Bilberry	Aloe vera	Parsley root & lf.	Elder flowers	Soy protein	Sage
Kelp & sea vegetables	Lemon balm	Marshmallow root	Burdock root	Peppermint	Rose hips
Chamomile	Nettles	Plantain	Fenugreek seed	Papaya leaf	Comfrey root
Ginger root	Thyme	Yarrow	Borage seed	Wheat bran	St. John's wort
Bee pollen	Spirulina	Fennel seed	Echinacea root	Wheat germ	Nettles
Barley grass	White pine bark	Watercress	Comfrey lf.	Sodium Ascorbate C	Chlorella

EXAMPLE FORMULAS OF ENHANCING YOUR PET'S BEAUTY COMPOUNDS:

AN OVERALL PET HEALTH COMPOUND		(A - 9010)	A SYSTEM STRENGTHENING DRINK COMPOUND		(SA - 8230)
Nutritional yeast	Barley grass	Spirulina	Miso	Borage seed	Nettles
Alfalfa	Garlic	Sodium Asc. C	Nutritional yeast	Yellow dock root	Horsetail
Lecithin	Soy protein	Rosemary	Soy protein	Oatstraw	Red raspberry
	Dandelion lf.		Alfalfa	Dandelion lf.	Fennel seed

SEE PAGE 1 FOR FORMULATING INSTRUCTIONS.

163

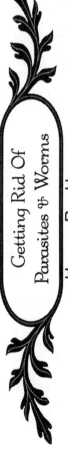

Getting Rid Of Parasites & Worms

Herbal Pet Health

Animals are constantly exposed to parasites from fleas and ticks, or from eating wild animals such as gophers and rats. A rundown animal with recurrent parasitic infestation indicates that immune resistance is low. Herbs can be a gentle, effective means of relieving parasite infestation. In our experience, the best method for expelling worms is to start by feeding a low fat, low carbohydrate diet for three days with no sweeteners or dairy products, to deprive the parasites of nutrients. Then put the animal on a 24 hour liquid diet with 1 teasp. of castor oil to clear the bowels. The next morning give herbal de-worming medicine. After an hour give another spoonful of castor oil and some slippery elm tea. Repeat the low fat and treatment for 3 days, adding oatmeal, garlic and honey syrup, acidophilus, and a little boiled fish. Check the stool for infestation at the end of a week, and repeat if necessary another week. The worms will be a weaker, and the animal's resistance much higher to remove remaining worms and eggs.

❧ ESSENTIAL CATEGORIES FOR VERMIFUGE & PARASITICIDE COMPOUNDS:

Laxative, Cleansing Herbs	Nutritive, Balancing Herbs	Vermifuge (worm expelling) Herbs	Vermicide (worm killing) Herbs	Herbs To Establish Digestive Integrity	Immune/Resistance Building Herbs
Butternut bark	Nutritional yeast	**Cascara sagrada**	**Black walnut**	**Acidophilus powder**	**Garlic**
Cascara sagarada	**Alfalfa**	**Gentian**	**Garlic**	Nutritional yeast	**Echinacea**
Slippery elm	Kelp & sea vegetables	**Mugwort**	**Thyme**	Miso	**Myrrh**
Fennel seed	**Bee pollen/Royal jelly**	**Senna**	**Aloe vera**	**Chlorella**	**Alfalfa**
Flax seed	**Oats**	**Wormwood**	Wormwood	Kelp/sea vegetables	**Nutritional yeast**
Garlic	Irish moss	**Tea tree oil**	Tea tree oil	**Spirulina**	Licorice root
Lemon balm	Parsley rt. & lf.	False unicorn rt.	Tansy	**Peppermint**	Pau d' arco
Senna	Nettles.	Pumpkin seed	**Comfrey rt & lf.**	Barley grass	**Mullein**
Ginger root	**Peppermint**	Dandelion rt.	**Flax seed oil**	**Dandelion rt. & lf.**	Onion

❧ ESSENTIAL HERBS FOR VERMIFUGE & PARASITICIDE COMPOUNDS:

Primary Herbs		Assisting & Complementary Herbs		Catalyst & Transporting Herbs	
Black walnut hulls	Butternut	Gentian rt.	Nettles.	Acidophilus powder	Lemon balm
Garlic	Fennel seed	Mugwort	Bee pollen/Royal jelly	Lecithin	Rosemary
Pumpkin seed	Alfalfa	Ginger root	Myrrh	Wheat bran	Watercress
Wormwood	Dandelion root & lf.	Comfrey rt & lf.	Echinacea	Wheat germ	Parsley rt. & lf.
Cascara sagrada	Butternut bark	Thyme	Peppermint	Sodium Asc. C	Red clover
Licorice root	Tea tree oil	Aloe vera	Senna	Borage seed	Fennel seed
Kelp & sea vegetables	Spirulina	Barley grass	Miso	Irish moss	Tansy
Flax seed oil	Pau d' arco	Oatstraw	Mullein	False unicorn	Dulse
Nutritional yeast	Slippery elm	Nutritional yeast	Soy protein	Chlorella	Onion

❧ EXAMPLE FORMULAS OF VERMIFUGE & PARASITICIDE COMPOUNDS:

A VERMIFUGE CAPSULE COMPOUND		(CD – 4200)	A VERMIFUGE COMPOUND		(CD - 8230)
Black walnut hulls	Fennel seed	Mugwort	Gentian rt.	Mugwort	Spirulina
Garlic	Cascara sagrada	Slippery elm	Wormwood	Slippery elm	Sodium Asc. C
Pumpkin seed		False unicorn	Butternut	False unicorn	Rosemary

A SYSTEM STRENGTHENING DRINK COMPOUND		(SA - 8230)
Nutritional yeast	Kelp	Barley grass
Alfalfa	Wheat bran	Garlic
Lecithin	Wheat germ	Soy protein
	Comfrey lf.	Dandelion lf.

See page 1 for formulating instructions.

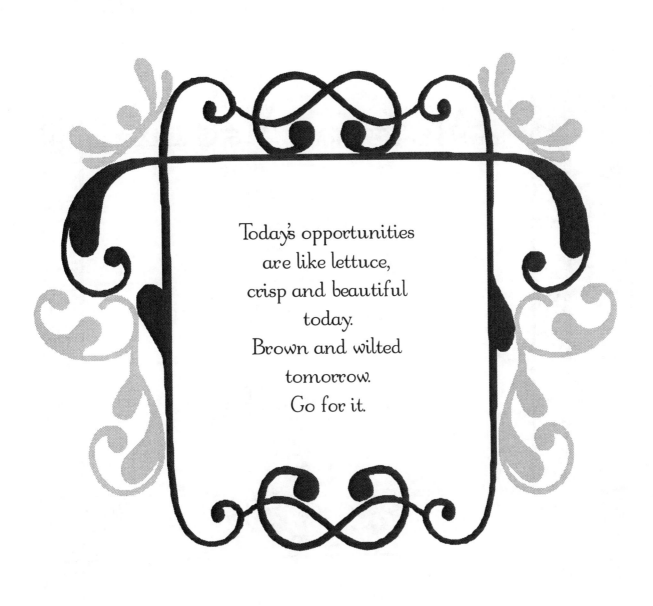

Today's opportunities
are like lettuce,
crisp and beautiful
today.
Brown and wilted
tomorrow.
Go for it.

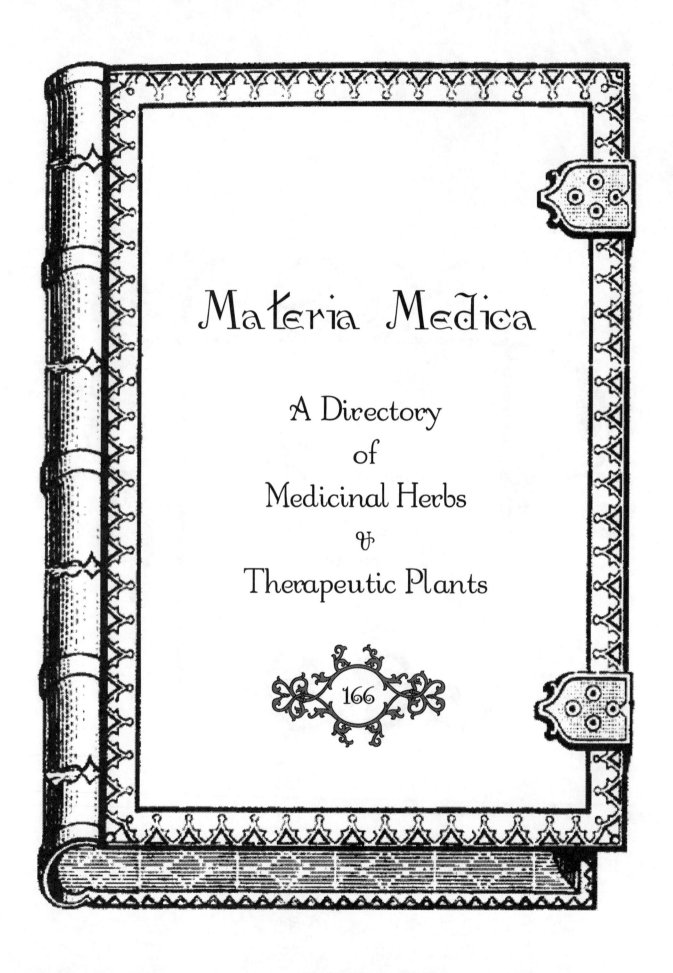

Materia Medica

A Directory

of

Medicinal Herbs

&

Therapeutic Plants

166

A Modern Materia Medica

This modern materia medica directory catalogues medicinal herbs and other therapeutic plants, such as sea vegetables, grasses and micro-algae, that are readily available to the herbal remedy consumer today. We have worked extensively with most of these plants over the last twenty years at Crystal Star Herbal Nutrition. Listing is by the most commonly used name, with alternate names where relevant. The botanical species is also given. Widely available Chinese, Ayurvedic and rainforest culture herbs are included if we have had experience with them. Since this is a medicinal directory, only those plants with recognized healing properties are catalogued. Cosmetic, potpourri, and culinary herbs and spices are omitted. Profile information is brief, with only the most significant properties and characteristics represented.

A short reference glossary of herbal properties and functions follows this section.

ABUTILON: *Malva verticillata* (Dongkuizi) - **Part used**: seeds. **Effective forms**: powder. **Therapeutic profile**: A sweet and cold herb used in TCM to regulate urination, promote lactation, and to moisten the intestines. **Primary uses**: used to treat dysuria and edema in combination with *poria* and *white atractylodes*; helpful for painful urination and blood in the urine. **Secondary uses**: used in combination with amomum fruit and ricepaper pith to treat obstructed lactation and breast distention; helpful as a moisturizing agent for constipation due to excessive dryness.

ACANTHOPANAX BARK: *Acanthopanax gracilistylus* (Wujiapi) - **Part used**: bark. **Effective forms**: decoction, capsule. **Therapeutic profile**: A bitter herb that takes action on the liver and kidneys and is used in TCM to dispel wind and dampness, strengthen the tendons and bones, and to improve urination. **Primary uses**: as an antispasmodic for rheumatism and pain in the limbs, edema, and soreness, weakness and pain in the lumbar region and the knees.

ACIDOPHILUS: *Lactobacillus acidophilus* - **Part used**: dried powder. **Effective forms**: capsules, food and drink supplement. **Therapeutic profile**: part of the friendly flora in the digestive tract. All beneficial bacteria produce enzymes that aid digestion and improve transit time in the colon. More than 400 species of bacteria are estimated to inhabit our digestive tracts - beneficial (friendly), pathogenic (hostile) and neutral bacteria. Acidophilus helps keep the overgrowth of yeasts such as candida albicans in check. Acidophilus is found in the form of a probiotic powder, in cultured vegetaables and cultured milks. **Primary uses**: important to strengthening and maintaining a strong immune system; may help to detoxify harmful substances by binding with some of the unwanted substances, causing them to be excreted.

AGAR AGAR: *Gelidium amansii* - **Part used**: algae. **Effective forms**: powder, flakes and fluid extract. **Therapeutic profile**: has the property of absorbing moisture and putrifactive material in the intestinal tract. **Primary therapeutic use**: for constipation, may be mixed in breads and cereals for a more laxative effect, or put into herbal formulas for intestinal lubrication and bulk.

AGASTACHE: *Pogostemon cablin* (Huoxiang) - **Part used**: aerial parts. **Effective forms**: combination capsules. **Therapeutic profile**: used in TCM to stop vomiting, and to dispel summer heat. **Primary uses**: indicated for abdominal distention, nausea, vomiting and poor appetite. May be useful in treating summer excess wind and cold symptoms like chills, fever, headache, nausea, vomiting or a feeling of excessive fullness.

AGRIMONY: *Agrimonia eupatoria* (Xianhecao) - **Part used**: entire herb. **Effective forms**: tea, suppository and extract. **Therapeutic profile**: a tonic, astringent and bitters herb, specifically stimulating to the liver for strength and increasing bile flow. Also a tonic that strengthens and tones the muscles of the body. A useful diuretic because it allows fluids to pass more readily through the kidneys. Used in TCM to stop bleeding, relieve dysentery and to kill parasites. **Primary uses**: for appendicitis (along with calendula); for childhood diarrhea and urinary incontinence. In TCM, used mainly to treat cough with blood, vomiting with blood, hematuria, epistaxis, bloody stool and uterine bleeding. **Secondary uses**: for childhood indigestion, chronic appendicitis, and colitis; as a suppository with cocoa butter to expel tapeworms, and tighten hemorrhoids. In TCM, used as a vaginal cleanser and detoxifier, in which cotton balls are soaked in a strong decoction and inserted into the vagina overnight once a week to treat trichomonas vaginitis with itching.

167

❧ AILANTHUS BARK: *Ailanthus altissima* (Chunpi)- **Part used:** bark, stem. **Effective forms:** decoction. **Therapeutic profile:** used in TCM to clear heat and dry dampness, treat hemorrhaging and to kill parasites. **Primary uses:** to treat diarrhea, and dysentery in combination with *coptis root, scutellaria root and costus root.* **Secondary uses:** used to treat leukorrhea in combination with *phellodendron;* indicated for uterine hemorrhaging in combination with *tortoise plastron, white peony root and scutellaria root.* **Contra-indications:** use in 3-5 gram dosage.

❧ AJWAN: *Opium graveolens* - **part used:** fruit. **Effective forms:** infusion, powder. **Therapeutic profile:** an Ayurvedic herb used to vitalize prana (life energy); revives obstructed metabolic functions; improves digestion as well as enthusiasm). **Primary uses:** used mainly to treat colic, gas and indigestion; valuable for colds, coughs and flu. **Secondary uses:** has a role in addressing *Candida albicans* yeast overgrowth; used to treat asthma, laryngitis and bronchitis. **Contra-indications:** not to be used in cases of hyperacidity or Pitta type imbalances, and ulcers.

❧ ALARIA: *Atlantic wakame* - **Part used:** leaf and midrib. **Effective forms:** broth, salad or soup garnish. **Therapeutic profile:** a highly nutritional sea vegetable, particularly rich in B vitamins, beta carotene, and organic calcium. **Primary uses:** as part of an absorbable mineral supplement. **Secondary uses:** as part of an iodine therapy combination.

❧ ALFALFA: *Medicago sativa* - **Part used:** leaf and seed. **Effective forms:** tea, capsule, alcohol extract. **Therapeutic profile:** a highly nutritive herb, rich in carotene, vitamin K, chlorophyll, amino acids, octacosonal and a full spectrum of minerals and trace minerals. Beneficial for all ailments because of its vitality and nutrient properties which are balanced for complete absorption. **Primary uses:** support for arthritis, rheumatism and osteoporosis; to stimulate removal of inorganic mineral deposits from the blood; as a blood clotting agent in counteracting internal bleeding from ulcers; as a phyto-estrogen precurser during menopausal hormone changes. **Secondary uses:** for indigestion and attendant problems such as colitis; in reducing blood sugar levels; in lowering cholesterol and in the prevention of tooth decay.

❧ ALISMATIS RHIZOME: *Alisma orientalis* (Zexie)- **Part used:** dried rhizome. **Effective forms:** decoction, capsule. **Therapeutic profile:** the rhizome is used in TCM to transform dampness and promote water metabolism. **Primary uses:** indicated for dysuria, turbid urine, edema, retention of phlegm and fluids. **Secondary uses:** has a role in the treatment of diarrhea and profuse leukorrhea.

❧ ALLSPICE: *Pimenta dioica* - **Part used:** berry. **Effective forms:** tea. **Therapeutic profile:** a pleasant tasting digestive spice, and an aromatic stimulant and carminative for the gastro-intestinal tract, resembling cloves in its action. **Primary uses:** to dispell flatulence, gas and indigestion and as a flavoring agent. **Secondary uses:** as part of a "spring tonic" formula and as an addition to other tonics and purgatives.

❧ ALOE VERA: *Aloe vera* - **Part used:** gelatinous interior of the leaf. **Effective forms:** juice, gel, poultice. **Therapeutic profile:** a contact healing herb that promotes rapid cell regeneration from wounds, rashes, burns and skin problems of all kinds. Aloe vera has antibacterial and antifungal activity, antiviral effects, immune enhancement, anti-allergy and anti-inflammatory aspects. **Primary uses:** as an external healing gel for infective and fungal skin conditions, burns, cuts, wounds, poison ivy and oak; juice, externally, as an eyewash for scleroderma and dry eyes; juice, internally, as a laxative and bowel toning agent. The juice is also used internally to treat peptic ulcers, as a gastrointestinal tonic, and for arthritis. It shows great promise when administered in the early stages of AIDS. **Secondary uses:** as an anti-biotic for internal infection and ulcers, to inhibit replication of viruses, and as a vermifuge for intestinal parasites. **Contra-indications:** should not be taken internally during pregnancy or breastfeeding. Evaporated aloe concentrate is a purgative. Do not use for more than 7 days at a time

❧ AMARANTH: *Amaranthus spp.* - **Part used:** leaf, flowers and seed. **Effective forms:** decoction; leaves and seed; can be taken as food. Used as a survival food by the Indians and is currently available in health food stores as a nutty tasting grain. **Therapeutic profile:** a highly nutritional herb, rich in iron, vitamin C, calcium and protein; contains phosporus, potassium, thiamine, riboflavin and niacin. **Primary uses:** to lessen irritability of the tissues in gastroenteritis or stomach flu. **Secondary uses:** topical application can reduce tissue swelling; astrong decoction can be used to remove worms or other parasites from the digestive tract.

❧ AMBER: *Pinus spp.* (Hupo)- **Part used:** powder obtained from ground, dried resin. **Effective forms:** powder, pills. **Therapeutic profile:** traditionally used in Chinese medicine to invigorate the blood and release stagnation, to calm and tranquilize the mind, and promote urination. **Primary uses:** used with *jujube seed* and *knotweed*

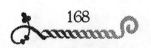

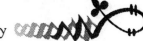

for palpitations, insomnia and sleep disturbed by excessive dreaming. **Secondary uses**: indicated for urinary tract disorders including frequent urination, painful urination, and blood or gravel in the urine. **Contra-Indications**: do not use as a decoction.

AMLA FRUIT: *Phyllanthus emblica* - **Part used**: fruit. **Effective forms**: jelly. **Therapeutic profile**: In Ayurveda, Chyavan Prash is an indispensable, high vitamin C, herbal jelly based on the Amla fruit - a general tonic which strengthens the blood. **Primary uses**: a blood strengthener in cases of debility; an excellent tonic for the eyes, improving nearsightedness. **Secondary uses**: also used as part of a cleansing regimen.

AMOMUM FRUIT: *Amomum vilosum* (Sharen)- **Part used**: root. **Effective forms**: decoction, capsule. **Therapeutic profile**: used in TCM to promote ch'i circulation and transform dampness; also an effective agent to calm a hyperactive fetus in the womb. **Primary uses**: indicated for dampness blocking the spleen and stomach or chi stagnation manifested by abdominal pain and distention, lack of appetite, vomiting, nausea and diarrhea. **Secondary uses**: considered effective for morning sickness and a restless fetus.

ANEMARRHENA RHIZOME: *Anemarrhena asphodeloides* (Zhi mu) - **Part used**: rhizome. **Effective forms**: dried, cleaned rhizomes baked with salt. **Therapeutic profile**: an antibiotic Chinese herb used to drain fire and to clear heat; helps treat high fever, irritability, thirst and delirium. **Primary uses**: to treat night sweats, irritability, low-grade fevers and bleeding gums. **Secondary uses**: has application in the treatment of nocturnal emissions and abnormally elevated sex drive. **Contra-Indications**: not be used except under the care of a qualified health practitioner - overdoses of this herb may cause a sharp drop in blood pressure; not to be used for diarrhea due to weakness of the spleen.

ANGELICA: *Angelica archangelica* - **Part used**: root. **Effective forms**: capsules, tea, bath, wine infusion. **Therapeutic profile**: an anise-like digestive agent, bronchial aid, and emmenagogue. Rich in coumarins, and a good sorce of flavonoids. **Primary uses**: to stimulate appetite and assimilation of food; as an expectorant to relieve inflammatory conditions of bronchitis, pleurisy and pneumonia; and also for flatulent dyspepsia. **Secondary uses**: a soothing phyto-hormone herb for menstrual cramping.

ANISE SEED: *Pimpinella anisum* - **Part used**: dried seed. **Effective forms**: tea, oil ointment. **Therapeutic profile**: a highly aromatic licorice-flavored seed, used as a digestive and bronchial aid. It has expectorant, antispasmodic, carminative, antimicrobial, aromatic and galactogogue activity. **Primary uses**: in throat-coating, soothing cough teas (expectorant and antispasmodic actions help relieve a persistent, irritable cough), digestive, and enzyme-stimulating blends. **Secondary uses**: as an aromatic adjunct to an allergen-neutralizing or bronchial-opening formula; as a secondary stimulant for inadequate breast milk; externally as an oil ointment for treating scabies and controlling lice.

ANISE, STAR, Chinese: *Illicium verum* - **Part used**: dried seed and pod. **Effective forms**: tea. **Therapeutic profile**: a highly aromatic seed with enzyme-enhancing properties. A digestive stimulant, and analgestic. **Primary uses**: in a digestive tea and for seasoning. Warms the abdomen, dispels gas, regulates energy, treats belching, vomiting, abdominal pains, and hernia. Used in the Orient as a remedy for colic and rheumatism. **Secondary uses**: as a pleasant flavoring for teas with bitter herbs.

ANNATTO: *Bixa orellana L.* - **Part used**: leaves and pulp surrounding the seeds. **Effective forms**: tea and extract. **Therapeutic profile**: an alcohol extract of dried annatto fruit and leaf has in vitro activity against Escherichia coli and Staphylococcus aureus. Test results with animals have found hypotensive and muscle relaxant activity. Annatto leaves contain flavonoids and the seeds contain carotenoids. **Primary uses**: leaves are used for diarrhea and dysentery. **Secondary uses**: a cool wash is used for sores, rashes and infected bites; an herbal leaf bath is used to treat swellings. The pulp is used as a natural flavoring and coloring agent.

APRICOT SEED: *Prunus armenica, (Xing Ren)* - **Part used**: crushed kernels. **Effective forms**: combination capsules, tea. **Therapeutic profile**: a lung tonic and expectorant; an anti-carcinogenic source of laetrile. Used in TCM to stop cough and relieve asthma; to moisten intestines and move stool. **Primary uses**: for bronchitis, emphysema, and a dry, hacking cough; as a support for cancerous tumor reduction. Used in TCM for coughs and asthma; and in combination with *hemp seed* and *dong quai* for constipation. **Secondary uses**: as a demulcent in a laxative formula; in cosmetics for its softening action on the skin. **Contra-Indications**: apricot seeds contain natural prussic acid - small doses are beneficial, large doses of 50 to 60 seeds can be lethal, especially to infants.

APPLE: *Malus spp.* - **Part used:** fruit. **Effective forms:** fresh and stewed fruit. **Therapeutic profile:** fresh apples are cleansing for the system with a mild laxative action. Other actions include tonic, digestive and liver stimulant, diuretic, anti-rheumatic and antiseptic. **Primary uses:** a good source of vitamins and minerals for anemia and debility. Ripe apples have been used as laxatives; unripe ones to counter diarrhea. **Secondary uses:** can reduce blood cholesterol levels.

ARAME: *Eisenia bicyclis, Japanese kelp* - **Part used:** leaf. **Effective forms:** broth, dried soup or salad sprinkle, bath. **Therapeutic profile:** mild sweet tasting sea vegetable, rich in proteins, minerals (high in calcium and iron), trace minerals, carotenes and B vitamins. The brown algae family (including arame, hijiki, kombu and wakame) contains alginic acid/sodium alginate, which binds and expels radioactive substances and heavy metals from the body. Sea vegetables have a propensity to bind with and neutralize various heavy metals. The brown sea vegetables bind excess strontium and iron. **Primary uses:** as part of a highly absorbable mineral blend, particularly one for iodine therapy. Arame adds nutritional value to the diet and helps to protect against radiation and environmental pollutants. **Secondary uses:** for alkalinity, and easily absorbed potassium.

ARBORVITAE SEED: *Biota orientalis* (Baiziren)- **Part used:** seeds. **Effective forms:** capsules. **Therapeutic profile:** indicated in TCM to nourish the blood and tranquilize the mind; moistens the intestines to ease the movement of feces. **Primary uses:** indicated for insomnia, irritability, palpitations and anxiety. Used with *ginseng, schizandra* and oyster shell for night sweats; effective against constipation due to dryness of intestines. **Contra-indications:** not to be used when loose stools or diarrhea is present.

ARECA SEED: *Areca cathecu* (Binglang) - **Part used:** dried seed. **Effective forms:** capsules, decoction. **Therapeutic profile:** used in TCM to promote circulation of chi in the body. An effective vermifuge and diuretic. **Primary uses:** used with *pumpkin seed* to kill tapeworms in the intestines; used in combination formulas to fight abdominal distention and constipation. **Secondary uses:** may be useful for edema and swollen and painful legs.

ARNICA FLOWERS: *Arnica Montana* - **Part used:** flower. **Effective forms:** externally only as an ointment or lotion; (safe internally when taken as a homeopathic remedy). **Therapeutic profile:** soothing, anti-inflammatory activity, with antibacterial action. Encourages healthy reabsorption of internal bleeding in bruises and sprains. **Primary uses:** to reduce pain, swelling/inflammation of sprains; a specific for bruises. **Secondary uses:** for rheumatic and inflammatory pain, such as phlebitis and shingles. **Contra-indications:** do not apply to broken skin.

ASHWAGANDHA: *Withania somnifera* - **Part used:** root. **Effective forms:** extract, capsule, decoction. **Therapeutic profile:** referred to as a "female ginseng," ashwagandha is an Ayurvedic, tonic adaptogenic herb used since ancient times to promote health and vitality. Regularly used to enhance immunity, and treat inflammation; thought to act as an aphrodisiac, especially for women. **Primary uses:** used to treat debility (including lack of sexual libido, and female sterility and infertility) and most degenerative diseases; studies show ashwagandha helps relieve aches and pains associated with arthritis; also shows promise in treating cancer. Ashwagandha is a specific in treating chronic fatigue syndrome, Epstein Barr virus and other auto-immune diseases, including AIDS. **Secondary uses:** used to treat loss of memory and nervous disorders; significantly reduces the incidence of stress-induced ulcers; used to treat male impotence, low sperm count and premature ejaculation. An antibiotic and antifungal against some pathogens. Considered to be an effective energy tonic for vegetarians. **Contra-indications:** Ashwagandha should not be used during colds, flus or acute fevers.

ASTRAGALUS ROOT: *Astragalus membranaceus, (Huang Chi)* - **Part used:** root. **Effective forms:** liquid and powdered extract, tea. **Therapeutic profile:** an organ toning and gland balancing herb, particularly for the spleen, kidneys, adrenals and lungs; stimulating to the immune system through induction of interferon (killer cells). **Primary uses:** as an antiviral specific in immune/resistance building formulas; to increase overall energy and build resistance to weakness and disease. Helps reduce the incidence and shorten the course of the common cold. **Secondary uses:** as a supporting herb to enhance the activity of other energy and immune response herbs; as a toning diuretic herb for kidney inflammation; for chronic, non-healing sores.

ATRACTYLODIS ROOT: *Atractylodis ovata, (Pai Shu)* - **Part used:** root. **Effective forms:** tea. **Therapeutic profile:** a gentle organ-toning herb with particular benefit for the kidneys, spleen and pancreas. **Primary uses:** as a beneficial diuretic that will not exhaust the kidneys. **Secondary uses:** as an astringent herb in controlling diarrhea, stomach bloating and gastro-enteritis.

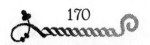

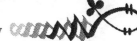

BALA: *Sida cordifolia* - **Part used**: root, leaves and seeds. **Effective forms**: powder, extracts. **Therapeutic profile**: A commonly prescribed aphrodisiac in Ayurvedic medicine, bala contains the alkaloid ephedrine. Regarded as cooling, tonic, astringent and stomachic, it has strong broncho-dilating properties but with less potential for misuse than ma huang, its TCM cousin. **Primary uses**: a cardiac tonic; routinely prescribed by Ayurvedic physicians for asthma, bronchial spasms and coughs. Indicated for asthma and chronic fevers. **Secondary uses**: used to treat male and female sexual dysfunction; may have use in treating nerve problems such as neuralgia and facial paralysis; may have a role in treating sciatica and rheumatism. A helpful addition to a weight loss formula where thermogeneic properties are needed.

✻ BANANA: *Musa acuminata* - **Part used**: fruit. **Effective forms**: easily digested tonic food. **Therapeutic profile**: moderate anti-tuberculosis activity has been demonstrated in vitro for Mycobacterium tuberculosis. Anti-ulcer activity has been shown with lab rats. Antibacterial activity has been shown against *Bacillus cereus, Bacillus coagulans, Bacillus stereothenmophilus,* and *Clostridium sporegenes* with a water extract of banana. **Primary uses**: easily digested tonic food often used as first choice for infants and invalids. Eaten alone is helpful for ulcers and gastritis. **Secondary uses**: eating only well-ripened bananas for 24 hours is useful for diarrhea.

✻ BANCHA GREEN TEA: (See KUKICHA TWIG for therapy)- the young green leaves of the tea plant.

✻ BARBERRY: *Berberis vulgaris* - **Part used**: bark of the root and stem. **Effective forms**: tea, capsules, liquid extract, tincture. **Therapeutic profile**: a bitter tonic herb beneficial to the liver for blood purification and bile formation; also a tonic, purgative and antiseptic. **Primary uses**: as part of a liver and/or gallbladder cleansing/tonifying formula, with mild laxative activity; for poor skin cases of acne, psoriasis, eczema and herpes, where constipation and malabsorption are the cause. **Secondary uses**: as a digestive and assimilation aid; as a vermifuge for some internal parasites; as a balancing spleen herb.

✻ BARLEY GRASS: *Hordeum vulgare* - **Part used**: stem and juice. **Effective forms**: as a drink, capsules and extract. **Therapeutic profile**: a nutritive herb, high in chlorophyllins, and anti-oxidant activity. It contains many components that strengthen and maintain the immune system. It has a cleansing effect on the cells, normalizing metabolism and neutralizing heavy metals like mercury. When barley juice is added to damaged cells, their DNA rapidly repairs the damage and, in the process, boosts the cells' ability to prevent cancer-type diseases from taking hold. Japanese scientists have shown that daily use of green barley juice helps to reverse many aspects of the aging process. **Primary uses**: a "superfood" used as a tonic and regenerating drink; as a chlorophyll-containing aid to the digestive system. **Secondary uses**: nutrient-rich, daily maintenance and sugar balance, especially in cases of hypoglycemia and diabetes; as part of a weaning formula to help dry up mother's milk.

✻ BASIL: *Ocinum basilicum (Tulsi)* - **Part used**: leaf. **Effective forms**: tea. **Therapeutic profile**: its actions include: antidepressant, antiseptic, stimulates the adrenal cortex, prevents vomiting, tonic, carminative, febrifuge, expectorant, soothes itching; an aromatic digestive stimulant. **Primary uses**: as a diarrhea control aid. **Secondary uses**: fresh rub on insect bites to reduce itching and inflammation, combine juice with an equal quantity of honey for a wash for ringworm and itching skin and for coughs.

✻ BAY CEDAR: *Guazuma ulmifolia* - **Part used**: bark and leaf. **Effective forms**: tea, tincture and wash. **Therapeutic profile**: a leaf extract of dried leaf showed in vitro cytotoxic activity against 9KB cancer cells, giving a 97.3% inhibition of cell growth. The leaf tincture exhibits *in vitro* antibacterial activity against *Bacillus subtilis* and against E. coli. **Primary uses**: the tea is used for dysentery and diarrhea; for prostate problems and as an aid to childbirth. **Secondary uses**: used as a wash for skin sores, infection, and rashes.

✻ BAY LEAF: *Laurus nobilis* - **Part used**: leaf. **Effective forms**: broth, tea, bath, oil. **Therapeutic profile**: an aromatic herb beneficial to the stomach and intestinal tract. Its actions include: stimulant, carminative, emmengogue, diaphoretic, emetic. **Primary uses**: the tea is used as a remedy for gas, flatulence and indigestion. **Secondary uses**: as a soothing agent for sore throat and cough, and as an alkalizing aid for an over-acid system. Oil of bay is used externally for sprains and bruises. The tea is useful for hysteria, amenorrhea, and colic.

✻ BAYBERRY: *Myrica cerifa* - **Part used**: bark of the root. **Effective forms**: tea, douche, capsules, gargle. **Therapeutic profile**: a strengthening hormone balancer for female organs; astringent activity for venous congestion, and inflamed mucous membranes; circulatory stimulant; promotes sweating. **Primary uses**: a specific when used with cayenne in controlling profuse and painful menstruation. Reduces toxic waste accumulations and growths in the female genito-urinary tract. **Secondary uses**: as a gargle for sore throat and bleeding gums, and relief of sinus and adenoid problems; with other spices, as part of an effective natural tooth powder; for diarrhea from stress causes. It may be used in the treatment of colds and feverish conditions.

BEAR PAW FERN: *Phlebodium decumanum* - **Part used**: root. **Effective forms**: decoction. **Therapeutic profile**: known to contain carotenoids, flavonoids, and steroids. **Primary uses**: decoction has been used as a remedy for stomach ulcers, pain, gastritis, and chronic indigestion. Belize herbalists (Rainforest) recommend drinking the tea for the beginning stages of cancer, for pain in later stages, and for high blood pressure.

BEE POLLEN: Part used: pollen granules. **Effective forms**: as is, in a drink, capsules. **Therapeutic profile**: a highly nutritive, tonic substance rightly known as a "superfood." Completely balanced for vitamins, minerals, proteins, carbohydrates, fats, and all essential amino acids. Use only unsprayed pollen for therapeutic applications. **Primary uses**: as part of a full spectrum body rejuvenating formula, particularly for the extra nutritional and energy needs of athletes and those recuperating from illness; for general healthy blood building. Builds resistance to diseases, helps to boost healing powers and provides the body with energy. **Secondary uses**: for management of pollen and seasonal allergy symptoms; as part of a wound healing combination.

BEET ROOT: *Beta vulgaris rubra* - **Part used**: root. **Effective forms**: capsules. **Therapeutic profile**: a scouring herb/food, particularly effective for the kidneys. **Primary uses**: as part of a kidney cleansing formula. The juice is anti-inflammatory and blood cleansing. **Secondary uses**: cleansing toxic wastes to help liver and spleen function; to encourage healthy blood cell formation.

BETH ROOT: *Trillium pendulum* - **Part used**: root. **Effective forms**: capsules, extract. **Therapeutic profile**: helps restore normal nerve supply to the organs in the thorax. **Primary uses**: for coughs, bronchial problems and hemorrhages from the lungs. Controls excessive menstruation and excessive vaginal discharges. An excellent remedy for diarrhea and dysentery.

BILBERRY: *(Huckleberry, Blueberry) Vaccinium myrtillus* - **Part used**: berry and leaf. **Effective forms**: capsules, extract. **Therapeutic profile**: a strong but gentle nutritive, astringent herb rich in flavonoids, carotene, vitamin E, and anthrocyanosides to fortify vascular activity and arterial weakness; particularly effective for strengthening the eyes. **Primary uses**: in compounds for night blindness/eyesight improvement; in formulas for anemia; as a sugar regulant for diabetes. **Secondary uses**: for vascular support, such as for varicose veins or easy bruising; a hematonic for kidney malfunction, and urinary stones; as an aid in treating diarrhea; as a nutritive tonic. Recommended for use during pregnancy.

BIRCH BARK: *Betula alba* - **Part used**: inner bark, leaves. **Effective forms**: tea. **Therapeutic profile**: a digestive bitters, wintergreen-flavored herb, with anti-rheumatic and diuretic activity. Also has anti-inflammatory, antiseptic and tonic actions. **Primary uses**: in arthritic and urinary pain combinations as well as removing excess water from the body. **Secondary uses**: externally as a wash applied to eczema and psoriasis inflammation; as part of a combination to treat intestinal worms; as an effective natural toothbrush (used as a twig frazzled at one end) with properties that prevent tooth decay. The bark placed against the skin will ease muscle pain.

BISTORT: *Polygonum bistorta* - **Part used**: root. **Effective forms**: powder, fluid extract. **Therapeutic profile**: is a powerful astringent and reduces phlegm. **Uses**: powdered root steeped is a successful treatment for diarrhea, dysentery and hemorrhages from the lungs and stomach. A decoction is used as a gargle for throat and mouth infections and as a douche for leukorrhea. The ground root mixed with echinacea, myrrh and goldenseal makes an excellent dressing for wounds and cuts.

BITTER APRICOT: *Prunus armeniaca* - **Part used**: ripe kernel. **Effective forms**: capsule. **Therapeutic profile**: an Ayurvedic herb is noted for its antispasmodic, expectorant properties, acting in the body on the lungs and large intestine. **Primary uses**: indicated for coughs, asthma and most respiratory conditions. **Secondary uses**: also used for constipation (when there is dryness.) **Contra-indications**: slightly toxic - take in moderation as directed by a qualified health practitioner.

BLACK COHOSH: *Cimicifuga racemosa* - **Part used**: root. **Effective forms**: extract, capsules. **Therapeutic profile**: a phyto-estrogen herb, with anti-spasmodic, diuretic and hormone-balancing qualities. Exerts vascular effects and reduces luteinizing hormone (LH) levels, implying a significant estrogenic effect. **Primary uses**: as a

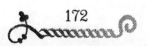

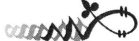

specific in female toning compounds, to relieve menstrual cramps and uterine disorders, encourage estrogen balance, and during the last weeks of pregnancy, to facilitate childbirth. Relieves hot flashes, depression and vaginal atrophy. Used in the treatment of arthritic, neurological, and rheumatic pain. Increases natural fertility by regulating hormone production after discontinuing the birth control pill. **Secondary uses:** as part of a formula for ringing in the ears; as a muscle relaxant; as an anti-spasmodic in lung and mucous conditions; for the aching experienced in osteo-arthritis. **Contra-indications:** avoid during the first eight months of pregnancy.

❧ **BLACK HAW:** *Viburnum prunifolium* - **Part used:** bark of root and stem. **Effective forms:** tea, capsules. **Therapeutic profile:** an antispasmodic similar to cramp bark, with strong muscle relaxant and sedative activity. Also has emmenagogue and tonic properties. **Primary uses:** as a specific for threatened miscarriage and false labor (eases cramps and contractions in the pelvic organs); useful for painful menstruation; in a formula for stress and nervous tension. Valuable in chronic uterine inflammation, congested uterus and leukorrhea. **Secondary uses:** to help lower blood pressure in hypertension cases.

❧ **BLACK WALNUT:** *Juglans nigra* - **Part used:** hulls, leaf, bark. **Effective forms:** extract, infusion, capsules, tea, skin wash. **Therapeutic profile:** a manganese-rich herb with broad spectrum activity from many parts of the plant; a strong anti-fungal, with laxative, astringent, blood cleansing, vermicide and tonic properties. Rich in organic iodine and tannins which provide antiseptic qualities. **Primary uses:** as a specific for effective treatment of intestinal worms; as an anti-fungal in cases of *candida* yeast overgrowth, ringworm, scabies and thrush; as a blood cleanser with effectiveness for eczema and for all toxic blood conditions, acne and psoriasis; as part of a laxative/purgative for chronic and stubborn constipation or diarrhea. **Secondary uses:** as an antiseptic to treat herpes, impetigo, canker sores and boils; in the treatment of systemic poison oak toxin. **Contra-indications:** avoid during pregnancy.

❧ **BLACKBERRY:** *Rubus fruticosus* - **Part used:** leaves, root bark, unripe berries. **Effective forms:** tea. **Therapeutic profile:** contains vitamins A and C; also contains iron, calcium, riboflavin, niacin and some thiamine; root has astringent properties. **Primary uses:** the tea can dry up sinus drainage; an infusion of unripe berries is useful for vomiting and loose bowels. **Secondary uses:** the tea has been used for dysentery and for giving vigor to the whole body.

❧ **BLADDERWRACK:** *Fucus vesiculosis* - **Part used:** leaf and stem. **Effective forms:** bath, tablets. **Therapeutic profile:** a sea vegetable rich in natural mineral salts, carotene and iodine; a nutritive metabolic stimulant and thyroid tonic; an anti-rheumatic and anti-inflammatory; also an anti-tumor and anti-fungal. An excellent weight-reduction aid. **Primary uses:** a thyroid stimulant; as part of an iodine therapy formula; as part of a weight loss formula where an underactive thyroid is the reason for the weight problem. Also a healthy oxygen supplier which increases the body's ability to burn fat through exercise. Useful as part of an adrenal stimulant formula; stamina is boosted, which allows cells to consume energy more efficiently. Has been found beneficial for nephritis, bladder inflammation, cardiac degeneration and menstrual problems. **Secondary uses:** internally, and externally in a bath for rheumatoid arthritis, (keeps inorganic minerals in solution instead of as deposits in the joints).

❧ **BLESSED THISTLE:** *Cnicus benedictus* - **Part used:** leaves. **Effective forms:** tea, capsules. **Therapeutic profile:** a bitters tonic and astringent herb useful for female hormone balance and circulation. Contains the B-complex vitamins, manganese, calcium, iron, phosphorus, and potassium. **Primary uses:** in female balancing formulas to regulate menstruation; to enrich mother's milk during lactation. Useful for headaches in menopause problems. An excellent tonic for stomach and heart; aids circulation and helps a wide variety of liver problems. Strengthens memory by bringing oxygen to the brain. **Secondary uses:** as a liver tonic for indigestion and increased circulation; as a diaphoretic to induce sweating for body cleansing.

❧ **BLOODROOT:** *Sanguinaria canadensis* - **Part used:** root. **Effective forms:** tea, tincture, ointment, gargle. **Therapeutic profile:** an expectorant and anti-spasmodic herb with primary effectiveness for respiratory problems. Also has tonic and antibacterial actions. **Primary uses:** to relieve and heal bronchitis, pneumonia, asthmatic coughing and sinus congestion; with bayberry as a snuff powder for the treatment of nasal polyps and rhinitis. **Secondary uses:** as a gargle to prevent oral plaque build-up; as an anti-fungal ointment applied directly to eczema, ringworm, and venereal warts and sores; as an anti-fungal tincture applied directly to skin cancers, nail fungus and other skin disorders. **Contra-indications:** contains the poisonous alkaloid, sanguinarine and other alkaloids. In toxic doses causes burning in the stomach, intense thirst, paralysis, vomiting, faintness, vertigo, collapse, and intense prostration with dimness of eyesight. Avoid during pregnancy.

BLUE COHOSH: *Caulophyllum thalictriodes* - **Part used:** root. **Effective forms:** capsules, tea, poultice. **Therapeutic profile:** an antispasmodic, female organ tonic and menstrual regulant. It also has antibacterial properties and complementary properties for the nerves. Contains vitamins E and B-complex, calcium, magnesium, phosphorus and potassium. **Primary uses:** as part of a PMS formula to tone uterine and organ tissue; to stop false labor and miscarriage; (used at the start of labor to insure easier dilation and birth). **Secondary uses:** as a poultice and emergency remedy for bee and poisonous insect sting reactions; as a remedy for spasmodic cough and asthma. **Contra-indications:** avoid during all but the last five weeks of pregnancy.

BLUEBERRY LEAF & BERRIES: *Vaccinium myrtillus* - Huckleberry (See BILBERRY)

BLUE FLAG RHIZOME: *Iris versicolor or I. germanica L.* - **Part used:** the rhizome. **Effective forms:** tincture, tea. **Therapeutic profile:** promotes bowel movement, clears toxins, removes lymph congestion & stops vomiting, promotes bile flow, reduces liver congestion, promotes detoxification, promotes expectoration, resolves phlegm & relieves couging, promotes menstruation, reduces swellings and tumors, stimulates pancreas and thyroid. **Primary uses:** as part of a formula for hepatitis, lymphoma, acute liver infections and congestion, spleen and liver enlargement, acute gastritis, chronic arthritis, chronic eczema, acute bronchitis, dysmenorrhea, uterine fibroids, soft swollen glands. **Secondary uses:** also used for chronic constipation, thyroid and pancreas deficiency.

BLUE VIOLET: *Viola odorata* - **Part used:** leaf, flowers. **Effective forms:** tea. **Therapeutic profile:** an anti-carcinogen, stress and fever reliever, and expectorant. Certain actions of violet have an affinity for reaching places only the blood and lymphatic fluids penetrate so they can have a positive effect in these areas. Contains vitamins A and C. **Primary uses:** for fevers and skin eruptions in children; for stress and tension headaches. An effective healer for internal ulcers. **Secondary uses:** counteracts diarrhea. Found useful both internally and externally for tumors, boils, abscesses, pimples, swollen glands and malignant growths. Useful in difficult breathing such as with asthma and bronchitis.

BORAGE: *Borago officinalis* - **Part used:** leaf and seed oil. **Effective forms:** extract, tea, capsules. **Therapeutic profile:** a gland renewing herb that acts particularly on exhausted adrenals, and also provides a source of critical essential fatty acids for prostaglandin balance. Acts on the kidneys to dispose of feverish catarrh; soothing to the mucous membranes of the mouth and throat. Contains potassium and calcium. **Primary uses:** as an adrenal tonic, helps restore vitality during recovery from illness. **Secondary uses:** as a galactagogue to stimulate the flow of breast milk. The tea is useful as an eyewash for sore eyes.

BOSWELLIA TREE: *Boswellia serrata* - **Part used:** gum, resin, fruit and stem. **Effective forms:** extract. **Therapeutic profile:** an anti-inflammatory Ayurvedic plant which produces a diuretic and demulcent gum used to treat a variety of female ills and blood sugar disturbances. **Primary uses:** to stimulate menstruation; resin is used as a mild sedative and pain reliever for arthritis. **Secondary uses:** fruits and stems are used to lower blood sugar.

BUCHU: *Barosma betulina* - **Part used:** leaves. **Effective forms:** capsules, extract and tea. **Therapeutic profile:** an antiseptic, diuretic and diaphoretic herb, best known as a remedy for urinary disorders including cystitis and prostate related problems. **Primary uses:** for chronic inflammation of the bladder, irritation of the urethra, uric acid problems, diabetes in the first stages, urine retention, and cystitis of the bladder. Used to treat enlargement of the prostate gland and burning urine. **Secondary uses:** in fever remedies. **Contra-indications:** do not use for serious kidney infections or problems, since buchu can be irritating to the kidneys over the long term.

BUCKTHORN: *Rhamnus frangula* - **Part used:** bark, berries. **Effective forms:** tea, capsules. **Therapeutic profile:** a gentle, non-habit forming laxative and diuretic herb effective for constipation, liver congestion, and cleansing through sweating. Helps stimulate bile. **Primary uses:** in bowel regulation combinations, (particularly for children). **Secondary uses:** as part of a vermifuge formula to expel intestinal worms; to control growth of warts. The bruised leaves applied to a wound will stop bleeding. An ointment of the herb helps relieve itching.

BUGLEWEED: *Lycopus virginicus* - **Part used:** whole herb. **Effective forms:** fresh herb or extract. **Therapeutic profile:** a specific in removing and neutralizing heavy metal poisons, and environmental pollutants. A cardiac tonic when an over-active thyroid is the cause. Contains compounds that contract mucous membrane tissues and reduce fluid discharges. Lowers the pulse and lessens its frequency, resembling the action of digitalis. **Primary uses:** in a detoxification formula against radiation and heavy metals. Helpful in relieving pain. **Secondary uses:** for irregular heartbeat and palpitations. Useful for the irritation of coughs and equalizes circulation.

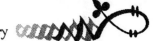

BUPLEURUM: *Bupleurum scorzoneraefolium, (Chai Hu)* - **Part used**: root. **Effective forms**: tea, capsules, extract. **Therapeutic profile**: an analgesic, anti-inflammatory herb effective in detoxifying the liver, and for menopausal symptoms. Other actions include: energy tonic, antibacterial, stimulates bile flow. **Primary uses**: as a liver cleanser, toner and strengthener; for menstrual cramping; to help reduce blood cholesterol levels. **Secondary uses**: as part of a muscle toning formula; for dizziness and headaches caused by anxiety and/or eyestrain; as part of an immune-enhancing formula.

BURDOCK: *Arctium lappa* (Niubangzi) - **Part used**: root, raw or baked fruit. **Effective forms**: tea, capsules, compress. **Therapeutic profile**: the root is a strong liver-purifying, hormone-balancing herb, with particular value for skin, arthritic, and glandular problems. Contains up to 45% inulin which is the reason for most of its curative actions. Inulin is important in the metabolism of carbohydrates. Burdock aids the pituitary gland in releasing an ample supply of protein to help adjust hormone balance in the body. Contains measureable amounts of vitamin C and iron, some vitamin A, bioflavonoids, E, B-complex, PAPA and small amounts of sulphur, silicon, copper, iodine and zinc. The fruit is used in TCM to release toxins and bring rashes to the surface, and also to disperse wind-heat and benefit the throat. **Primary uses**: the root is used as a specific in all blood cleansing and detoxification combinations; as an important anti-inflammatory and anti-infective for serious female conditions such as endometriosis inflammation, and excess fluid retention; as a specific for antihistimine activity in cases of histimine reactions, and eruptive skin problems such as acne and eczema; as a primary herb in a formula for gout to excrete uric acids. An invaluable help in all cases of female glandular imbalance. The fruit is used in combination formulas for sore throat; used to encourage skin rashes to come to the surface; good for most excess heat conditions including swelling, carbuncles and mumps. **Secondary uses**: as an alkalizer for acidic conditions such as arthritis, herpes, kidney and bowel inflammation; externally as a compress to reduce bruising, boils, and canker sores; as part of a purifying formula for viral warts and venereal disease.

BUTCHERS BROOM: *Ruscus aculeatus* - **Part used**: root. **Effective forms**: tea, capsules. **Therapeutic profile**: a flavonoid-rich, blood thinning herb, used to improve circulation and strengthen vein structure. Its properties include vasoconstricting action, toning a sluggish venous system and reducing capillary fragility. Has an enzymatic effect which reduces pain and swelling, anti-inflammatory, insufficient circulation to the extremities is reversed and improves circulation problems involving the retina. **Primary uses**: as an anti-thrombosis agent in cases of phlebitis and arterioscleriosis; in formulas for treatment of varicose veins and hemorrhoids. Good for all circulation disorders. Very useful for post-operative recovery especially with prolonged and heavy bleeding, when anti-coagulant therapy was used or with phlebitis patients. **Secondary uses**: as a diuretic herb for cellulite release, to relieve heaviness in the legs. **Contra-indications**: should only be used short term (1 week to 1 month), so that blood chemistry can achieve its own balance.

BUTTERBUR ROOT: *Petasites hybridus* - **Part used**: root. **Effective forms**: tincture, decoction, liniments, salves, compresses. **Therapeutic profile**: promotes sweating, reduces fever, promotes eruptions, promotes expectoration, relieves coughing, stops spasms and relieves pain, promotes and harmonizes urination and menstruation, benefits skin, reduces infection and clears toxins, promotes tissue repair. **Primary uses**: as part of a formula for the acute stages of colds or flu, chronic bronchitis, eruptive fevers, gastritis, gallstone cramping, asthma, and spasmodic dysmenorrhea. **Secondary uses**: helps in cases of tension headache, promotes more regular urination and menstruation, benefits skin, restores heart, and helps heal chronic skin infections and weeping or running ulcers or sores. **Contra-indications**: do not use in pregnancy as it stimulates the uterus.

BUTTERNUT: *Juglans cinerea* - **Part used**: bark of the root. **Effective forms**: capsules, tea. **Therapeutic profile**: a bitters herb and mild laxative effective for intestinal worms and parasites. Effective as part of a treatment for liver disorders (homeopathy). Increases the manufacture and secretion of bile and increases the activity of glands in the walls of the intestinal tract. **Primary uses**: as a specific in a gentle formula for chronic constipation and liver congestion; as part of a skin cleansing formula to release acid wastes. **Secondary uses**: as a vermifuge for internal worms; as part of natural pest control when the strong tea is poured around plants in the garden.

CABBAGE: *Brassica oleracea* - **Part used**: leaves. **Effective forms**: a food, juiced, decoction. **Therapeutic profile**: anti-inflammatory, anti-bacterial, anti-rheumatic, heals tissues by encouraging cells to proliferate, liver decongestant. Constituents include vitamins A, B$_1$, B$_2$, C minerals, amino acids, fats. **Primary uses**: since ancient Greek times as a digestive remedy, a joint tonic, and for skin problems and fevers. Recent clinical trials have demonstrated its effectiveness for treating stomach ulcers. **Secondary uses**: used externally on wounds, ulcers, inflammations, arthritic joints, acne and other skin conditions.

CALAMUS: *Acorus calamus* - **Part used:** dried rhizomes. **Effective forms:** tea. **Therapeutic profile:** a bitters tonic for treatment of gastro-intestinal disorders; a specific for regeneration of speech and brain impairment after a stroke. The root oil is antibacterial. Studies show serum cholesterol, serum triglyceride, and blood fibrinogen lowering activity while increasing fibrinolytic activity. **Primary uses:** in a digestive improvement formula where gastric ulcers and flatulence are particular problems. **Secondary uses:** with gotu kola as part of a tonic for the nervous system. **Contra-indications:** avoid use during pregnancy.

CALENDULA: (marigold) *Calendula officinalis* - **Part used:** flower. **Effective forms:** tincture, compress, tea, bath, ointment, lotion. **Therapeutic profile:** a soothing but powerful astringent for skin and wound healing, with a wide variety of uses both internal and external; effective against bruises, sprains, bleeding cuts and inflamed wounds; as a gastro-intestinal healer. Also an antiseptic, antifungal, anti-inflammatory, menstrual regulator; stimulates bile production. **Primary uses:** as a specific for inflammatory gastric problems, including ulcers, diverticulitis, gallbladder inflammation, and gastritis; as an antiseptic in skin healing formulas for burns, inflammatory eruptions such as measles, chicken pox, bruises, sprains, etc.; as a strong anti-fungal both internally and externally for thrush, candida albicans yeasts, athlete's foot, etc. The tincture is useful for stagnant liver problems, including sluggish digestion. **Secondary uses:** as an emmenagogue to regulate delayed or painful menstrual periods; for the tightening of varicose vein tissue. Use an infusion for mouth ulcers and gum disease.

CANADA SNAKEROOT: (Wild ginger); *Asarum canadense, (Xi Xin)* - **Part used:** whole plant. **Effective forms:** tea. **Therapeutic profile:** a strong emmenagogue, pungent-warm stimulant, spasmolytic, diaphoretic and abortifacient, (traditionally used as part of a birth control program). **Primary uses:** as a tea for one week before the menstrual period is due to promote menses and regulate conception. Useful for easing labor and enhancing contractions. Increases estrogen. **Secondary uses:** relieves lung spasms and congestion (promotes expectoration, resolves phlegm and relieves coughing). Promotes sweating, opens the sinuses and relieves pain.

CARAWAY SEED: *Carum carvi* - **Part used:** seed. **Effective forms:** powder mixed in water or juice, oil. **Therapeutic profile:** an aromatic digestive aid. A powerful antiseptic, especially useful in relieving toothaches. Applied to the skin, it acts as an anesthetic. Caraway contains the B-complex vitamins, is high in calcium & potasium and contains smaller amounts of magnesium, silicon, zinc, lead, iodine, copper, cobalt and iron. **Primary uses:** as a relieving, carminative drink for indigestion, gas and flatulence; helps to settle the stomach after nausea or indigestion; helps to increase mother's milk. **Secondary uses:** as gentle relief for uterine cramping. Useful for mucus in the lungs.

CARDAMOM: *Eletarria cardamomum (Bai dou kou)* - **Part used:** seeds. **Effective forms:** powder in capsules, seeds in a tea or drink, oil. **Therapeutic profile:** a digestive aid effective for gas and flatulence relief. A good nerve restorative; has circulatory stimulating action. Promotes expectoration. **Primary uses:** a specific in a digestive aid combination. Generates strength and restores the nerves. Helps relieve depression. **Secondary uses:** as part of a warming, anti-mucous, lung tonifying formula; relieves coughing and opens the sinuses.

CARROT: *Daucus carota*- **Part used:** root vegetable, seed. **Effective forms:** capsule, powder, extract, root vegetable, juice. **Therapeutic profile:** a highly nutritious, cleansing, therapeutic vegetable containing high amounts of carotene, a precursor to vitamine A, and calcium and magnesium. **Primary uses:** in formulas to address failing vision, alterative properties make carrot very useful (especially in juice form) to aid in liver function for hepatits and other liver dsfunction. Can improve resistance to infections; has particular use in healing internal ulcers. **Secondary uses:** has potential in the treatment of anemia because it increases red blood cell count. Carrot seeds have diuretic properties making them useful for treating urinary retention. Use the wild root as a specific for urinary stones.

CASCARA SAGRADA: *Rhamnus purshiana* - **Part used:** dried bark. **Effective forms:** tea, capsules. **Therapeutic profile:** a bitters tonic for the liver and gall bladder, and non-habit forming tonic laxative. Has hormone-like oils which promote peristaltic action in the intestinal canal. Increases the secretions of the stomach, liver, and pancreas. Is effective for normalizing the gall ducts and aids the body to rid itself of gallstones. Contains B-complex, calcium, potassium, manganese, traces of tin, lead, strontium and aluminum. **Primary uses:** as a specific for chronic constipation and flatulence from gas. Useful for hemorrhoids because of poor, flaccid bowel structure or constipation. Very cleansing to the colon; also helps rebuild colon functions. **Secondary uses:** as part of a formula to expel intestinal worms; as a night time regularity aid with nervine and sleep-promoting ability.

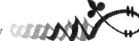

CASTOR OIL: *Ricinus communis* - **Part used**: only oil from the seed. (The seed itself, if taken internally is fatally poisonous). **Effective forms**: *only* the oil, as a purgative, compress and poultice. **Therapeutic profile**: a laxative that also helps draw toxicity from the liver; an effective compress and poultice ingredient for drawing out infective growths. An excellent emollient with lubricating properties. Castor oil packs enhance the function of the thymus gland and the other component parts of the immune system, making the immune system more effective in protecting the body. **Primary uses**: internally as a purgative for chronic constipation; externally as a compress or rub on the abdomen to draw out toxins from the liver and gallbladder. **Secondary uses**: externally as a compress or poultice to draw out infective growths such as cysts, warts, and ganglions; as a rub for bruises and sprains. Externally the oil is good for various cutaneous complaints, such as ringworm, itch, etc.

CATNIP: *Nepeta cataria* - **Part used**: leaves and tops. **Effective forms**: tea, enema, tincture. **Therapeutic profile**: a gentle but powerful diaphoretic for colds, flu, fever and respiratory problems, especially useful for children. A soothing carminative to the gastrointestinal tract and a mild tonic. It is a member of the mint family and like peppermint has been shown to have antibiotic properties. It stimulates appetite before meals - after meals it stimulates digestion. It also has a sedative effect on the nervous system. Helps overcome fatigue and improves circulation. Called nature's "Alka-Seltzer, " catnip is high in vitamins A, C and the B-complex; contains magnesium, manganese phosphorus, sodium and sulphur. **Primary uses**: a specific, with natural anti-biotic properties, for cold and flu remedies; for digestive problems, abdominal cramping and colic in infants; for the treatment of diarrhea. **Secondary uses**: effective as a relaxant for insomnia, and anti-spasmodic for a wide variety of childhood diseases; an effective enema in the elimination of disease-causing bacteria and mucous accumulation from the bowel. The tea is used also for headaches and stomach aches. (Catnip contains a volatile oil which is attractive to cats, causing them to cavort playfully while attempting to saturate their entire bodies with the distinctive aroma of the plant. Catnip put into a cotton sock makes a wonderful, natural cat toy!)

CAYENNE: *Capsicum annum* - **Part used**: fruit. **Effective forms**: capsules, tincture, gargle, compress, wash. **Therapeutic profile**: a highly aromatic, carotene-rich digestive herb and heart tonic with anti-bacterial and anti-viral qualities; a central system catalyst and circulatory stimulant in many compounds. Often called the purest and best stimulant in the herb kingdom. Rich in vitamins A, C, iron, calcium and potassium, it contains vitamin B-complex, magnesium, phosphorus, and sulphur. **Primary uses**: as a specific in heart muscle regulation, to strengthen all parts of the circulatory system and to normalize blood pressure; as a specific in digestive formulas to control gas, flatulence and upset stomach; to increase proper digestive enzyme secretions when there has been pleasure drug, prescription drug or alcohol abuse; as a warming agent for arthritic, lower back and rheumatic pain; a specific in breaking up mucous congestion in colds, flu, bronchitis, respiratory and cleansing formulas; to treat shock, and to prevent the onset of shock (as in a heart attack or stroke). **Secondary uses**: as a hemostatic both externally and internally to stop bleeding, and fight infection; externally, as an antiseptic wash, or a stimulating compress; as a gargle to heal a sore throat. Can rebuild tissue in the stomach and heals stomach and intestinal ulcers. Acts as a transporter and catalyst, carrying other herbs in a formula quickly to the central system of the body and throughout the body, while increasing their effectiveness.

CEDAR BERRY: *Juniperus monosperma* - (See JUNIPER BERRY)

CELANDINE HERB: *Chelidonion* - **Part used**: whole herb, root. **Effective forms**: fresh juice, freeze dried extract, tincture, infusion. **Therapeutic profile**: promotes bile flow and bowel movement, reduce liver congestion, removes accumulaton and relieves fullness, stimulates heart and circulation, restores coronary circulation, circulates chi, loosens constraint and stops spasms, relieves wheezing and coughing, promotes sweating, reduces fever, relieves pain, promotes urination, drains fluid congestion and relieves edema, resolves toxicosis, promotes tissue repair and inflammation, reduces tumors, benefits skin, strengthens and clears vision. **Primary uses**: as part of a formula for jaundice and liver malfunction headaches and migraines; helpful in formulas for chronic hepatitis and gallstones, coronary disease edema and gout. **Secondary uses**: for respiratory problems, like spasmodic coughing, asthma, cold or flu onset, remittent fevers, wounds, sprains, running ulcers or sores, eye inflammation, tumors, stomach and skin eruptions and cancers; also relieves toothache.

CELERY (WILD): *Apium graveolens* - **Part used**: root, seeds. **Effective forms**: powder, extract, root can be eaten raw or made into broths. **Therapeutic profile**: has carminative, diuretic, nervine stimulant and tonic properties. **Primary uses**: is used for incontinence of urine, dropsy, rheumatism, neuralgia and as an aid in ridding the body of excess acid. Whole celery can be used to treat kidney ailments, arthritis and rheumatism.

CENTAURY: *Erythraea centaurium* - **Part used:** leaf. **Effective forms:** extract, tea. **Therapeutic profile:** a bitters herb, beneficial as a stomach cleanse, vermifuge, blood purifier and an excellent tonic. **Primary uses:** in a bitters combination for sluggish digestive activity, and for nutrient assimilation in cases of anorexia nervosa. Centaury's ability to promote appetite and strengthen the digestive system is useful during convalescence, especially for muscular rheumatism. Strengthens the bladder of the elderly and also helps prevent bed-wetting. **Secondary uses:** externally applied as a weak tea for skin spots and discoloration, and as a clearing eyewash. Acts as a diffusive stimulating tonic to the heart, stomach, liver, generative organs and the nervous system.

CEREUS: *Cereus grandiflorus* - **Part used:** stem, flower. **Effective forms:** stem, flower. **Therapeutic profile:** produces nutritive support for the entire nervous and muscular structure of the heart. Enhances cardiotonic effects and has antidepressant effects. A nervous restorative and regulator for sympathetic nervous balance and cerebral circulation. **Primary uses:** for cardiac deficiency and to reduce risk of heart failure; for cerebral deficiency, and adrenal deficiency. **Secondary uses:** for chronic nervous depression, irritability, menopausal syndrome, edema, and skin eruptions. **Contraindications:** do not use where there is high blood pressure.

CHAMOMILE: *Matricaria recutita* - **Part used:** flowers. **Effective forms:** tea, gargle, bath and steam, mouth-wash and eyewash, extract. **Therapeutic profile:** a soothing tonic herb with absorbable calcium, that improves digestion and assimilation and relaxes nervous tension. An anti-inflammatory and anti-fungal, effective internally and externally for these conditions. Helps promote a hormone which helps rejuvenate hair and skin texture; helps in mental alertness. High in calcium and magnesium, it contains potassium, iron, manganese, zinc, azuline and some vitamin A. **Primary uses:** a specific in formulas for insomnia, and stress; soothes a nervous stomach, relieves indigestion, gas and flatulence, and calms shattered nerves; as part of a digestive formula where there are ulcers, gastritis orpoor enzyme activity. **Secondary uses:** in a calming formula for menstrual pain and nerve stress; as a calmative during drug withdrawal. Speeds wound healing both internally and externally; to overcome fungal infections; as a mouthwash for gingivitis or thrush; as an eyewash for conjunctivitis and inflamed eyes. As a steam or inhalation for nasal congestion; as a gargle for sore throat; in healing skin treatments.

CHAPARRAL: *Larrea tridentata* - **Part used:** leaf. **Effective forms:** capsules, tea, mouthwash. **Therapeutic profile:** a strong anti-oxidant, blood purifier, anti-tumor agent, pain-killer, antiseptic and one of the best herbal antibiotics used for major disease healing and rebuilding; a detoxifying agent for chemicals, heavy metals and hydrocarbons. Historically used to remove residues of LSD out of the system, helping to eliminate hallucinogenic recurrences. High in protein, potassium and sodium, it also contains measureable silicon and sulphur. **Primary uses:** as a specific in a lymph cleansing formula for treating cancer, leukemia, melanoma and malignant tumors; as an anti-infective and anti-biotic; in the treatment of arthritis and other acidic conditions, such as acne and skin dermatitis; as a liver and urethral tract cleanser; as part of a bowel cleansing and rebuilding combination to tone and normalize peristalsis; in a program to overcome drug addiction, especially from hallucinogenic drugs. **Secondary uses:** to treat venereal disease; as part of a vermifuge formula to expel intestinal worms; as a mouthwash to prevent tooth decay. **Contra-indications:** avoid during pregnancy, or if there is already serious liver damage.

CHASTE TREE BERRIES: *Vitex agnus-castus* - **Part used:** berries. **Effective forms:** capsules, extract. **Therapeutic profile:** an ancient herb widely-used for women's hormone imbalance and menstrual disorders; an organ and hormone affecting herb that stimulates progesterone production, and regulates menstruation. Chaste tree helps create an effect in women that leads to a balancing of the ratio of the hormones estrogen and progesterone by acting on the regulatory hormones in the pituitary gland, helping the whole endocrine system to operate efficiently at a "master" regulatory level. **Primary uses:** in formulas to help alleviate PMS symptoms and a host of menstrual abnormalities; to reduce recurring fibroid cysts of the ovaries and uterus; to ease menstrual water retention, and to help overcome suppressed or irregular periods; also for pre-menstrual mouth herpes. **Secondary uses:** to promote an abundant supply of mother's milk during lactation; for eliminating some unpleasant side effects of lowered estrogen production, such as mid-cycle bleeding during menopause; for post-menopause symptoms such as hot flashes, water retention and low blood sugar. **Note:** For best results take *vitex* for 4 to 6 months on alternating months. **Contra-indications:** useful for its positive impact on infertility, but should not be used once a women becomes pregnant. Use of vitex with along synthetic hormone therapy is not recommended.

CHIA SEED: *Salvia hispanica* - **Part used:** seed. **Effective forms:** food supplement. **Therapeutic profile:** a delicious addition to a fiber or protein drink to stimulate bowel elimination. It is a demulcent and very nutritious. **Primary uses:** in a sweet candy or fiber bar, or nutritional drink to promote gentle regularity.

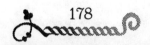

❧ **CHICHIBE:** Sida rhombifolia L. - **Part used:** leaf and root. **Effective forms:** decoction, poultice. **Therapeutic profile:** antibacterial and antifungal activity has been shown. **Primary uses:** for burning in urine, stoppage of urine, gonorrhea, and as an expectorant to loosen dry coughs. **Secondary uses:** the mashed root is used for sprains.

❧ **CHICKWEED:** Stellaria media - **Part used:** leaf. **Effective forms:** tea, capsules, oil. **Therapeutic profile:** a diuretic, alkalizing, chemistry-balancing herb; has antiseptic properties when exposed to the blood, and has been called an effective anti-cancer agent. Rich in vitamin C, B-complex, iron, copper, calcium, and sodium, it also contains vitamin D, manganese, phosphorus and zinc. **Primary uses:** as a body-balance herb for a weight loss formula; for water retention during PMS. To alkalize the body from an over-acidic condition caused by excess red meat, drug or synthetic steroid intake. Valuable for treating blood toxicity, fevers, and inflammation. **Secondary uses:** useful for stomach ulcer and inflamed bowels because of its mucilage elements; a soothing oil for skin eruptions or eczema; as a rub for arthritis or gout.

❧ **CHICORY:** Chicorium intybus - **Part used:** root. **Effective forms:** dry-roasted grain coffee substitute, tea. **Therapeutic profile:** a non-caffeine herb that when dry roasted has energy raising properties. It is rich in vitamins A, B, C, G, K, and P. **Primary uses:** the tea helps eliminate unwanted phlegm from the stomach and is good for an upset stomach. Helps uric acid conditions of gout, rheumatics and joint stiffness. **Secondary uses:** as a wash for boils and sores. Sap of the stems is useful for poison ivy and sunburned skin.

❧ **CHINCHONA:** Cinchona calisaya - **Part used:** bark. **Effective forms:** extract. **Therapeutic profile:** contains quinine, which suppresses cell enzymes and acts as a disinfectant in cases of malaria and rheumatism. It is a good tonic. **Primary uses:** an effective preventive for influenza; strengthening to the stomach in convalesence, and on the central nervous system. **Secondary uses:** for remittent and intermittent fevers.

❧ **CHITRAK:** Plumbago zeylanica- **Part used:** root. **Effective forms:** capsule, paste **Therapeutic profile:** an Ayurvedic herb known for its alterative, decongestant, carminative and astringent properties, acting in the body on the digestive and respiratory sytems, and the spleen and stomach. **Primary uses:** useful for digestive ailments including diarrhea, poor absorption, gas, indigestion, abdominal distention and hemorrhoids. Small doses can help stimulate the appetite. **Secondary uses:** used topically on enlarged glands, paralytic affections, rheumatism, scorpion stings and certain skin diseases. May have use in the treatment of hysteria and hernia. **Contra-indications:** excess use of the root can cause abortion and large dose can cause death; use a low dosage 100-250mg as directed by a qualified health practitioner; may also irritate the skin when used externally.

❧ **CHLORELLA:-** **Part used:** dried powdered plant. **Effective forms:** tablets, capsules, as a drink. **Therapeutic profile:** a nutritive micro-algae superfood, rich in chlorophyllins, proteins, anti-oxidants, vitamin B, beta carotene and zinc; an anti-viral immunostimulant, (especially toward neutralizing the AIDS virus). A whole body tonic and regenerative. **Primary uses:** a revitalizing drink, particularly after illness or surgery; as part of a blood building and liver support combination; as an anti-biotic and anti-carcinogen to inhibit growth and development of toxic bacteria; as an intestinal deodorizer. Restores and enhances the immune system, rebuilding health and resistance to disease. **Secondary uses:** to accelerate tissue cell activity, especially in cases of low red blood cell count; to check and regulate heavy menstrual flow. An aid to sugar balance in cases of hypoglycemia and diabetes.

❧ **CHRYSANTHEMUM:** Chrysanthemum morifolium, (Chu Hua) - **Part used:** flower. **Effective forms:** tea. **Therapeutic profile:** a rejuvenative herb with anti-inflammatory and anti-biotic properties. **Primary uses:** as part of a combination for inflammatory chest, headache, fever and flu congestion. **Secondary uses:** as a rejuvenating eyewash for inflamed eyes, dry eyes, blurred vision and spots before the eyes; as a part of longevity and colds and flu combinations. Helps reduce blood pressure.

❧ **CILANTRO:** Coriandrum sativum- **Part used:** leaves. **Effective forms:** in foods. **Therapeutic profile:** an alterative, cooling Ayurvedic herb used in many popular culinary dishes as a flavor addition and a pungent digestive aid. Diuretic properties make this herb useful for urinary problems. Acts favorably on the circulatory and respiratory systems. **Primary uses:** used primarily to loosen mucous congestion and relive hay fever. **Secondary uses:** may have application in relieving edema, urinary stones, skin diseases and genital herpes.

❧ **CINNAMON:** (Cassia), Cinnamomum cassia - **Part used:** bark, twigs, oil. **Effective forms:** tea, decoction, tincture, capsules. **Therapeutic profile:** a warming stimulant for digestive improvement, with mild circulatory stimulation. The twigs and bark are carminative to promote sweating; they act as a warming digestive remedy, antispasmodic, antiseptic, tonic and uterine stimulant. Cinnamon oil is a potent antibacterial, antifungal and uterine stimulant. **Primary uses**: as part of an enzyme-producing formula for better digestion. Tincture in a little hot water is useful for colds and chills. **Secondary uses**: as an astringent against diarrhea; to relieve nausea; as a mild catalyst to transport herbal constituents throughout the body. Putting 4 to 5 drops of the oil in boiling water and inhaling the steam is useful for coughs and respiratory irritation. A good spice to use for taste in any children's tea.

CITRONELLA: Part used: oil derived from the grass and the entire plant. **Effective forms**: soap, tea, spray, dentifrice, and external oil. **Therapeutic profile**: a reed-shaped grass with antibacterial, insecticide, fungicidal, and antiseptic properties. **Primary uses**: used in natural sprays to ward off insects including mosquitos and ticks; citronella oil is a great addition to any camper's supplies. **Secondary uses**: indicated in the treatment of skin infection and funguses - has some activity very similar to tea tree oil. **Contra-indications**: Some people are allergic to the oil or find it irritating to the skin: essential oils can be dangerous, never use undiluted or internally without expert advice.

CLEAVERS: (Bedstraw) *Galium aparine* - **Part used**: leaf and herb. **Effective forms**: tea, compress, skin wash. **Therapeutic profile**: an alterative, astringent, diuretic, antipyretic, laxative, cleavers is a lymphatic tonic with valuable diuretic properties. Used to dissolve kidney stones and urinary sediment. **Primary uses**: as part of a bladder/kidney combination for overcoming infection and water retention; as a lymphatic tonic for swollen glands, particularly for tonsillitis and adenoids; as a body cleanser for skin diseases such as eczema and psoriasis. Helps clean the blood and strengthen the liver. **Secondary uses**: used to help break fevers, it is an anti-inflammatory to counteract venereal disease. Used externally as a compress for malignant tumer growths; as a skin wash for sunburn and freckles.

CLOVES: *Syzygium aromaticum* - **Part used**: flower bud and oil. **Effective forms**: tea, oil. **Therapeutic profile**: has antiseptic, aromatic, carminative, stimulant, anodyne, anti-emetic and aphrodisiac properties. A stimulating spice for the digestive system. Increases circulation of the blood. It is one of the most powerful germicidal agents in the spice or herb kingdom. Cloves contain vitamins A, C, the B-complex, potassium, phosphorus, calcium, magnesium and sodium. **Primary uses**: as a catalyst for energy combinations; for indigestion, especially where there is belching and nausea. **Secondary uses**: as an aid to correct kidney malfuntion; the oil, directly placed on an aching tooth can bring almost immediate relief of toothache; as a specific in stopping hiccups and vomiting during a cold. Good for bad breath.

CODONOPSIS: *Codonopsitis lanceolate* - **Part used**: root. **Effective forms**: tea, capsules. **Therapeutic profile**: a Chinese herb with ginseng-like properties that enhances vital, deep level energy in the organs. **Primary uses**: in an over-all energizing formula. **Secondary uses**: in a combination to rebuild liver and spleen strength. Often used as part of a formula for arthritis.

COIX SEED: *Coix lachryma-jobi L. var* (Yiyiren): **Part used**: seed. **Effective forms**: 10-30g capsules. **Therapeutic profile**: used in Traditional Chinese medicine to transform dampness and promote water metabolism; helps clear heat and eliminates pus. **Primary uses**: for spleen deficiency problems such as edema, dysuria and diarrhea in combination with *alismatis rhizome* and *white atractylodes*. **Secondary uses**: coix has application in problems related to accumulation of damp-heat and stagnation of chi and blood such as lung and intestinal abscesses.

COLEUS FORSKOHLII: *Labiatae* (perennial member of the mint family) - **Part used**: root. **Effective forms**: capsules. **Therapeutic profile**: contains a unique substance called forskolin which activates an enzyme (adenylate cyclase) which in turn increases the amount of cyclic adenosine monophosphate (cAMP) in cells. Cyclic AMP is an important cell regulating compound. **Primary uses**: clinical applications show Coleus forskohlii is effective in a number of conditions, such as eczema (atopic dermatitis), asthma, psoriasis, angina and hypertension. **Secondary uses**: has a long history of use in Ayurvedic medicine includes the treatment of cardiovascular disease, ezema, abdominal colic, respiratory disorders, painful urination, insomnia, and convulsions.

COLLINSONIA: (See STONE ROOT)

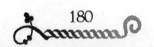

COLTSFOOT: *Tussilago farfara* - **Part used:** leaves and herb. **Effective forms:** tea. **Therapeutic profile:** an expectorant and anti-spasmodic herb for respiratory system treatment. Contains a high percentage of mucilage and saponins which have disinfectant and anti-inflammatory effects to help respiratory problems. Rich in vitamins A and C, it also contains calcium, potassium, zinc, vitamin B$_{12}$ and B$_6$. **Primary uses:** as part of combinations for asthma, chronic and acute bronchitis, hacking cough and sore throat. A chest and lung expectorant, it has a soothing effect on the throat as well as on the brains' cough-activating mechanism. **Secondary uses:** as a healant for emphysema symptoms; as a tea to arrest diarrhea; externally as a compress for boils, bruises and sores.

COMFREY: *Symphytum officinale* - **Part used:** root and leaf. **Effective forms:** tea, green drink, capsules, compress, poultice, extract, douche. **Therapeutic profile:** a soothing mucilaginous astrigent and toning herb, rich in allantoin (an agent which promotes cell proliferation), with impressive wound and bone healing properties both internally and externally; especially useful for irritation and inflammatory conditions. One of the few plants that can produce vitamin B$_{12}$ from the cobalt in the soil. **Primary uses:** as the healing and tissue building part of a combination for stomach and duodenal ulcers, bowel inflammations and colitis; as a specific for asthmatic, lung and bronchial inflammation; as part of a colds and flu combination to lower fever and soothe coughs. Effective as an anti-viral for staph and strep; as a specific for bone, cartilage, tendon and muscle rebuilding; as a soothing healer for cystitis, bladder and prostate infection. An effective hemostatic to stop internal hemorrhaging from the lungs and urethral system; internally for excessive menstruation, and externally for bleeding cuts and wounds. **Secondary uses:** as part of a blood cleansing tonic; externally, as a poultice for bone knitting and fractures; as a compress or poultice for cuts, burns, varicose veins, and chest congestion; as part of a douche for vaginal yeast infections; as treatment for swelling from insect bites and stings; as part of a green drink providing measureable amounts of chlorophyll, calcium, vitamin C, beta carotene, vitamin B$_{12}$ and allantoin. **Contra-indications:** although used for thousands of years safely and effectively, recent investigation shows comfrey species to contain hepatotoxic pyrrolizidine alkaloids (PA's), such as echimidine. Whether this is from environmental toxins or is naturally present in the plant, *but neutralized by other plant substances, has not been determined.* Until a safe source can be guaranteed, comfrey should not be used during pregnancy. I recommend using an organically grown source for a very short limited time, or using comfrey externally until more information on these alkaloids is known.

CONTRA HIERBA: *Syngonium podophyllum* - **Part used:** leaves. **Effective forms:** decoction. **Therapeutic profile:** plants in this family (*Araceae*) often contain calcium oxalate crystals which if taken internally, can be irritating to internal tissue and even toxic. **Primary uses:** used warm as a wash for skin conditions, sores, dry skin, fungus, itching, rashes, and bruises. **Secondary uses:** a 7 day alcohol leaf extract is used externally for rheumatism, arthritis, pains and swellings. **Contra-indications:** taken intenally can cause irritation and toxic reactions.

COPTIS ROOT: *Coptis chinensis franch* (Huanglian): **Part used:** dried root. **Effective forms:** decoction and capsule. **Therapeutic profile:** commonly employed in TCM to clear heat and dry dampness and to reduce fire and dispel toxins. **Primary uses:** in combination with *evodia fruit* for vomiting due to liver fire; in combination with *bamboo shoots* for vomiting due to fire in the stomach. Indicated for diarrhea and dysentery. **Secondary uses:** in the treatment of boils, carbuncles and furuncles; for febrile diseases with symptoms such as fever, irritability, loss of consciousness and delirium. **Contra-indications:** use with caution as large dosages weaken the stomach.

CORIANDER: *Coriandrum sativum* - **Part used:** leaves and seeds. **Effective forms:** tea. **Therapeutic profile:** actions include stimulant, aromatic and carminative. An effective digestive-stimulant spice that helps relieve diarrhea. **Primary uses:** as part of a combination to correct stomach upset, indigestion and gas. **Secondary uses:** relieves diarrhea and strengthens the urinary tract; to help relieve colic and diarrhea in children.

CORNEL FRUIT: *Cornus officinalis* - **Part used:** fruit. **Effective forms:** decoction. **Therapeutic profile:** an Ayurvedic tonic herb for the liver and kidneys; used primarily for its obstructive, antihypertensive, antiperspiration, astringent, diuretic properties. **Primary uses:** used to control high blood sugar, diarrhea, dizziness, tinnitus and insomnia. **Secondary uses:** helps treat excessive menses, excessive perspiration, excessive urination, vaginal discharges, and seminal emissions. **Contra-indications:** not to be used when there is constipation.

CORNFLOWER or **CYANI:** *Centaurea cyanus* - **Part used:** leaf, seed and petals. **Effective forms:** powder. **Therapeutic profile:** a plant traditionally used by the Plains Indian tribes for its nervine properties, and properties similar to blessed thistle. **Primary uses:** as an antidote for snakebite, insect bites and stings. Also used as an aid for nervous disorders, infectious diseases, fevers, and indigestion. **Secondary uses:** water distilled from petals is used for weak eyes. The dried powder is used to accelerate bruise healing.

❧ **CORNSILK:** *Zea mays* - **Part used:** stigmas from the female flowers. **Effective forms:** tea, capsules. **Therapeutic profile:** a soothing diuretic, effective for many bladder and kidney dysfunctions. Has a cleansing effect on the circulation of urea and it will cleanse the cystic membrane in cystic catarrh. Rich in vitamin K, it also contains vitamin B, PABA and silicon. **Primary uses:** as a specific for cystitis, urethral and prostate inflammation; as part of a formula to dissolve kidney stones and sediment; as a specific diuretic to relieve fluid retention. **Secondary uses:** in a combination to treat bedwetting in children.

❧ **CORYDALIS TUBER** : *Corydalis turtschaninovii* (Yanhusuo): **Part used:** dried pieces of the rhizome. **Effective forms:** capsules, decoction. **Therapeutic profile:** used in TCM to invigorate the blood and promote chi circulation and to stop pain. **Primary uses:** relieves pain due to ch'i and blood stagnation in combination with *sichuan chinaberry, Chinese angelica root, chuanxiong rhizome, frankincense and myrrh.*

❧ **COUCHGRASS:** *Agrophyron repens* - **Part used:** root. **Effective forms:** tea. **Therapeutic profile:** a diuretic herb with some anti-biotic properties for control of bladder, kidney, and urinary infections. Rich in vitamins A, C, the B-complex, silicon, potassium and sodium. Also contains magnesium and calcium. **Primary uses:** as a specific for urinary, bladder, kidney and urethral infections to relieve sediment and inflammation; as part of a cleansing combination for gallstones, kidney stones. **Secondary uses:** as an aid in dissolving the crystalline deposits of gout and bursitis. Makes a good spring tonic.

❧ **CRAMP BARK:** *Viburnum opulus* - **Part used:** bark, berries. **Effective forms:** extract, capsules, tea. **Therapeutic profile:** a powerful anti-spasmodic and relaxant for cramping, muscular and menstrual pain. An excellent relaxant to the ovaries and uterus. Contains potassium, calcium and magnesium. The berry, sometimes used like cranberries, is rich in vitamins C, bioflavonoids and K, along with some minerals. **Primary uses:** a specific for menstrual cramping; to arrest threatened miscarriage. **Secondary uses:** an astringent to reduce excessive periods associated with menopause; as a muscle relaxant for cramping.

❧ **CRANBERRIES:** *Vaccinium macrocarpon* - **Part used:** juice. **Effective forms:** tea, capsules. **Therapeutic profile:** an alkalizer that creates an unfavorable environment for urinary infecting bacteria. Recent studies show components in cranberry juice reduce the ability of *E. coli* to adhere to the lining of the bladder and urethra. This may be the most important factor in cranberry juice's positive effects in bladder infections. Cranberry juice also reduces the amount of ionized calcium in the urine by more than 50% in patients with recurrent kidney stones. **Primary uses:** a specific in formulas for bladder infection. **Secondary uses:** a cleansing agent for candida albicans.

❧ **CRANESBILL:** *Geranium maculatum* - **Part used:** root. **Effective forms:** tea, vaginal suppository, astringent powder. **Therapeutic profile:** an astringent herb effective for diarrhea, internal bleeding, hemorrhoids and duodenal ulcers. Also has important hemostatic/styptic properties. **Primary uses:** as part of a balancing combination to control excessive menstrual flow; in control of hemorrhoidal bleeding; for cessation of diarrhea and dysentery; a safe, effective astringent bitters herb for gastrointestinal problems. **Secondary uses:** as a direct application to stop bleeding; as a vaginal suppository or douche for leucorrhea, flaccid tissue and common yeast infection. Useful for all excessive chronic mucous discharges.

❧ **CUBEB BERRIES:** *Piper cubeba* - **Part used:** berries. **Effective forms:** capsules, tea. **Therapeutic profile:** a diuretic, expectorant, stimulant, carminative herb. **Primary uses:** as part of an anti-inflammatory formula for chronic urethral problems, venereal disease and discharge. **Secondary uses:** for help in hemorrhoid control. Also used for leucorrhoea, cystitis, urethritis, abscesses of the prostate gland, piles and chronic bronchitis.

❧ **CUCUMBER:** *Cucumis sativa* - **Part used:** fruit. **Effective forms:** juice. **Therapeutic profile:** a food diuretic, useful internally and externally in treating poor skin conditions. Cooling, healing and soothing to an irritated skin, whether caused by the sun or the effects of a cutaneous eruption. **Primary uses:** a gentle, skin clearing herb; a diuretic drink. **Secondary uses:** as part of a treatment for tapeworm infestation, followed by a cathartic.

❧ **CULVER'S ROOT:** *Varoniscastrum virginicum* - **Parts used:** root. **Effective forms:** capsules, extract. **Therapeutic profile:** A popular medieval herb, culver's has a tonic effect on the liver and stomach. Contains measureable amounts of potassium and magnesium. **Primary uses:** as part of a formula for intestinal indigestion, purifies the blood, and removes catarrhal obstructions and congestions. Also used to aid diarrhea, fevers and food poisoning.

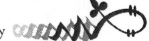

DAMIANA: *Turnera diffusa* - **Part used:** leaf. **Effective forms:** tea, extract, capsules. **Therapeutic profile:** a mild aphrodisiac and tonic for the central nervous and hormonal systems. **Primary uses:** a specific in compounds to treat frigidity in women and impotence in men; as a body tonic and energizer; it has stimulating properties and has been used for nervousness, weakness and exhaustion; as part of an anti-depressant. As part of a hormone balancing formula for both sexes; for delayed menstruation in young girls. One of the most popular and safest of all plants claimed to restore the natural sexual capacities and functions. **Secondary uses:** as part of a formula to relieve constipation and bloating; for irritation of urinary/urethral passages.

DANDELION LEAF: *Taraxacum officinale* - **Part used:** leaf, fresh and dried. **Effective forms:** tea, salad herb, capsules. **Therapeutic profile:** an effective diuretic, high in potassium and vitamins A and D. Dandelion greens are richer in vitamin A than carrots, and exceed the vitamin B, C and D content of most other traditional vegetables. **Primary uses:** a specific in a formula to relieve water retention, especially if due to high blood pressure; as part of a liver and gall bladder tonic for congestion and jaundice. Adding dandelion leaf to the diet helps improve the enamel of the teeth. **Secondary uses:** as part of a formula to overcome anemia and "tired blood."

DANDELION ROOT: *Taraxacum officinale* - **Part used:** root. **Effective forms:** capsules, extract, tea. **Therapeutic profile:** a source of natural potassium, has a high inulin content; an excellent liver cleansing and toning herb; soothing, healing properties for the digestive system and bowel inflammation. All glands involved with the digestive system respond rapidly and effectively to dandelion root. **Primary uses:** a specific for liver cleansing and healing, including serious liver conditions such as hepatitis, jaundice and cirrhosis; to stimulate bile secretion, and enzyme therapy; as part of a bowel cleansing and toning formula; as part of a combination to reduce high blood pressure and its resultant edema. **Secondary uses:** an aid to weight loss and cholesterol reduction through improved liver activity; as part of a formula for arthritis and rheumatism because the roasted root increases uptake of organic calcium by the body. (If you drink a lot of phosphate containing, calcium-blocking commercial sodas, dandelion root tea several times a week can help you keep from losing precious calcium.)

DENDROBIUM: *Dendrobium nobile Lindl.* (Shihu): **Part used:** dried stems. **Effective forms:** capsule, extract, decoction. **Therapeutic profile:** used to tonify yin and clear heat; also used to promote the production of body fluids and nourish the stomach. **Primary uses:** in TCM for febrile disease with symptoms such as dry or red tongue and excessive thirst; used in fevers related to yin deficiency and excessive heat. **Contra-indications:** Cook dendrodium before adding other herbs to the decoction.

DEVIL'S CLAW: *Harpagophytum procumbens* - **Part used:** root. **Effective forms:** capsules, extract, decoction. **Therapeutic profile:** an anti-inflammatory and blood cleansing herb with prostaglandin balancing activity, specifically used for joint pain relief. Has the abillity to cleanse deep into the muscles and tissue walls, with natural cleansing agents that clean the system of toxic impurities. **Primary uses:** as a specific for inflammation and pain of arthritic and rheumatic conditions; to reduce elevated cholesterol levels and uric acid in the blood. Studies have shown that regular use of the devil's claw tea helps hardened vascular walls to become more elastic with a generalized feeling of strength. **Secondary uses:** to relieve inflammatory liver and gall bladder problems. Good for a spring cleanse for the most important organs, lymph and blood.

DIKAMALI: *Gardenia florida* - **Part used:** fruit resin. **Effective forms:** paste, decoction. **Therapeutic profile:** used in Ayurveda to soothe Pitta imbalances, especially of the liver and spleen. Noted for alterative, anthelmintic, antiseptic and antispasmodic properties. **Primary uses:** as a decoction for dentition, fever, gas, nervous disorders, obesity, round worms and skin problems. **Secondary uses:** as a topical paste for sores and toothache

DILL SEED: *Anethum graveolens* - **Part used:** seeds. **Effective forms:** tea, rice wine infusion. **Therapeutic profile:** a gentle remedy for children' upsets, and nursing mothers. **Primary uses:** the herb of choice for flatulence or colic in infants and children's upset stomach (steep an ounce of powdered seed in 2 cups rice wine with 2 TBS. of chamomile flowers for two weeks. Strain and give 1 teasp. at a time - or mix powdered seed with a little honey, and give to an infant on your fingertip); to promote the flow of breast milk. Dried leaves are used as a healthful condiment. Fresh leaves are used in salads - a little goes a long way. **Secondary uses:** chew seeds for bad breath.

DONG QUAI: *Angelica sinensis*, (Tang Keui) - **Part used:** root. **Effective forms:** capsules, extract, tea. **Therapeutic profile:** a blood purifying, warming tonic herb with ginseng-like properties, effective for female problems. Increases hormone uptake by the body. Widely used as a phyto-hormone regulator to "keep the female system female." Has a tranquilizing effect on the central nervous system and nourishes the brain cells. Possesses nutritive constituents for the female glands, and helps to strengthen all internal body organs and muscles. Contains vitamin A, B$_{12}$ and E. **Primary uses:** for relief of many menstrual/menopause problems and female PMS imbalance; for infertility; for vaginal dryness; for hot flashes, headaches, breast soreness, premenstrual gas, and low blood sugar caused by hormone imbalance; an anti-spasmodic and circulation stimulant. **Secondary uses:** a strengthener for the blood to counteract anemia; as part of a blood balancing formula to help ringing in the ears, heart palpitations, and blurred vision. Also beneficial to men for prostatic disorders as it supports deficient testosterone secretion. Useful in aiding recovery from an accident if internal bleeding and body bruises exist. **Contra-indications:** not advised during the first two tri-mesters of pregnancy.

DRAGON'S BLOOD: *Daemonorops draco Bl.* (Xuejie) - **Part used:** resin secretion from fruit and stems. **Effective forms:** capsules. **Therapeutic profile:** in TCM to stop hemorrhaging and to aid in the healing of wounds; relieves pain; removes stagnation in blood. **Primary uses:** externally for hemorrhages due to external injuries; combine with *frankincense* and *myrrh* to be used externally for chronic ulcers; indicated for swelling and pain. **Contra-indications:** used only when there are signs of blood stagnation.

DULSE: *Rhodymenia palmata* - **Part used:** whole leaf and stem. **Effective forms:** tea, salad or soup sprinkle, in a mineral drink. **Therapeutic profile:** a potent sea vegetable with highly absorbable mineral and protein content. All sea vegetables contain radio-protective properties. Red sea vegetables, such as dulse are the most effective at binding plutonium. **Primary uses:** for its high mineral, iron, calcium or potassium content as part of a protective formula against radiation and environmental pollutants. **Secondary uses:** as a nutritive drink or food addition.

ECHINACEA ANGUSTIFOLIA: *Echinacea angustifolia* - **Part used:** root and leaf. **Effective forms:** extract, capsules, tea, ointment. **Therapeutic profile:** a powerful immuno-modulating, blood purification herb (often called the "King of the Blood Purifiers") with anti-biotic, anti-septic and anti-inflammatory activity. Improves lymphatic filtration and drainage. Gentle for all ages and health constitutions, yet very effective, increasing production and activity of white blood cells against pathogenic organisms. Contains vitamins A, E, and C, iron, iodine, copper, sulphur and potassium. **Primary uses:** as a specific in any formula to overcome bacterial infection and toxicity; a primary herb in any formula to rebuild and strengthen immune defenses; an anti-tumor agent; a specific in bladder, kidney and prostate infection control; as a primary herb in a formula for pelvic infectious disease.; as an anti-fungal for candidiasis; for treating venereal disease, such as syphilis and gonorrhea, and as a douche for vaginal infections. **Secondary uses:** as part of a general blood, gland and lymph cleansing combination for allergy symptoms, tonsillitis and respiratory disease prevention; for breast soreness. As an effective mouthwash for toothache, strep throat, mouth and gum disease; as an anti-inflammatory tonic for rheumatoid arthritis.

ECHINACEA PURPUREA: *Echinacea purpurea* - **Part used:** root and whole herb. **Effective forms:** capsules, extract, tea and antiseptic cream. **Therapeutic profile:** an anti-microbial infection fighter and blood purifier against staph and strep viruses; an effective anti-biotic lotion to help heal septic cuts, wounds and sores. Both echinacea purpurea and angustifolia are famous worldwide for their antibacterial, antiviral and antifungal properties. Cultivated purple coneflower is usually *E. purpurea*, although some pracititioners consider *E. angustifolia* to be more potent. **Primary uses:** in a formula with *echinacea angustifolia* in antibiotic combinations, for its particular vasodilating and lymph/circulatory clearing activity; with *echinacea ang.* as part of a maintainence and preventive formula for eczema and herpes. **Secondary uses:** as a bowel and colon detoxifier, and as part of a vermifuge for internal parasites; as effective control for systemic reactions to poison oak and venomous bites; for staph infections such as impetigo and nail fungus.

ELDER; *Sambucus nigra* - **Part used:** leaves, berries, flowers, bark. **Effective forms:** tea, herbal wine, oil, ointment, tincture, juice. **Therapeutic profile:** a plant high in vitamin C and flavonoids, used chiefly as a "spring cleaning" agent for detoxification from winter's chronic colds and flu; an expectorant and sweating herb for respiratory problems. An anti-inflammatory, elder increases blood circulation and can reduce fever when needed. Contains vitamin A, C and bioflavonoids. **Primary uses:** a specific detoxifier for colds, flu and upper respiratory congestion; as part of a skin cleansing formula. **Secondary uses:** to relieve stopped up ears due to upper respiratory congestion; as an ointment for tumors; the ointment or oil for burns, cuts, scratches and chapping.

ELECAMPANE: *Inula helenium* - **Part used:** root. **Effective forms:** capsules. **Therapeutic profile:** a bitters, expectorant and anti-bacterial for relieving chronic respiratory congestion and infections. One of the richest sources of natural insulin and therefore helpful for the pancreas. Contains calcium, potassium and sodium.

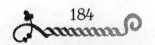

Primary uses: a specific in formulas for colds, flu, coughs and bronchial, and asthma congestion; for treating emphysema and tuberculosis. Helpful for intestinal worms, retention of water and to lessen tooth decay and firm the gums. **Secondary uses:** to strengthen poor digestion by keeping the intestines clear of excess mucous.

❧ **ELEUTHERO:** (Siberian ginseng), *Eleutherococcus senticosus, (Wujiashen)* - **Part used:** root. **Effective forms:** tea, liquid and powdered extract, capsules, herbal wine. **Therapeutic profile:** an excellent general tonic and nutritive herb, stimulating to the circulatory/cardiac system; exhibits many of the rejuvenative, adaptogen properties of panax ginseng in terms of energy, endurance and balance, along with antispasmodic and antirheumatic actions. Less heating than Asian ginseng and may be more suitable for those who find Korean ginseng too stimulating. **Primary uses:** in tonic and energy formulas against depression and fatigue, especially when rebuilding system strength after exhaustion; as part of an immune rebuilding compound to increase body resistance to disease; effective in lowering blood pressure and cholesterol, stimulating adrenal function, and raising sexual vitality. Increases mental alertness and work output. **Secondary uses:** for relief of arthritis and congestive problems, such as heart disease and chronic respiratory ailments; for hypoglycemia symptoms. **Contra-Indications:** avoid during pregnancy, if you have high blood pressure, or when taking major drug medication.

❧ **EPHEDRA:** *Ephedra sinica, (Ma huang)* - **Part used:** aerial parts. **Effective forms:** tea, capsules extract. **Therapeutic profile:** a strong nervine stimulant, heart stimulant and broncho-dilator, particularly effective for opening air passages, stimulating circulation, and counteracting fatigue. It contains some vitamin B_{12}, cobalt, and copper. **Primary uses:** for relief of asthma, allergy, bronchitis, sinusitis, and other respiratory congestive conditions; effective against environmental allergies such as hayfever; a "dieter's" herb to reduce fatigue, stimulate thermogenesis (calorie burning) and allay hunger. **Secondary uses:** in balancing formulas for circulatory stimulation; as a part of a natural energy formula; for relieving congestion in migraine headaches and bloating; in the treatment of low blood pressure. **Contra-Indications:** Do not use if there is hypertension, high blood pressure, heart disease, thyroid disease, diabetes or difficulty in urination due to enlargement of the prostate gland. Also should not be used in patients on anti-hypertensive or antidepressant drugs.

❧ **EPSOM SALTS:** *Sodium sulphate* - **Part used:** salts. **Effective forms:** eyewash, gargle, bath, foot bath, compress. **Therapeutic profile:** a bowel cleansing purgative; a soothing, bath for muscle strain. **Primary uses:** a cathartic cleanser for the elimination system, often used on the first day of a serious fast. A bath for aching muscles and strained ligaments. **Secondary uses:** a gargle for sore throat; a neutralizing wash for abscesses and skin ulcers; as an eyewash for conjunctivitis. **Contra-Indications:** Do not use internally during pregnancy.

❧ **EUCALYPTUS:** *Eucalyptus globulus* - **Part used:** leaf. **Effective forms:** tea, an external oil, steam, ointment. **Therapeutic profile:** a measurable source of rutin, eucalyptus has strong antiseptic properties, effective internally for colds, flu and sore throats, and externally for chest congestion, and sore muscles. An antispasmodic, stimulant, febrifuge, and expectorant, it reduces blood sugar levels and expels worms. **Primary uses:** internally and externally for asthma and respiratory congestion relief. **Secondary uses:** a sports medicine rub for pain relief; for pets to ward off fleas, ticks and mites.

❧ **EUCOMMIA BARK:** *Eucommia ulmoides oliv.* (Duzhong) - **Part used:** bark. **Effective forms:** decoction. **Therapeutic profile:** used in TCM to tonify the kidneys and liver; strengthens bones and tendons; calming to fetus. **Primary uses:** Used with *psoralea fruit* and *walnut seed* for soreness and pain in the lower back and knees; indicated for impotence due to deficient kidneys. **Secondary uses:** to prevent spontaneous abortion and restlessness of fetus with symptoms such as lower abdominal pain and uterine bleeding during pregnancy.

❧ **EUPATORIUM:** *Eupatorium fortunei Turcz.* (Peilan)- **Part used:** aerial parts. **Effective forms:** tea or capsule. **Therapeutic profile:** in TCM to transform dampness and to release summer-heat. **Primary uses:** indicated for epigastric and abdominal distention and fullness, nausea, vomiting and poor appetite. **Secondary uses:** for fevers with symptoms such as stifling sensation in the chest, lack of appetite, low-grade fever and sallow complexion.

❧ **EVENING PRIMROSE:** *Oenothera biennis* - **Part used:** flower oil. **Effective forms:** capsules. **Therapeutic profile:** a GLA (Gamma Linoleic Acid) rich herb to enhance prostaglandin balance. **Primary uses:** as part of a hormone balancing program to control PMS, menopausal problems, infertility, and other glandular malfunctions - especially prostate problems for men; as part of a program for serious degenerative diseases such as M.S. and muscular dystrophy. GLA supplied from evening primrose can be an important dietary supplement to increase prostaglandin production in treating essential fatty-acid deficiencies. **Secondary uses:** for skin beauty and health; to help prevent hangovers and cell damage from drugs and alcohol; for breast soreness.

EYEBRIGHT: *Euphrasia officinalis* - **Part used:** leaf. **Effective forms:** tea, capsules, eyewash, extract. **Therapeutic profile:** an anti-bacterial and astringent herb, effective in maintaining optical system health; a specific anti-catarrhal for sinusitis and other congestive states. Stimulates the liver to clean the blood and relieve conditions that effect clarity of vision and thought. Antiseptic properties fight eye infections. Strengthens all parts of the eye and provides an elasticity for nerves and optic devices responsible for sight. Also useful for inflammations because of its cooling and detoxifying properties. Rich in vitamins A and C; contains B-complex, vitamin D, E, iron, silicon, and traces of iodine and zinc. **Primary uses:** a specific in combinations to treat eye problems, such as conjunctivitis, cataract formation, glaucoma, weak eyesight and eyestrain; to help remove cysts caused by chronic eye inflammation; externally for rapid relief of redness and swelling in conjunctivitis. **Secondary uses:** as part of a decongestive allergy formula; as part of a liver cleansing and stimulating formula.

FALSE UNICORN: (Helonias), *Chamaelirium luteum* - **Part used:** root. **Effective forms:** capsules, tea. **Therapeutic profile:** a toning diuretic effective for the female reproductive system and genito-urinary problems. It contains strong antiseptic properties. High in vitamin C, it contains copper, sulphur, cobalt, molybdenum and traces of zinc. **Primary uses:** as an estrogen precursor in female formulas to balance menstrual irregularities and pain, and for cases of infertility; for uterine strength against miscarriage; as a diuretic in kidney/bladder combinations. Used to help correct almost all of the problems associated with the female and male reproductive organs. **Secondary uses:** internally and externally as a vermifuge (like pumpkin seeds) for the removal of tapeworms.

FENNEL: *Foeniculum vulgare* - **Part used:** seed. **Effective forms:** tea, extract, oil. **Therapeutic profile:** an aromatic anti-inflammatory herb with digestive and diuretic abilities. Helps stabilize the nervous system and moves waste material out of the body; anticonvulsive, pain-relieving and mucus-countering. Contains potassium, sulphur and sodium. **Primary uses:** an important part of anti-gas, laxative/diuretic and weight loss formulas; as part of a regeneration formula from the effects of radiation and chemotherapy; as part of a compound for bladder or prostate infection; as a tea and wash to relieve conjunctivitis and inflammation of the eyelids. **Secondary uses:** as part of a combination to enrich quantity and quality of mother's milk; externally, the oil as part of a relief rub for muscle or rheumatic aches and strains.

FENUGREEK: *Trigonella foenum-graecum* - **Part used:** seed. **Effective forms:** tea, capsules, poultice. gargle. **Therapeutic profile:** a soothing, mucilaginous herb used for metabolic dysfunction and to alleviate mucous congestion in both respiratory and waste elimination systems. Softens and dissolves hardened masses of accumulated mucus, and helps expel mucus and phlegm from the bronchial tubes. Also helps expel toxic waste through the lymphatic system. Contains lecithin, a lipotropic (fat dissolving) substance, which dissolves cholesterol. Has antiseptic properties and fights infections in the lungs. Rich in vitamins A and D, in several important minerals, and protein. Contains vitamins B_1, B_2 and B_3, choline, and iron. **Primary uses:** a specific to remove phlegm and soothe mucous membranes in the lungs and gastrointestinal tract; a lecithin-containing herb for a cellulite control formula to help dissolve fatty substances; as part of a fiber drink to expel wastes and toxic mucous; in a combination to regulate insulin production and blood sugar use; as part of a digestive aid formula. **Secondary uses:** to bring down fever; to draw infection from boils and abscesses; as a gargle for sore throat.

FEVERFEW: *Tanacetum parthenium* - **Part used:** leaf and flower. **Effective forms:** extract, tea. **Therapeutic profile:** an anti-inflammatory and vasodilating herb particularly useful as a remedy and preventive for migraines. Enhances the secretion of inflammatory and allergic mediators such as histamine and serotonin. Feverfew has a favorable effect on blood platelets to inhibit platelet aggregation. Exerts a tonic effect on vascular smooth muscle, so that the combined action on smooth muscle and platelets contributes to its effectiveness in the prevention and treatment of migraine headaches. Contains high amounts of iron, niacin, manganese, phosphorus, potassium and selenium. Also contains vitamin A, C, silicon, sodium and zinc. **Primary uses:** a specific in the treatment of migraines, cluster headaches and neuralgia; as part of a long term formula to relieve arthritic inflammation. **Secondary uses:** as part of a relief combination for painful or sluggish menstruation; as part of a formula for tinnitus or vertigo. **Contra-indications:** do not use when pregnant - may start uterine contractions.

FIGWORT: *Scrophularia nodosa* - **Parts used:** herb and root. **Effective forms:** powder. **Therapeutic profile:** provides hormone-like materials into the system which helps soothe the digestive organs and clean the kidneys.

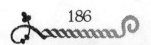

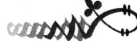

Primary uses: as a poultice for ulcers, piles, scrofulous glands in the neck, sores and wounds, and toothache. As part of a circulatory correction formula to treat and reduce varicose veins. **Secondary uses:** as a skin medication for eczema, scabies, tumors and rashes.

FLAX: (Linseed), *Linum usitatissimum* - **Part used:** seed. **Effective forms:** tea, oil, poultice. **Therapeutic profile:** mucilagenous seeds with high Omega-3 oils (flaxseed is the world's richest source of omega-3 oils); effective as a laxative and stool softener; and as a soothing agent in inflammatory respiratory problems. Flaxseed oil is unique because it contains both of the essential fatty acids (alpha linolenic - an omega-3 fatty acid and linoleic acid - an omega-6 fatty acid) in appreciable amounts; also contains calcium and potassium. **Primary uses:** as part of a fiber laxative combination; in a pulmonary or bronchial relief formula. Contains Omega-3 fatty acids with their beneficial effect in cardiovascular disease, inflammation reduction, allergies and cancer. One tablespoon of flaxseed oil a day is an excellent way to supplement essential fatty acids into one's diet. **Secondary uses:** as a poultice to relieve abscesses, boils, shingles, psoriasis outbreakes and other skin swellings.

FO-TI: *Polygonium multiflorum, (Ho-Shou-Wu)*; Multiflower Knotweed (Ayurveda) - **Part used:** root/tuber. **Effective forms:** tea, extract, capsules. **Therapeutic profile:** a liver and blood tonic to restore energy and vigor; a long-term immune system tonic. It has been found to have sedative effects, anti-cancer properties, anti-fever, and beneficial effects on fertility and other female functions involving ovulation and corpus luteum formation. It has been found to reduce hypertension, blood cholesterol levels and the incidence of coronary heart disease among individuals prone to these conditions; increases red blood cell count and reduces blood fat; a tonic for the endocrine glands. Has properties comparable to *panax ginseng*. **Primary uses:** as part of a liver, kidney and general organ strengthening formula, particularly where there is exhaustion or serious deficiency; as part of a formula to restore fertility. Useful for neurasthenia, insomnia, sweating, dizziness, and tuberculous adenopathy; used for seminal emission and vaginal discharge. **Secondary uses:** as a counter measure to many of the effects of aging, such as loss of hair color, and muscle tone; helps reduce high cholesterol levels and coronary disease; good for weakness, backache, aches and pains of the knee joint, neurasthenia and traumatic bruises.

FRANKINCENSE: *Boswellia carterii* - **Part used:** resin. **Effective forms:** externally in a liniment, an oil for aromatherapy. Has some antibacterial effects. **Therapeutic profile:** an antiseptic agent for relief of septic sores, abscesses, carbuncles, etc. **Primary uses:** in a liniment for rheumatic and arthritic pain, and to draw infection from septic sores. **Secondary uses:** as an incense to clear and calm the mind and ease anxiety.

FRINGE TREE ROOT BARK: *Chionanthus virginicus* - **Part used:** the root bark. **Effective forms:** tincture, decoction, washes, compresses. **Therapeutic profile:** a cholagogue stimulant addressing stagnation of all the organs directly involved in digestion, as well as heat and damp heat in the liver and spleen. The restorative property extends to all the upper digestive organs, and includes hepatic and spleenic enlargement, as well as local venous blood congestion. Encourages bowel movement, reduces fever and inflammation, promotes bile flow, reduces liver congestion, restores the pancreas, promotes tissue repair. **Primary uses:** for acute liver and gastric infections, remittent fever, liver congestion, jaundice, spleenic and hepatic enlargement, pancreatitis, and exhaustion due to chronic illness, or diabetes. **Secondary uses:** for ulcers, and injuries with inflammation.

FUMITORY HERB: *Fumaria officinalis* - **Parts used:** the leafy herb. **Effective forms:** infusion, tincture. **Therapeutic profile:** a remedy to remove obstruction and promote detoxification, it excells in conditions of general toxicosis with toxin and mucus acumulation. **Primary uses:** in a formula for liver congestion, stagnant blood, jaundice, deficient or excessive bile flow. **Secondary uses:** also for dysmenorrhea, and cyclical skin conditions.

GALANGAL: *Alpina galanga* - **Part used:** root. **Effective forms:** tea. **Therapeutic profile:** a ginger-like herb effective for indigestion, flatulence, motion sickness and nausea. Its actions include stimulant and carminative. **Primary uses:** as part of an enzyme-stimulating combination for better food assimilation; as a part of a remedy to allay seasickness. **Secondary uses:** as a cardiac tonic. Helps carry an herbal formula through the body.

GARDENIA: *Gardenia jasminoides, (Zhi Zi)* - **Part used:** fruit. **Effective forms:** tea. **Therapeutic profile:** an anti-inflammatory agent that promotes basic healing processes. Has antibacterial and antifungal effects. **Primary uses:** in a combination to relieve jaundice and liver congestion. **Secondary uses:** in a formula to promote healing of stomach ulcers.

GARLIC: *Allium sativum* - **Part used:** bulb. **Effective forms:** oil, capsules, extract, poultice, enema and implant, food. **Therapeutic profile:** an allicin-containing universal anti-biotic and anti-fungal, effective for internal and external infections; effective against viruses, and both staph and strep bacteria. Garlic is highly nutritive, immune system enhancing, and strengthens the body against allergens and pollutants. Supports development of beneficial intestinal flora while killing pathogenic organisms. An excellent disease preventive, containing allicin, vitamins A, C, B₁, potassium, zinc, iron, selenium, sulphur, calcium, manganese, copper. **Primary uses:** as a specific in all anti-biotic, anti-fungal, and antiseptic formulas; as a preventive agent for many types of cancer and other degenerative disease; as an anti-tumor agent to inhibit tumor growth; to equalize blood pressure and reduce blood fats, (a specific for reducing LDL cholesterol and raising HDLs); effective in killing and expelling intestinal parasites; as part of many detoxification combinations, particularly those involving digestive or waste elimination malfunction; as a specific in a formula to kill candida yeasts; as part of a general system tonic against pollutants and allergens. Garlic is useful in the treatment of a variety of infectious conditions, where enhancing immune function is desired; also in cardiovascular applications. **Secondary uses:** as an enema for detoxification and to expel worms; as a poultice to detoxify infected sores and wounds; helps regulate blood sugar; as a liver stimulant for bile production; as part of a compound to re-establish beneficial flora in the digestive tract; as a douche against vaginitis and leucorrhea.

GENTIAN: *Gentiana macrophylla, (Qin Jiao)* - **Part used:** rhizomes. **Effective forms:** tincture, tea. **Therapeutic profile:** a digestive bitters and blood cleanser. One of the best stomach tonics, gentian stimulates circulation and strengthens the system. High in iron, it contains B-complex, especially inositol and iron. Also contains manganese, silicon, sulphur and zinc. **Primary uses:** as part of a liver cleansing combination to stimulate digestive enzymes and bile production, especially after illness; as a specific for pelvic inflammatory disease (PID), and virally caused venereal infection. It is useful for strengthening the pancreas, spleen and the kidneys. **Secondary uses:** in the treatment of trichomonas and HPV; as part of a formula for sluggish digestion.

GINGER: *Zingiber officinale* - **Part used:** rootstock. **Effective forms:** tea, tincture, capsules, syrup, gargle, compress. **Therapeutic profile:** a warming circulatory stimulant and body cleansing herb, with excellent effectiveness for cramping, indigestion, nausea, coughs, sinisitis and sore throat. Ginger has adaptogenic, antioxidant, thermo-regulatory (to alleviate the severity of a fever), anti-inflammatory, and anti-aggregatory properties. It also contains anti-ulcer constituents. Ginger has been shown to stimulate the growth of the beneficial Lactobacillus species while also being inhibitory to pathogenic (unfriendly) bacteria. **Primary uses:** as a catalyst in all formulas where circulation to the extremities is needed, (as in arthritis); for conditions of inflammation (as in arthritis); for respiratory and lung/chest clearing combinations; in digestive system stimulants and alkalizers for clearing gas; as an aid in promoting menstrual regularity and relief from cramping and sluggishness; for all kinds of nausea, motion sickness and morning sickness; as a direct compress with cayenne to stimulate venous circulation. Ginger is useful in warming the body and relieving the "chills" caused by the common cold as it reduces fever. **Secondary uses:** as a catalyst in nervine and sedative formulas; as a gargle and part of a sore throat syrup; as a diaphoretic where sweating is needed for removing toxic wastes; as a stimulant to the kidneys for extra filtering activity; externally as a compress for muscle pulls and ligament strains. *Note: Modern medicine is now suggesting regular intake of aspirin to prevent life-threatening strokes and heart attacks. The justification is that aspirin inhibits a specific enzyme and makes the blood less prone to dangerous clotting. Ginger not only inhibits this same enzyme but it does so without side effects. Including ginger in the daily supplement routine is far safer than aspirin while ginger also offers a host of other benefits.*

GINKGO BILOBA: *Ginkgo biloba* - **Part used:** leaf. **Effective forms:** liquid and powdered extract, capsules, tea. **Therapeutic profile:** a longevity herb, it increases blood flow to the brain, resulting in an increase in oxygen and glucose utilization, with great success in overcoming many unpleasant symptoms of aging, such as memory loss, lack of awareness, depression, and ringing in the ears (tinnitus); a high source of quercitin; has an antioxidant, scavenging effect on free radicals; a vaso-dilator to increase the supply of blood to the bodies vital tissues and organs, such as the brain and heart; and is membrane stabilizing. Also blocks a common allergic substance in our body called platelet-activating factor (PAF). **Primary uses:** as a specific in anti-aging and regenerative compounds for loss of memory and senility; in cardiac protection formulas against stroke and atherosclerosis; for hearing disorders and vertigo where blood flow is poor in the ears. Ginko soffers significant protective action against the development of Alzheimer's disease, hearing loss and strokes. **Secondary uses:** to overcome environmental stress, and improve circulatory and nervous system function.

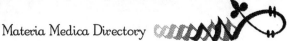

✖ **GINSENG:** (Panax, Chinese & American, (red and white) *Panax quinquefolium (xi yang shen)* - **Part used:** root. **Effective forms:** tea, capsules, liquid and powdered extract. **Therapeutic profile:** the most effective and stimulating of all tonic herbs, ginseng has measureable amounts of germanium, and can provide stimulation to all body systems, allowing rebuilding from stress, fatigue, inherent weakness, and nutritional deficiencies. Particularly nourishing to the male reproductive organs, blood and circulatory systems. Ginseng is useful for women as a stimulant for brain and memory centers, and as a phytohormone source to help control menopausal hot flashes and other symptoms. New tests show ginseng has properties that help bind to estrogen receptor sites to help prevent hormone-driven breast cancer. **Primary uses:** in regenerative and energizing formulas, for increased foundation energy, strength and vitality; for increased concentration and memory; helpful to older people recuperating from debilitating disease. Used in China for fevers and for exhaustion due to chronic, wasting diseases, such as tuberculosis. Also helps coughs related to lung weakness. **Secondary uses:** in heart and circulatory combinations to normalize blood pressure, and reduce arteriosclerosis; as part of a sugar-balancing formula for hypoglycemia. **Contra-indications:** avoid during pregnancy, if there is high blood pressure, high blood sugar, or thyroid disease.

✖ **GINSENG:** (Korean white) *Panax ginseng (ren shen)* - **Part used:** root. **Effective forms:** capsules, tea, extract. **Therapeutic profile:** a potent tonic for energy and rejuvenation. Strengthens the immune system and decreases fatigue. Replenishes *chi* (energy), especially in the spleen and lungs. Research has identified steroidal components similar to human sex hormones. **Primary uses:** to help increase brain and memory center function; to energize and regenerate after shock, illness or exhaustion. **Secondary uses:** to counteract high triglyceride levels and heart weakness. It is useful to take Panax ginseng for one month in the fall to strengthen the body for winter.

✖ **GINSENG:** *(Imperial wild) (Ching Chun Bao)* - **Part used:** root. **Effective forms:** tea, capsules, extract. **Therapeutic profile:** usually designated as the "king of ginsengs," these roots are old with a great deal of panax concentration; extremely rare and expensive. Roots are usually ten or more years old when harvested. **Primary uses:** the strongest representer of ginseng stimulating tonic effects; usually part of a male regeneration and stimulating combination formula. Often chewed before athletic contests or workouts.

✖ **GINSENG:** (PRINCE) *Pseudostellaria heterophylla, (Pai Zi Shen)* - **Part used:** root. **Effective forms:** tea. **Therapeutic profile:** a tonic and stimulating herb with ginseng-like properties. **Primary uses:** as a fast-acting stimulant after fatigue, and effective appetite suppressant during dieting. **Secondary uses:** as an oral tonic, especially where there has been depletion and wasting; especially beneficial for wasting dryness of the lungs. **Contra-Indications:** Should not be used in persons with acute disease, high fever and severe inflammations.

✖ **GINSENG:** Siberian *(See Eleuthero)*

✖ **GINSENG:** (Tienchi) *Panax pseudoginseng* - **Part used:** root. **Effective forms:** tea, liniment, compress. **Therapeutic profile:** a Japanese herb with ginseng-like tonic properties, valuable for its ability in acute conditions to curtail internal bleeding from injuries and wounds. Internally, to dissolve blod clots and circulatory obstructions. **Primary uses:** as a blood and cardiac tonic particularly for athletes that greatly increases stamina without overtonification; as a hemostatic for hemorrhaging and abnormal bleeding (may be taken internally or applied directly); to keep circulation clear in cases of embolism and phlebitis. **Secondary uses:** as an external hemostatic linament for sprains and injury trauma.

✖ **GLAUBER'S SALT :** *Sodium sulfate* (Mangxiao) - **Part used:** sodium sulfate. **Effective forms:** capsules. **Therapeutic profile:** used in TCM to soften stool and encourage bowel movements; to clear heat. **Primary uses:** used in combination with *rhubarb* for constipation; indicated for sore throat, ulcerated mouth, red eyes and boils (used externally). **Contra-Indications:** Do not use during pregnancy.

✖ **GLUCOMANNAN:** *Amorphophallus konjak* - **Parts used:** root. **Effective forms:** powder. **Therapeutic profile:** Glucomannan is taken from the Konjac root (from the same family as the yam). High in fiber (100 percent natural fiber without calories), and is excellent for cleaning the digestive system. Contains vitamins A, C, niacin, B_1 and B_2, as well as calcium, magnesium, phosporus, potassium, sodium, iron, zinc, selenium, manganese and silicon. **Primary uses:** valuable for gastrointestinal problems (since lack of fiber is a major cause for gastrointestinal disorders). Helps reduce cholesterol, maintain regularity and promotes bowel health. A specific for normalizing blood sugar levels. Absorbs toxic substances produced during digestion and the waste removal process, and eliminates them before they can be absorbed into the blood stream. Aids weight control because it expands to about 50 times its original volume when used with a glass of water.

GOKSHURA: *Tribulis terresris* - **Part used:** entire plant, particularly fruit and root. **Effective forms:** decoction, infusion, powder, medicated oil. **Therapeutic profile:** used in Ayurvedic medicine for many urinary tract disorders; strengthens reproductive system (esp. post partum). Considered an effective kidney tonic; rejuvenating to Pitta and calming to Vata. **Primary uses:** indicated as an effective agent in treating urinary complaints and kidney disorders, including hematuria, chronic cystitis, cholecystitis, nephritis, and edema. Used in formulas for bladder and gall stones and kidney stones; **Secondary uses:** helpful for venereal/reproductive diseases such as enlarged prostate, genital herpes, HIV/AIDS, poor semen quality, impotence and infertility.

GOLDENROD: *Solidago viraurea* - **Part used:** dried herb, leaves and flowers. **Effective forms:** tea, infusion, gargle, extract. **Therapeutic profile:** a specific for flu and upper respiratory catarrh, it is also useful for laryngitis and gas. **Primary uses:** as part of an anti-inflammatory combination for colds and flu. **Secondary uses:** as an anti-inflammatory antiseptic for bladder infection; astringent and diuretic properties make it especially good for bladder stones; indicated for weak digestion; also used as a gargle for throat infection.

GOLDENSEAL: *Hydrastis canadensis* - **Part used:** leaf and root. **Effective forms:** tincture, capsules, tea, wash, douche, poultice. **Therapeutic profile:** a primary antibiotic and antiviral herb, used to fight infections of all kinds; a source of natural insulin; a hemostatic to control both external and internal bleeding; an alterative, with tonic and laxative properties make it a useful agent in digestive disorders. **Primary uses:** a specific in any lymph cleansing, anti-biotic combination for infections. In eczema and psoriasis formulas; to help stop excessive menstrual bleeding, and mid-cycle bleeding; in cold, flu and upper respiratory combinations; as a specific for amoebic dysentery; as part of a formula for diabetes control; for urinary tract inflammation. **Secondary uses:** to heal stomach ulcers, colitis and other gastric/bowel inflammation; indicated for chronic constipation; especially useful for hemmorrhoids and other chronic inflammation of the colon and rectum; as a mouthwash for cankers, mouth and gum sores; as an eyewash for conjunctivitis or other eye infection; as a skin wash for skin cancers, open sores, ringworm and dermatitis; an excellent aid during childbirth; works excellent as a douche for most vaginal infections. **Contra-indications:** Avoid during pregnancy because of uterine muscle stimulation.

GOTU KOLA: *Centella asiatica* - **Part used:** tops, root and leaf. **Effective forms:** tea, infusion, tincture, capsules, extract. **Therapeutic profile:** a memory and rejuvenating brain tonic used to overcome depression, increase longevity, heart and nerve health. **Primary uses:** a specific in all brain and memory stimulation formulas, such as learning disabilities or Alzheimer's disease; as a specific in any energizing, mental burn-out, or weight loss compound. A specific in formulas for fat metabolism and cellulite release. Indicated for many neurotic disturbances; in anti-aging formulas; to increase healthy circulation; in a thyroid support formula to counteract depression and fatigue. A specific for nerve regeneration when recovering from disease. **Secondary uses:** as part of a formula to alleviate menopause imbalance and pain; with wild yam as part of a spermacidal contraceptive combination; neutralizes blood acids; used to lower temperature. **Contra-indications:** avoid during pregnancy or hyper-thyroid conditions.

GRAPE SEED: and other sources of procyanidolic oligomers (PCOs), also known as oligomeric proanthocyanidin complexes (OPCs). PCOs (also referred to as proanthocyanidins and procyanidins) are one of the most beneficial groups of plant flavonoids and exist in many plants. Commercially available sources include extracts from grape seeds and the bark of the maritime pine. The term Pycnogenol is a registered trademark and refers to the PCO extracted from the bark of the French maritime pine. **Part used:** extract from such plants as grape seed, pine bark, lemon tree bark, cranberries and citrus peel. **Effective forms:** capsules. **Therapeutic profile:** potent antioxidant and free radical-scavenging effects; has ability to increase intracellular vitamin C levels; decrease capillary permeability and fragility; inhibit destruction of collagen; and prevent the release and synthesis of compounds that promote inflammation and allergies. **Primary uses:** an important free radical scavenger (free radical damage is linked to the aging process and virtually every chronic degenerative disease including heart disease, arthritis and cancer), capillary fragility and easy bruising, atherosclerosis prevention, diabetes, macular degeneration and diabetic retinopathy, varicose veins and wound healing. **Secondary uses:** an important part of a formula for PMS and other dysmenorrhea symptoms, especially for the woman over 40 who is still menstruating heavily. *Note: Although both grape seed and pine bark extracts are excellent sources of PCOs only grape seed extract contains the gallic esters of proanthocyanidins the most active free radical scavenging PCOs.*

🌿 **GRAVEL ROOT:** (Queen of the Meadow) *Eupatorium purpureum* - **Part used:** root. **Effective forms:** capsules, infusion, decoction. **Therapeutic profile:** a diuretic herb with the ability to dissolve stones and sediment. **Primary uses:** in formulas for kidney and gallstone removal, for relief of prostate and urethra sediment and inflammation; used to treat frequent nightime urination, fluid retention and hematuria (blood in the urine). **Secondary uses:** to help dissolve the systemic inorganic crystalline deposits of gout, rheumatism and arthritis; also helpful in nerve rebuilding combinations.

🌿 **GREEN TEA:** *Camellia sinensis* - **Parts used:** leaf bud and leaf. **Effective forms:** tea. **Therapeutic profile:** contains polyphenols which possess outstanding therapeutic action (antioxidant and anticancer properties). The major polyphenols in green tea are flavonoids (catechin, epicatechin, epicatechin gallate, epigallocatechin gallate and proanthocyanidins). Epigallocatechin gallate is considered as the most significant active component. Both green and black tea come from the same plant, however green tea is produced by lightly steaming the fresh-cut leaf while black tea leaves are allowed to oxidize. The oxidation of black tea causes enzymes present in the tea to convert polyphenols to compounds with much less activity. Green tea polyphenols inhibit cancer by blocking the formation of cancer-causing compounds such as nitosmines, suppressing the activation of carcinogens, and detoxifying or trapping cancer-causing agents. **Primary uses:** as antioxidant supplementation and an agent for cancer prevention. An excellent liver cleanser to help in all detoxification programs that involve the liver; (especially effective for an annual spring body cleanse - should be used in the morning for best results). **Secondary uses:** as part of a formula to stimulate thermogenesis for increased calorie burning and weight control. Helpful as a digestive stimulant. *Note:* some population studies indicate that *heavy black tea* consumption may *increase* the risk for certain cancers.

🌿 **GRINDELIA:** (Gum weed) *Grindelia squarrosa* - **Parts used:** flowering top and leaves. **Effective forms:** tea, compress, syrup and tincture, powder and extract. **Therapeutic profile:** internally, a relaxant for the heart; externally, soothing for burns, rashes, blisters and skin irritations. High in selenium, it also contains traces of lead, arsenic, tin, cadmium and zinc. **Primary uses:** as part of a respiratory and bronchial combination to control spasmodic coughing, nasal congestion and asthma symptoms. **Secondary uses:** as an antidote compress for poison oak dermatitis, and skin rashes. May be used for all skin disorders. Useful for asthma spasms and whooping cough, and for broncial irritations and nasal congestion. **Contraindications:** should not be used when the heart is weak. High selenium content makes grindelia mildly toxic in large doses; the resin in grindelia is considered to be hard on the kidneys and should only be used for acute ailments.

🌿 **GUIACUM:** *Guaiacum officinale* - **Part used:** heart-wood, resin and bark. **Effective forms:** tea and capsules. **Therapeutic profile:** a resinous wood with anti-rheumatic and anti-inflammatory activity. Has gentle expectorant properties. **Primary uses:** a specific for osteo-arthritis and rheumatoid arthritis, and a preventive for gout. **Secondary uses:** a specific in treating syphilis; useful in treating influenza and inflamed respiratory conditions.

🌿 **GUAR GUM:** *Cyamopsis tetragonoloba* - **Part used:** legume. **Effective forms:** powder in a drink, capsules. **Therapeutic profile:** a mucilaginous fiber herb, similar to apple pectin, with sugar balancing and fiber laxative qualities. When taken before meals, guar gum is thought to reduce the appetite and delays the emptying of the stomach. **Primary uses:** as part of a fiber drink for healthy bowel activity and weight loss. **Secondary uses:** as part of a formula for diabetes control to flatten the blood sugar curve. **Contra-Indications:** may cause flatulence and diarrhea due to increased bacterial fermentation in the colon.

🌿 **GUARANA:** *Paulina cupana* - **Part used:** seed. **Effective forms:** capsules, tea. **Therapeutic profile:** a traditional stimulant plant containing natural guaranine, effective as an energizing stimulant. **Primary uses:** in energy and endurance formulas, to overcome fatigue; helpful for hangovers and menstrual headaches. **Secondary uses:** used in weight loss combinations to increase metabolic rate and help the body metabolize fat as fuel; increases body temperature in sedentary people; may be toxic to *E.coli* and *Salmonella* pathogen species.

🌿 **GUDUCHI:** *Tinospora cordifolius* - **Part used:** stem, leaves and roots. **Effective forms:** cold infusion, tincture and extract. **Therapeutic profile:** a bitter, cooling herb, considered a valuable rejuvenative tonic in Ayurveda; used for intestinal irritation and other digestive problems; an alkalizer indicated for over-acid conditions. **Primary uses:** to relieve cold and flu fevers, as a mild diuretic urinary problems including seminal weakness and overly acid urine. Also used for malabsorption, chronic diarrhea, food allergies, and stomach irritation. **Secondary uses:** Ayurvedic uses guduchi to strengthen the immune system, and for Pitta type arthritis, gout, and rheumatism.

GUGULIPID: *Commiphora mukul* - **Parts used**: resin. **Effective forms**: extract of the soluble portion of the resin (soluble portion contains gugulipid - insoluble portion contains toxic gum carbohydrates) A standardized extract known as gugulipid is usually regarded as the most beneficial in terms of safety and effectiveness for medicinal purposes. **Therapeutic profile**: the soluble portion has significant cholesterol-lowering and anti-inflammatory activity. **Primary uses**: a valued Ayurvedic botanical medicine used for rheumatoid arthritis and lipid disorders. **Secondary uses**: used in the treatment of obesity and other disorders of fat processing, including its ability to lower cholesterol and triglyceride levels and promote weight loss.

GURMAR: *Gymnema sylvestre* - **Part used**: whole plant. **Effective forms**: extracts. **Therapeutic profile**: an Ayurvedic herb used to treat diabetes since the sixth century; helps repair damage to the pancreas, increasing its output of insulin to near normal levels. Research shows that *gymnema* reduces blood sugar levels after sugar consumption. Molecular structure is similar to sugar and can block absorption of up to 50% of dietary sugar calories; both sugar and *gymnema* are digested in the small intestine, but the larger molecule of gymnema cannot be fully absorbed. Therefore, if taken before sugar, the gymnema molecule blocks the passages through which sugar is normally absorbed, and fewer sugar calories are assimilated. A person who eats a 400 calorie, high sugar dessert only absorbs 200 of the sugar calories when taking *gymnema* - the remaining sugar is eliminated as waste. **Primary uses**: used to treat diabetes and hyperinsulinism; helps repair damage to the liver and kidneys.

HARITAKI: *Terminalia chebula*- **Part used**: dried fruit. **Effective forms**: decoction, gargle, powder. **Therapeutic profile**: A bitter, laxative and expectorant, this Ayurvedic herb used to soothe Vata and act as a tonic to the body's sytems, particularly the nervous and respiratory system. Also a tonic to the brain and nerves, regulates the colon, improves digestion, absorption. Raises voice and vision quality. **Primary uses**: used as a gargle for coughs, hoarse voice and hiccoughs; indicated to regulate colon in cases of constipation and diarrhea; indicated for asthma. **Secondary uses**: a helpful addition in a program to combat hemorrhoids (Vata type); used for Parkinson's disease and Multiple Sclerosis as a nerve rebuilder and nourisher in Ayurveda. **Contra-indications**: Not to be used during pregnancy, dehydration, excess pitta conditions, and severe exhaustion and emaciation.

HAWTHORN: *Crataegus oxyacantha* - **Part used**: leaf, berry, and flower. **Effective forms**: extract, tea, capsules. **Therapeutic profile**: a tonifying, high bioflavonoid herb for the heart and circulatory system, with vaso-dilating and heart muscle strengthening activity; effective in reducing high blood pressure and arterial plaque. **Primary uses**: for all cardiac tonic combinations to regulate and strengthen the heart, tone venous structure, and to provide a definite feeling of well-being through blood pressure and cholesterol reduction. **Secondary uses**: strengthens vein and capillary structure; acts as a digestant for better food assimilation (especially meat); stimulates appetite; useful in the treatment of diarrhea and abdominal distention. Take the tea for nervous disorders and insomnia.

HEAL ALL: (Self heal) *Prunella vulgaris* - **Part used**: the dried herb. **Effective forms**: tea, wash, gargle, lotion. **Therapeutic profile**: a soothing, anti-inflammatory, antioxidant herb particularly useful for treating infected skin conditions and healing inflamed wounds. **Primary uses**: as a specific in a wound healing combination; as part of a soothing healant used externally and internally for eczema and psoriasis. **Secondary uses**: as a gentle astringent lotion for diarrhea, hemorrhoids and hemorrhaging; used for fevers, hepatitis, jaundice, high blood pressure and edema; as part of a soothing tea and gargle for sore throats.

HEMP SEED: *Cannabis sativa L.* (Huomaren)- **Part used**: seed. **Effective forms**: tea, capsules. **Therapeutic profile**: used in TCM to lubricate the intestines and move stool. **Primary uses**: used for constipation and hemorrhoids due to dryness and heat in the large intestine. **Contra-indications**: do not use when diarrhea is present.

HIBISCUS: *Hibiscus rosa-sinensis* - **Part used**: flowers. **Effective forms**: tea. **Therapeutic profile**: a refreshing, vitamin C and bioflavonoid-rich herb with laxative and tonic properties. **Primary uses**: in digestive and weight control formulas, especially for cellulite; used for mild intestinal and stomach complaints. **Secondary uses**: as a flavorful vitamin C source; as a tea flavoring to counteract bitterness of other herbs; has refrigerant properties that make it useful for fevers.

HIJIKI: *Hijikia fusiform* - **Part used**: dried leaf. **Effective forms**: in broth or a mineral drink, and as food flavoring and condiment. **Therapeutic profile**: a Japanese sea vegetable rich in protein, calcium, iron, carotenes, B vitamins and trace minerals. **Primary uses**: as part of high mineral, and absorbable calcium supplement combinations. **Secondary uses**: as part of iodine and potassium therapy formulas.

HONEY LOCUST: *Gledista triacanthos* - **Part used:** aromatic pods. **Effective forms:** pills or lozenges, rectal suppository. **Therapeutic profile:** a cough suppressant and expectorant. **Primary uses:** as a lozenge to relieve coughs; to help clear the lungs and chest of phlegm. **Secondary uses:** to help revive consciousness after a stroke or epileptic seizure; as a rectal suppository for roundworms. **Contra-indications:** do not use during pregnancy.

HONEYSUCKLE: *Lonicera japonica, (Jin Yin Hua) (Shuang Hua)* - **Part used:** flowers. **Effective forms:** tea, tincture, decoction. **Therapeutic profile:** an antibiotic, lymph clearing, detoxification herb for acute and inflammatory conditions; effective against respiratory and flu infection. **Primary uses:** as part of a cleansing/strengthening combination for breast cancer; as part of a systemic cleanser for poison oak and other inflammatory poisons; as part of an acute treatment for colds, flu and fever. **Secondary uses:** in a formula for swollen inflamed throat; as part of a sweating mixture to cleanse from a flu or cold infection. Indicated in cases of rheumatism and rheumatoid arthritis. Use the tincture in cases of gastro-enteritis or diarrhea related to food poisoning.

HOPS: *Humulus lupulus* - **Part used:** female flowers. **Effective forms:** tea, tincture, aromatic bitter for beer, compresses, wash and capsules. **Therapeutic profile:** a sedative relaxant and restorative for the central nervous system. **Primary uses:** a specific in formulas for insomnia, to relax tension and anxiety. **Secondary uses:** a relaxing astringent for control of nervous colitis and stomach ulcers; to decrease delerium tremens and desire for alcohol; use a compress for varicose ulcers; use an infusion as a wash for ulcers, skin eruptions and wounds. **Contra-indications:** Avoid in cases of depression; the growing plant may cause contact dermatitis.

HOREHOUND: *Marrubium vulgare* - **Part used:** leaves and tops. **Effective forms:** tea, skin wash, cough syrup with honey. **Therapeutic profile:** a bitters, anti-spasmodic, demulcent herb that helps respiratory congestion through sweat cleansing and expectoration. **Primary uses:** an expectorant for cough, lung congestion, whooping cough and laryngitis; as a part of a formula for bronchitis. **Secondary uses:** as part of a cardiac tonic to normalize heart palpitations; as a wash for skin dermatitis conditions; also as a healer for skin wounds; a bitters digestive and hepatic tonic; a gentle circulatory stimulant; indicated for fevers, colds and coughs.

HORSE CHESTNUT: *Aesculus hippocastanum* - **Part used:** seed and bark. **Effective forms:** extract; ointment. **Therapeutic profile:** an astringent herb with high tannins and flavonoids to tone and strengthen tissue. **Primary uses:** a strengthener for veins and capillaries; as part of a formula for hemorrhoids, (may be applied directly to hemorroidal tissue); particularly to help improve the look and tone of varicose and spider veins. Moderates the menses; enriches the blood and removes congestion; as part of a formula for prostate enlargement. **Secondary uses:** as a direct application to leg ulcers; as protection against sunburn. **Contra-indications:** Use with caution - there are citations of poisonings in children who have ingested the seeds. Symptoms of poisonings include muscle twitching, weakness, vomiting, paralysis, diarrhea, dilated pupils, and lack of coordination.

HORSERADISH: *Armoracis lapathiafolia* - **Part used:** fresh and dried root. **Effective forms:** capsules, food condiment. **Therapeutic profile:** a high sulphur stimulating agent with diuretic, antibiotic, digestive and blood sugar balancing qualities; has a stimulating effect on the stomach and pancreas. **Primary uses:** fresh root, mixed with lemon or cider vinegar as an immediate and powerful mucous expectorant; dried root, as part of a hypoglycemia or diabetic formula to control blood sugar use; for relief of gout and arthritic pain. **Secondary uses:** fresh root, as part of a cold and flu combination to warm the body, relieve sinus ache, and release excess mucous; dried root, as part of a urinary infection relief formula;

HORSETAIL: (Shavegrass) *Equisetum hyemale* - **Part used:** dried stems and tops. **Effective forms:** tea, liquid and powdered extract, poultice, bath, eyewash. **Therapeutic profile:** a silica-rich herb that helps rebuild and provide elasticity to skin, hair and nails. Useful as a diuretic and tonic for body "spring cleaning" and detoxification. **Primary uses:** as a specific in any skin, hair, nails and eyes, or "cosmetic elements" formula; as part of a detoxification and body cleanse; as an astringent for diarrhea and dysentery; as part of a bone, cartilage, and connective tissue strengthening formula; as a toning astringent to treat incontinence in the elderly, and bed-wetting in children; as part of a compound to dissolve kidney stones, and relieve kidney congestion; the extract is a specific in prostate gland treatment (BPH). **Secondary uses:** as part of an herbal calcium and silica supplement; as part of a formula to expel internal parasites; helps healing and clotting of sores and wounds; externally as a compress for hemorrhoids and anal fissures. As an eyewash to relieve inflammation and conjunctivitis; as a bath for rheumatism and arthritic stiffness; strengthens the heart and lungs. Used to clear fevers and release nervous tension; horsetail acts as a blood coagulant and is useful for problems related to excessive bleeding

❧ HO-SHOU-WU: *(Fo-Ti) Polygonum multiflorum* - **Part used**: root. **Effective forms**: powder and extract. **Therapeutic profile**: has a toning effect on the liver and kidneys. A tonic for the endocrine glands with properties comparable to Panax ginseng. **Primary uses**: helps the nervous system; is effective as a part of any body healing and regeneration formula. Helpful as part of an anti-aging formula. **Secondary uses**: is useful for conditions of premature graying of hair, backache, aches and pains of the knee joint, neurasthenia and traumatic bruises.

❧ HYDRANGEA: *Hydrangea arborescens* - **Part used**: root. **Effective forms**: tea, capsules. **Therapeutic profile**: a diuretic herb particularly useful for prostate infection and inflammation; effective for arthritis swelling and kidney fluid retention. **Primary uses**: as a specific in a prostate healing formula, especially for urinary stones or sediment; as part of a compound to dissolve kidney stones, bladder stones and gravel. **Secondary uses**: for the fluid retention and swelling of arthritis, and bladder infections.

❧ HYSSOP: *Hyssopus officinalis* - **Part used**: dried aerial parts of the herb, essential oil, flowers. **Effective forms**: tea, capsules, extract, gargle. **Therapeutic profile**: wide ranging healing properties, including antispasmodic activity for pulmonary congestive disease, nervine effectiveness for epilepsy and hysteria, and stimulation for improved liver function. **Primary uses**: as a specific for asthma, colds, coughs and chest congestion; as a specific in a liver cleansing formula for gas and stomach irritation. **Secondary uses**: as a compress for bruises and wounds; as a gargle for sore throat; use the essential oil as chest rub for bronchitis. **Contra-indications**: avoid during pregnancy or if suffering from epilepsy. Use the essential oil as directed as it contains the ketone pinocamphone which causes convulsions in high doses.

ICELAND MOSS: *Cetraria islandia* - **Part used**: whole plant. **Effective forms**: tea, tincture. **Therapeutic profile**: a gentle demulcent tonic with high mucilage content, effective for irritated mucous membranes. **Primary uses**: it is a specific in treating gastric problems, such as heartburn and nausea; soothing to respiratory membranes in dry cough, and consumptive lung disease. **Secondary uses**: a mild laxative; for digestive malfunction such as malnourishment, anorexia and chronic diarrhea. As part of any sea plant formula for skin tone, cellulite or as a source of natural iodine and potassium.

❧ IMMORTAL ROOT: *Asclepias asperula, A. capricorna, A. syriaca* - **Part used**: root. **Effective forms**: decoction, tincture. **Therapeutic profile**: stimulating to the heart, lungs, circulation and uterus. Relaxant effect on the bronchi. **Primary uses**: for chronic bronchitis, asthma, pneumonia, cold and flu onset, remittent fevers, or coronary deficiency. **Secondary uses**: helps promote menstruation. **Contraindications**: do not use during pregnancy.

❧ INDIAN SNAKEROOT: *See SARPAGANDHA.*

❧ IRISH MOSS: *Chondrus crispus* - **Part used**: leaf and stem. **Effective forms**: broth, capsules. **Therapeutic profile**: a sea coast vegetable widely used for its natural gelling, emulsifying, and food stabilizing properties; also has soothing demulcent ability for the kidneys and lungs; and externally for the skin. **Primary uses**: in respiratory combinations for a soothing quality is needed to overcome inflammation, such as bronchitis; a soothing/coating agent for gastritis and stomach ulcers. **Secondary uses**: as a skin softener; as part of a mineral rich combination to overcome deficiencies; mild laxative properties make it a useful digestive aid.

JASMINE: *Jasminum officinale* - **Part used**: flower and leaves, essential oil for aromatherapy. **Effective forms**: tea. **Therapeutic profile**: an analgesic herb effective against inflammatory arthritic and rheumatic pain. **Primary uses**: as part of an arthritis pain formula. **Secondary uses**: to reduce inflammation of boils and abscesses; essential oil has an antidepressive, aphrodisiac-type effect, and eases female reproductive pain.

❧ JATAMANSI: *Nardostachys jatamansi* - **Part used**: rhizome and oil from the rhizome. **Effective forms**: tincture, infusion, oil. **Therapeutic profile**: considered a nerve strengthener and effective substitue for valerian root, jatamansi is an antispasmodic nervine indicated for a broad spectrum of nervous disorders; acting on the central nervous sytem, it soothes Pitta, combines well with gotu kola or cinnamon for nerve strengthening; also used with gotu kola to promote greater awareness. **Primary uses**: in Ayurveda, used to combat insomnia, mental disorders and hysteria, cerebral palsy, multiple sclerosis, paralysis and Parkinson's disease. **Secondary uses**: a helpful addition to fight migraine headaches, hypertension and dsymenorrhea (PMS).

❧ JEWELWEED: *Impatiens palida* - **Part used**: leaf and whole herb. **Effective forms**: tea, wash, decoction. **Therapeutic profile**: a high tannin herb with cathartic action. **Primary uses**: a specific in a formula to cleanse the

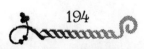

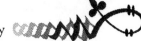

body of systemic toxins such as poison oak and sumac. **Secondary uses**: the fresh plant can be made into an ointment to treat hemorrhoids; the juice is helpful in removing warts, corns and reversing ringworm. **Contra-indications**: A powerful cathartic and emetic. Use with care internally.

JOJOBA: *Simmondsia chinensis* - **Part used**: nut oil. **Effective forms**: oil. **Therapeutic profile**: removes the embedded sebum around hair follicles and makes the scalp less acidic. Jojoba contains B-complex, vitamin E, silicon, chromium and is very high in iodine. It also has copper and zinc. **Primary uses**: is used to promote hair growth and relieve skin problems. When deposits of sebum collect around hair follicles, solidify and cause dandruff, hair loss and scalp disorders. Jojoba oil removes the sebum and contributes to healthy hair.

JUNIPER: *Juniperus communis* - **Part used**: dried berries. **Effective forms**: tea, oil, capsules. **Therapeutic profile**: a diuretic bitters stimulant that increases flow and congestion release from bladder and kidneys. **Primary uses**: a specific for chronic cystitis to remove acid and toxic wastes; helps dissolve kidney stones or prostate sediment; an adrenal stimulant; to treatment water retention; anti-inflammatory effects make it useful for chronic arthritis and gout. **Secondary uses**: because of its sugar regulant qualities, as part of a formula for diabetes or hypoglycemia. Carminative properties make the oil useful for indigestion and flatulence; berries have a stimulating effect on the appetite. **Contra-indications**: do not use during pregnancy; should be avoided during kidney disease as overstimulating and irritating to the tissue.

KAVA KAVA: *Piper methysticum* - **Part used**: root. **Effective forms**: tea, capsules. **Therapeutic profile**: an analgesic sedative used to relieve pain, nervousness and insomnia. **Primary uses**: as part of a mood elevating combination for stress relief and relaxation; helpful for many nervous disorders including anxiety and depression. As part of a pain relief sleep-inducing combination; relieves body stress after trauma or injury; improves cognitive function. **Secondary uses**: as an agent to help in remembering dreams; antiseptic properties make it useful in a douche and for urinary tract infections; heplful for cramps associated with muscular spasms; useful for neuralgia. **Contra-indications**: regular use of large doses may cause a build up of toxins in the liver; may cause inflammation of the body and eyes.

KELP: *Ascophyllum nodosum* - **Part used**: leaf and stem, whole plant. **Effective forms**: capsules, extract, food sprinkle, seaweed bath. **Therapeutic profile**: a sea vegetable rich in carotene, iodine, chromium and other minerals; with anti-biotic, cleansing and thyroid stimulating activity. **Primary uses**: as part of weight loss, pre-natal, gland/blood sugar balancing and iodine therapy compounds; excellent for skin balance and smoothness. Used in TCM to resolve phelgm and soften hardness; promotes water metabolism. **Secondary uses**: as part of an organ cleansing tonic because it is able to bind with toxic heavy metals in the intestines and carry them out; used as a blood purifier for rheumatism and atherosclerosis. Effective for growth of hair and nails. Relieves constipation. **Contra-indications**: use small amounts of kelp if you are on a salt restrictive diet, because kelp is high in sodium; some feel that excessive use of kelp over a long period of time may cause a goiter condition.

KOLA NUT: *Cola acuminata* - **Part used**: seed. **Effective forms**: capsules, in an extract or drink mix. **Therapeutic profile**: a powerful nervous system stimulant containing natural caffeine; heart tonic. **Primary uses**: as an effective short term stimulant for depression or exhaustion; as a naturtal thermogenesis stimulant for calorie burning in a weight loss program; as a specific for some kinds of migraines. **Secondary uses**: as part of a sexual energy stimulating formula to enhance the sexual experience, especially for women; for nervous debility. For diarrhea associated with convalescence; and as an appetite stimulant to aid in overcoming anorexia nervosa.

KOMBU: *Laminaria angustata* - **Part used**: leaf and stem. **Effective forms**: mineral broth or drink, extract, sea weed bath. **Therapeutic profile**: a good tasting sea vegetable, particularly rich in iodine, riboflavin and calcium and potassium. **Primary uses**: as part of a mineral bath or extract combination for iodine therapy and body cleansing. **Secondary uses**: as a food addition for iodine, protein and potassium supplementation.

KOMBUCHA: (tea kwass, Russian)- **Part used**: commercially prepared mixture from "mushroom": **Effective forms**: tea **Therapeutic profile**: not technically part of the fungi family, kombucha is instead a symbiotic culture of genus Saccharomyces yeast and xylinum bacteria. Believed to have detoxifying and antibiotic properties which address the body's systems, its fermentation is believed by many to contribute a variety of health benefits including the growth of friendly bacteria in the intestines. **Primary uses**: alleviates the symptoms of arthritis, cancer, chronic fatigue syndrome (CFS), constipation , gout, impotence, kidney stones, multiple sclerosis, obesity and PMS; effective in the treatment of arteriosclerosis. **Secondary uses**: may help reduce prematuring graying hair and facial wrinkles. **Contra-Indications**: Kombucha may develop mold and potential botulism spores which could cause illness or death. Proper handling and growing methods should be of primary concern.

KUDZU ROOT: *Pueratiae lobata, (Ko Ken)* - **Part used**: root. **Effective forms**: food starch thickener. **Therapeutic profile**: a mild tonic with the ability to replenish body fluids in the treatment of sugar imbalances, and colds, flu, intestinal problems, alcoholism and fever. **Primary uses**: neutralizes acidity in the body; as a starch thickener for stir fried vegetables or grains that when eaten can help regulate sugar use in the blood stream; when mixed with bancha tea and ginger as a remedy for acute colds, flu and fever; a hangover preventive. **Secondary uses**: as an aid to treating diarrhea; anti-alcohol effects of daidzin, one of kudzu's flavonoids, make it a specific for recovery from alcoholism.

KUKICHA TWIG: **Part used**: roasted twigs and stems. **Effective forms**: tea. **Therapeutic profile**: a mellow, soothing tea without the caffeine of bancha leaf, but with a rich nut-like flavor. **Primary uses**: as an alkalizing blood cleanser and aid in body uptake of calcium. **Secondary uses**: to relieve nausea and digestive upsets.

LADY'S MANTLE: *Alchemilla vulgaris* - **Part used**: leaves and flowers: **Effective forms**: tea, tincture, douche. **Therapeutic profile**: an astringent and emmenagogue to promote menstrual regularity. **Primary uses**: as part of a menstrual formula to reduce and control excessive bleeding, particularly in the beginning menopause years. **Secondary uses**: as an astringent for control and treatment of diarrhea; can be used as a douche for leucorrhea.

LADY SLIPPER: *Cypripedium pubescens* - **Part used**: root. *Note:* this is an endangered species - a protected plant in the wild. Only cultivated crop plants should be used. **Effective forms**: extract, tea, capsules. **Therapeutic profile**: a wide spectrum nervine, effective for all stress, tension and anxiety states. **Primary uses**: as a specific for all nerve, stress and tension formulas; as a mood elevator for depression; for nerve, muscle and headache pain. Take before retiring in cases of chronic insomnia and anxiety, and when "the brain just won't turn off" to allow sleep. **Secondary uses**: as a nerve food that may be used as needed for restlessness and stress. Mild antispasmodic properties make it useful in the treatment of neuralgia, epilepsy or tremors; helpful for nervous stomach conditions.

LAPACHO: *Tabebuia avellanedae* or *Tabebuia ipe* - Also known as Pau d'Arco. (See PAU D'ARCO.)

LAVENDER: *Lavandula vera* - **Part used**: flower. **Effective forms**: aromatherapy, tea, bath, oil, liniment. **Therapeutic profile**: a highly aromatic herb particularly useful for relief of stress, tension and depression headaches. **Primary uses**: as a nervine and relaxant particularly in a bath or in aromatherapy. **Secondary uses**: as a calmative part of a sleep tea or bath; as aromatherapy for depression; lavender oil is also used in many skin care products to address acne or sensitive skin, and hair care products for hair health, color and beauty; a few drops can be rubbed on the temple or forehead to relieve stress and tension headaches. **Contra-Indications**: The oil is only to be used as directed as large doses of it can cause death by convulsion.

LAVER: *Wild Atlantic nori* (See NORI)

LEDEBOURIELLA ROOT: *Radix ledebouriella divaricata* (Gui Zhi). **Part used**: root. **Effective forms**: tea. **Therapeutic profile**: a Chinese herb that expels wind and is indicated for blood deficiency and pain conditions. **Primary uses**: *gui zhi* is generally recommended for obstructions, headache (especially migraine), chills and body aches, flatulence and diarrhea. **Secondary uses**: may have use in regulating body temperature; inhibits some influenza viruses; may be useful as an antidote to arsenic poisoning.

LEMON BALM: *Melissa officinalis* - **Part used**: fresh and dried leaves, fresh aerial parts. **Effective forms**: tea, compress, ointment, essential oil. **Therapeutic profile**: a calming, sedating, diaphoretic herb. **Primary uses**: in a relaxing formula to treat nervousness, insomnia and depression; ointment succesfully used as a remedy for herpes; as a relaxing tonic for heart, circulatory and hypertension; as part of a formula for spasmodic hiatal hernia, and associated flatulence. **Secondary uses**: as an anti-spasmodic for calming respiratory catarrh. Use the tea for children when acute symptoms of colds and flu (especially fevers) begin; helpful for hyperactive children with digestive disturbances; as an afternoon tea with chamomile during a stressful day; use the ointment for repelling insects and healing insect bites. Use a compress for swelling and gout-like symptoms.

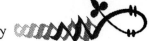

LEMONGRASS: *Cymbopogon Citratus* - **Part used:** leaf and stem. **Effective forms:** tea, oil. **Therapeutic profile:** a delicate aromatic herb useful for tonic and astringent properties. **Primary uses:** as part of a body "spring cleaning" program. **Secondary uses:** as a refreshing, pleasant tea that improves "medicinal tasting" herbs; traditionally used for colds; the oil can be used to cleanse oily skin.

LEMON PEEL: *Citrus limonia* - **Part used:** fruit peel. **Effective forms:** tea, hair rinse, syrup, bath. **Therapeutic profile:** a purifying digestive and cleansing agent, valuable for liver and spleen congestion. **Primary uses:** as part of a liver/kidney cleansing and detoxification combination; as a circulatory tonic. **Secondary uses:** as a syrup with garlic and honey for colds and flu; as a lightening hair rinse with water; as a flavor addition to counteract unpleasant tastes in medicinal teas. **Contra-indications:** be careful of sucking lemons or using lemon peel water over a long period of time - for some people it is so strong that it can eat away tooth enamel.

LEMON VERBENA: *Hippia citriodora* - **Part used:** leaf. **Effective forms:** tea, extract. **Therapeutic profile:** a mild digestive for upset stomach. **Primary uses:** as part of a drink to calm nausea, indigestion, and related sweating and palpitations. **Secondary uses:** the tea can be used for colds, fevers, asthma and spasms; an extract of the leaf has been useful as an antibiotic agent against *E. coli*, tuberculosis and staphylococcus aurea.

LICORICE: *Glycyrrhiza glabra, (Gan T'sao)* - **Part used:** root. **Effective forms:** tea, extract, capsules, gargle, syrup. **Therapeutic profile:** a wide-ranging, anti-inflammatory, anti-fungal, anti-spasmodic, anti-bacterial herb, extremely valuable for blood cleansing, nerve, endocrine and hormone support. A major source of phyto-hormone activity (especially estriol); very important for balancing women's hormones during menopause. (Some studies even indicate that licorice has breast cancer inhibiting qualities through its phytohormone properties.) Also effective for men against prostate hypertrophy. Important functions include effectiveness as a blood sugar regulant, a healant for gastro-intestinal conditions such as ulcers, and an adrenal nutrient that acts as a natural cortisone. **Primary uses:** a specific in a blood cleansing and detoxification tonic; a specific in a formula to regulate both hypoglycemia and diabetes; a specific in formulas to balance male and female hormones. To speed healing of mucous membranes in a treating ulcers; as a primary stimulant to the adrenal glands. Aas an anti-fungal in treating candida albicans yeast; as an anti-bacterial against staph and strep, and for acute bronchitis and severe congestion. **Secondary uses:** as a gargle for sore throat, cough and singer's throat; as part of an energy formula; as part of an emmenagogue to bring on suppressed menstruation. Helps strengthen digestion; helps detoxify poisons; to relieve abdominal pains and spasms. **Contra-indications:** avoid if there is high blood pressure.

LIGUSTICUM: *Ligusticum wallichii, (Chuan Xiong)* - **Part used:** root. **Effective forms:** tea, extract. **Therapeutic profile:** a blood purifying Chinese herb. **Primary uses:** as a specific to overcome anemia, especially when there is excessive menstrual bleeding. **Secondary uses:** combats emotional tension associated with pre-menstrual syndrome; to improve circulation.

LIGUSTRUM: *Ligustrum lucidum (Nu Chen Zi)* - **Part used:** berries. **Effective forms:** tablets, tonic tea. **Therapeutic profile:** an alterative herb with specific activity for the liver and kidney functions. **Primary uses:** to reduce viral and bacterial cells in the blood and skin layers; as part of an immune stimulant formula; widely used in China to combat the side effects of chemotherapy and radiation by restoring bone marrow production, enhancing the lymphatic system and increasing the number of white blood cells in patients undergoing radiation treatment. **Secondary uses:** as part of a formula against the symptoms of aging, such as early graying hair, blurry vision, tinnitus, and joint pain; used in formulas that address sexual weakness.

LILY OF THE VALLEY: *Convallaria maialis* - **Part used:** leaf, flower. **Effective forms:** infusion, tincture, washes, compresses. **Therapeutic profile:** a neurocardiac restorative and stimulant. Has antidepressant qualities. Contains a string of flavonoids that act favorably on capillary circulation. A cardiac stimulant with diuretic actions. **Primary uses:** in formulas for cardiac deficiency, edema and valvular diseases including cardiac asthma and concussion; for chronic nervous depression. **Secondary uses:** for cerebral deficiency and stroke, especially if it involves partial paralysis. For arteriosclerosis, rheumatism, tumors, infected wounds, bruises, and insect bites. **Contra-indications:** Caution, this herbs is reported to have toxic side effects. Symptoms include nausea, vomiting, diarrhea, dazedness; relatively small amounts of potentially toxic cardioactive glycosides in lily of the valley could be dangerous, especially to people on heart medications.

LINDEN: *Tilia Europaea* - **Part used:** flowers. **Effective forms:** tea. **Therapeutic profile:** a nervine and antispasmodic herb, particularly useful for respiratory problems and high blood pressure. **Primary uses:** in a combination to lower hypertension, and relieve migraine headaches. **Secondary uses:** as part of a feverish colds and cough combination; as a relaxant for stress and anxiety, particularly useful for children. The tea is often suggested as a way to make iron more available in the body for anemics.

LOBELIA: *Lobelia inflata* - **Part used:** leaf and herb. **Effective forms:** tea, capsules, extract, enema, smoking herb, poultice, emetic. **Therapeutic profile:** a powerful herb, both relaxing and stimulating depending on the form and amount used. A non-addictive smoking herb with action similar to that of nicotine. An anti-spasmodic expectorant, and anti-asthmatic emetic. **Primary uses:** a specific in "stop smoking" combinations to decrease the desire for tobacco; (lobeline salts in the body make nicotine taste terrible when smoked); a specific for bronchial asthma, both internally to calm spasms and open passages, and as an emetic to throw out mucous obstruction; the extract may be used as an emergency measure to revive a person who has overdosed on a narcotic or is in convulsions from epilepsy; as part of a combination for spasmodic lung and respiratory problems, such as croup or whooping cough. **Secondary uses:** as a nerve/muscle relaxant; as part of a diuretic to relieve bloating. As a blood cleansing treatment for syphilis. As a cardio-tonic in circulation formulas. In compounds to overcome reactions from poisonous insect bites and poison oak. As an enema in the treatment of mumps. For use in combinations to overcome drug withdrawal. The tincture is used externally in opthalmia, sprains, bruises and certain skin diseases. **Contra-indications:** avoid during pregnancy, and if there is a history of irregular heartbeat.

LOMATIUM: *Lomatium dissectum* - **Part used:** leaf and herb. **Effective forms:** extract, tea. **Therapeutic profile:** an anti-viral, anti-bacterial and immune stimulating herb. **Primary uses:** to overcome viral infections in flu, chronic fatigue, strep and staph infections; as a primary herb to combat Epstein Barr virus and chronic fatigue syndrome; may also have uses, along with St. John's wort, in the natural treatment of HIV viral infection. **Secondary uses:** for relief of respiratory and congestive conditions, such as colds, swollen glands and sore throats. **Contra-indications:** may cause itching or a rash after extended use over a period of time.

LOTUS ROOT: Part used: root. **Effective forms:** decoction, powder. **Therapeutic profile:** a cooling nervine used in Ayurveda to treat a variety of ailments; rejuvenating, soothes Pitta; nutritive tonic. **Primary uses:** used in Ayurvedic healing for coughs, neurosis and diarrhea.

LOVAGE: *Ligusticum levisticum (Gao Pen)* - **Part used:** root. **Effective forms:** tea, gargle. **Therapeutic profile:** an herb with emmenagogue and anti-spasmodic properties. **Primary uses:** as part of a menstrual regulating formula. **Secondary uses:** an abdominal and body aches relaxant; use as a mouthwash or gargle for sore throat; helpful for colic and flatulence; stimulates appetite.

LUNGWORT: *Pulmonaria officinalis* - **Part used:** leaf. **Effective forms:** tea, compress. **Therapeutic profile:** a gentle astringent, and expectorant, used to control excess mucous conditions, from lung and respiratory congestion to tumors and dysentery. **Primary uses:** for bronchitis and other upper-respiratory catarrh; as an astringent agent in cases of diarrhea and hemorrhoids. **Secondary uses:** for asthmatic cough, particularly in children; as a compress to reduce swelling from bruises, injuries and enlarged thyroid.

LYCII BERRY; *Lycium Chinensis, (Kao Chi Tza)* - **Part used:** berry. **Effective forms:** tea. **Therapeutic profile:** a tonic herb with particular strength for the liver, kidneys and pancreas; lycii berries nourish the blood and help reproductive secretions. **Primary uses:** as a part of a liver and kidney cleansing formula; in combinations to combat nephritis. **Secondary uses:** as part of a blood sugar balancing combination for diabetes. Indicated for impotence and nocturnal emission in men and boys. **Contra-indications:** avoid this herb if you have an inflammatory condition or digestive problems.

MAGNOLIA: *Magnolia liliflora, (Xin Yi Hua or Hou po bark)* - **Part used:** unopened buds, bark. **Effective forms:** tea, powder, extract. **Therapeutic profile:** a decongestant and analgesic herb. **Primary uses:** as part of a nasal and sinus decongesting formula; bark is primarily used for digestive complaints including flatulence, constipation, diarrhea and abdominal distention. **Secondary uses:** as a mild lung decongestant.

MA HUANG: (See EPHEDRA)- *Note:* Chinese ephedra (ma huang) is more powerful. Avoid during pregnancy, high blood pressure, heart or kidney disease.

MALVA, BLUE: *Malva sylvestris* - **Part used:** flowers, roots, and leaves. **Effective forms:** tea, bath, compress. **Therapeutic profile:** a soothing herb, widely used in "spring cleaning" tonics. **Primary uses:** as a cleansing

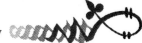

tonic for the respiratory and digestive systems. **Secondary uses:** as an astringent compress to draw out infections from abscesses, boils, etc. Use the tea for colds and coughs. *Note: Black malva flowers are for pot pourris and decorative use only. Do not take internally.*

❧ MANJISHTA: *Rubia cordifolia* - **Part used:** fruit, fresh and dried. **Effective forms:** paste, decoction, infusion. **Therapeutic profile:** noted for being the best Ayurvedic blood purifier: regulates the liver, spleen and kidneys; increases blood flow; helps to heal damaged tissue and broken bones. **Primary uses:** used in bleeding disorders, excessive menstruation; in formulas to dissolve gall and kidney stones. Useful for traumatic injuries, broken bones, rickets, and paralysis. **Secondary uses:** fruit is indicated in hepatic obstructions, jaundice and hepatitis.

❧ MARIGOLD: *Calendula officinalis* (See CALENDULA) - **Part used:** the herb. **Effective forms:** tincture and tea. **Therapeutic profile:** is high in phosporus and contains vitmins A and C. A useful herb to keep on hand as a first aid remedy, because it can address all manner of skin conditions from burns to abrasions. **Primary uses:** used to relieve earaches or as a tea for acute ailments, especially fevers. Useful for bleeding hemorrhoids; effective as a tincture when applied to bruises, sprains, muscle spasms, and ulcers. **Secondary uses:** has been used as a snuff to discharge mucus from the nose. Used as an aid for the heart and circulation and has an excellent effect as part of a combination to treat old or badly healed scars.

❧ MANDRAKE: *Podophyllum peltatum* - **Part used:** dried root. **Effective forms:** capsules, tincture for external use. **Therapeutic profile:** a powerful liver stimulant to produce bile flow; for the glands as an appetite suppressant; for the gastric process for digestion. Under study as a natural treatment for cancer - some tests have shown an ability to kill cancer cells. **Primary uses:** as a liver stimulant for metabolizing fats in a weight loss formula where there is congestion and constipation; topically as a dilute tincture for venereal and other wart removal. **Secondary uses:** as part of a formula for female sterility; as a wash for skin diseases. **Contra-indications:** use moderately and carefully; never use when pregnant; avoid in cases of Crohn's disease, colitis or irritable bowel syndrome.

❧ MARJORAM: *Origanum vulgare* - **Part used:** leaf, herb. **Effective forms:** tea, gargle, mouthwash, oil, lotion, extract. **Therapeutic profile:** a stimulating diaphoretic to help relieve colds, flu and fever. Also effective as a digestive aid. **Primary uses:** as a mouthwash and gargle for sore throat and irritated gums; to promote perspiration during colds and flu; to help gas and indigestion; as a tea to help bring on supressed menstruation and relieve associated congestive discomfort; externally as an antiseptic for cuts and wounds; as a throat coat and expectorant for coughs. **Secondary uses:** as a tea to relieve headaches (may also be rubbed on the temples); the oil for muscle and rheumatic pain; as a lotion to soothe insect bites and stings.

❧ MARSHMALLOW: *Althaea officinalis* - **Part used:** root, flowers, leaves. **Effective forms:** tea, capsules, compress, extract, syrup. **Therapeutic profile:** a mucilaginous calcium-rich herb to soothe and heal mucous membranes, for skin, lungs, digestive tract and bowel. **Primary uses:** a soothing agent in formulas for bronchitis, congestion and scratchy cough; a specific in treating allergy symptoms; a soothing diuretic for bladder and urethra inflammation; to help release and dissolve kidney stones; to increase and enrich mother's milk; externally to strengthen and soothe varicose veins; also used externally on wounds, burns, skin ulcers, boils, and to relieve abscesses. **Secondary uses:** an effective compress for varicose veins or dermatitis; a natural fiber to regulate bowel activity and increase colonic flora; as part of a vermifuge; as a tea to soothe the throat; as part of an herbal calcium formula; useful in treating gastritis and hiatal hernia.

❧ MAITAKE: *Grifola frondosa* - **Part used:** mushroom. **Effective forms:** tea, extract. **Therapeutic profile:** a potent anti-bacterial, anti-tumor, immuno-stimulant and anti-fungal. **Primary uses:** a program specific to overcome candida albican yeast overgrowth; to control nail fungus, athlete's foot and thrush conditions; anti-tumor properties make it useful against many cancers including Kaposi's sarcoma. **Secondary uses:** to kill staphylococcus virus. Useful in the treatment of diabetes, hypertension, and obesity.

❧ MEADOWSWEET: *Filipendula ulmaria* - **Part used:** leaf. **Effective forms:** infusion, tincture, eyewash and compress soaked in the tincture. **Therapeutic profile:** anti-inflammatory, anti-rheumatic, soothing digestive remedy, diuretic, promotes sweating. Constituents include salicylates, flavonoids, tannins, volatile oil, citric acid, mucilage. **Primary uses:** an infusion has been used for feverish colds, or rheumatic pains and for children's stomach upsets. The tincture may be added to remedies for gastric ulcers or excess acidity, such as licorice. Can be used with angelica or willow for arthritis. The compress soaked in the tincture can be applied to painful arthritic and rheumatic joints. The eyewash has been used for conjunctivitis and other eye complaints.

✿ **MILK THISTLE SEED:** *Silybum marianum* - **Part used:** seed. **Effective forms:** extract, capsules. **Therapeutic profile:** a bitter, tonifying, detoxifying herb for the liver, and specific for the gall bladder, with anti-oxidant properties to prevent free radical damage; indicated in cases of congestion of the liver, spleen and kidneys; stimulates protein synthesis to accelerate regeneration of damaged liver tissue. **Primary uses:** as a specific in a liver regeneration and rebuilding combination, particularly in cases of hepatitis, jaundice and cirrhosis; to increase the secretion and flow of bile from liver and gall-bladder; as a safe promoter of mother's milk. **Secondary uses:** as a liver protective when recovering from alcoholism, drug or dietary abuse, or from exposure to environmental pollutants that threaten liver health.

✿ **MISTLETOE:** (European species only) *Viscum album* - **Part used:** leaf. (*Never use berries.*) **Effective forms:** capsules. **Therapeutic profile:** a powerful nervine and cardiac depressant that acts on the vagus nerve. It should be used with care; used as a cardiac tonic and to stimulate circulation; vasodilating and anti-neoplastic properties. **Primary uses:** as a primary part of a formula for migraine headaches, especially when there is high blood pressure; to lessen nervous tachycardia; to reduce high blood pressure in general; in a formula to reduce arteriosclerosis and strengthen capillary walls. **Secondary uses:** as an anti-tumor agent. **Contra-indications:** stimulates uterine contractions, never use when pregnant.

✿ **MOTHERWORT:** *Leonuus cardiaca* - **Part used:** leaf, tops. **Effective forms:** capsules, tea, fomentation. **Therapeutic profile:** a heart tonic that improves blood flow; also used for treatment of female gland and hormone disorders. **Primary uses:** as a menstrual and uterine tonic to relieve cramping, delayed or stopped menses, and to support the female organs during menopause; a primary heart tonic for high blood pressure symptoms and palpitations; a specific in all stress-related heart disease. **Secondary uses:** as part of a hyperthyroid formula; to ease false labor pains; for hormone balance after discontinuing birth control pills. Use a hot fomentation made from the tea to relieve menstrual cramps; useful for many nervous disorders including cramps, convulsions, sleeplessness, gas and urine retention. May be used to treat swollen thyroid, neuralgia and nervous complaints.

✿ **MUGWORT:** *Artemisia vulgaris* - **Part used:** leaf. **Effective forms:** tea, capsules, herbal wine, sleep pillow, smudge stick, wash, poultice. **Therapeutic profile:** an emmenagogue to help regulate menstrual periods; a hemostatic that helps prevent miscarriage and excessive bleeding. Also a bitters tonic for digestion and liver function improvement. **Primary uses:** as part of any combination to relieve menstrual flow problems; used fresh as the primary part of a sleep pillow for REM sleep, and help in remembering dreams. **Secondary uses:** as a wash to relieve skin itching; as a treatment for intestinal parasites and worms; as an aromatherapy treatment to ease depression and nerves; useful in the treatment of kidney stones or gravel; drink the tea frequently for pain in the stomach or bowels, nervousness, and insomnia; apply it as a poultice for boils and abcesses.

✿ **MUIRA PAUMA:** *Liriosma ovata* (Potency wood) - **Part used:** balsam and root. **Effective forms:** capsules, extract. **Therapeutic profile:** a sexual stimulant; a tonic for the kidneys and adrenal glands; a nerve stimulant. **Primary uses:** a male toning herb to enhance libido, counteract impotence, and support organ regeneration. **Secondary uses:** as a treatment for female frigidity; also useful in treating neuralgia, paralysis and rheumatism.

✿ **MULBERRY:** *Morus nigra* and *M. alba* - **Part used:** berries, leaves, branch and twigs, root bark. **Effective forms:** tincture, infusion, mouthwash/gargle. **Therapeutic profile:** berries are tonic and laxative; leaves are anti-bacterial, promote sweating and expectoration; branch is antirheumatic, reduces high blood pressure and is analgesic; root bark is sedative, diuretic, expectorant, and lowers high blood pressure. **Primary uses:** berries are used as a tonic for weakness; in China as a tonic to nourish the blood and "chi." Black mulberry leaves, in Europe are used to stimulate insulin production in diabetes. White mulberry leaves in China are used for colds with fevers, headaches and sore throats and to cool liver heat, which can lead to sore eyes and irritability, and to cool the blood. Branch and twigs are analgesic and can reduce high blood pressure. Root bark is a good expectorant for coughs associated with "hot" conditions typified by thick, sticky yellow phlegm. **Secondary uses:** as a sedative and soothing agent to help asthma. **Contraindications:** avoid leaves and bark if the lungs are weak or "cold."

✿ **MULLEIN:** *Verbascum thapsus* - **Part used:** leaf and flower. **Effective forms:** tea, capsules, extract, oil, smoking herb, suppository, gargle. **Therapeutic profile:** an anti-spasmodic and astringent herb, effective for a wide range of respiratory problems and swollen membrane conditions. **Primary uses:** as a specific for bronchitis, environmental allergy symptoms, chest and sinus congestion, asthma, emphysema, and cough; as an expectorant to help loosen and remove mucous; the oil for ear infections when the eardrum is not perforated; both internally and as a suppository for hemorrhoids; infused oil can be applied externally as as salve for hemorrhoids, wounds, and eczema. **Secondary uses**: to reduce pain and swelling in the glands and joints; as part of a vermifuge; as an infusion gargle for throat problems.

MUSTARD: *Sinapis alba* - **Part used**: seeds. **Effective forms**: infusion, plaster or poultice. **Therapeutic profile**: is an excellent source of calcium, phosphorus and potassium. It contains vitamins, A B_1, B_2, B_{12} and C. Also contains sulphur, iron, cobalt and traces of manganese and iodine. A strong stimulating herb. **Primary uses**: helps promote appetite and stimulate the gastrate mucous membrane which helps in digestion. An infusion of the seed stimulates the urine and helps in delayed menstruation. A valuable emetic for narcotic poisoning because it empties the stomach without depression of the system. A valuable thermogenesis source for calorie-burning during a weight loss diet. **Secondary uses**: Used as a plaster for sore, stiff muscles in order to loosen them up and carry away the toxins that cause the muscles to tighten.

MYRRH: *Commiphora molmol* (Mo Yao) - **Part used**: gum resin. **Effective forms**: capsules, extract, gargle, ear oil, liniment, wash. **Therapeutic profile**: a digestive stimulant with potent antiseptic and anti-pathogenic properties for stomach, lung and bronchial problems; raises white blood cell levels for immuno-modulation; myrrh destroys putrification in the intestines and prevents the absorption of toxins in the blood. **Primary uses**: a specific for ulcers and inflamed mucous membranes; part of a formula for diabetes; an important part of antibiotic combinations; clears bronchial, sinus and respiratory catarrh; a gargle or topical application for mouth and gum sores and sore throat; an oil specific for repelling fleas and harmful "kissing bugs"; useful in treating chronic diarrhea, lung problems and body weakness. **Secondary uses**: as part of a tooth brushing powder for bad breath or pyorrhea; as an ear oil; an anti-fungal immune stimulant for thrush or candida yeast infection; as an emmenagogue to bring on suppressed menstruation; a liniment for wounds and abrasions; use as a wash for skin disease and wounds. **Contra-indications**: do not take in large amounts or over a long period of time without a break.

N EEM: *Azadirachtea indica* - **Part used**: whole plant. **Effective forms**: oil, paste, lotion, soap, shampoo, extract, capsule, tea, gargle, douche, ear drops. **Therapeutic profile**: a potent antibacterial, Neem is generally recommended for cosmetic problems and to ward off insects. Neem seed oil is reported to have antidiabetic, spermicidal, antifungal, alterative and antifertility effects. **Primary uses**: as a natural insect control agent for farmers and campers. Excellent in the treatment of psoriasis and eczema, relieving the itchiness and pain while reducing the scale and redness of patches; has potential in the treatment of diabetes, reducing the need for insulin by 30 to 50 % for nonketonic, insulin fast and insulin-sensitive diabetes; antifungal properties make neem very useful in the treatment of jock itch, athlete's foot, ringworm, yeast infections (including vaginal), thrush and diaper rash; reduces fevers. Topically as a cream to fight STD's, including gonorrhea, syphilis, chlamydia, herpes, and genital warts. Use the tea as a douche to combat candida. Use the water extract of neem leaves to treat parasites (including lice, scabies, intestinal worms), malaria, encephalitis, and chagus disease. **Secondary uses**: use topically to treat infections, wounds, arthritis and skin diseases (including Kaposi's sarcoma - an accompanying disease of AIDS). Included in natural toothpastes to fight periodontal disease (including gingivitis, pyorrhea, cavities and toothaches; may be helpful in the treatment and prevention of AIDS, cancer, heart disease and herpes when taken orally; gargle with a neem mouthwash to heal and soothe a sore throat; use the oil in ear drop preparations to relieve inflammation, pain and fight infection; use as a tea for migraines and hypertensive headaches. Use neem-based shampoos for dandruff and itchy scalp. Use the tea to prevent kidney problems, enhance circulation, and detox after blood poisoning.

NETTLES: *Urtica dioica* - **Part used**: leaf. **Effective forms**: tea, capsules, extract. **Therapeutic profile**: a widely applicable astringent, alkalizing, high chlorophyll, blood purifying, diuretic herb; useful as a mineral rich tonic and thyroid balancer for fatigue, an anti-arthritic, to stop excess bleeding, diarrhea and dysentery, and for inflammatory skin conditions. Effective for childhood diseases. **Primary uses**: a specific in bladder infection formulas, including cystitis and kidney infection. Nettles inhibit prostate activity and is helpful in the treatment of benign prostatic hyperplasia (BPH); a specific mucous cleanser for asthma relief and lung congestion; relieves mucous congestion of the colon; to check hemorrhage of the uterus, nose, lungs, and rectum; as rich organic mineral nourishment in arthritic pain formulas; the leaves are a good tonic for anemia as nettles draw iron and other minerals from the soil. **Secondary uses**: externally, to clean wounds and ulcers; for childhood eczema and diarrhea; as a tincture for hypothyroid conditions to increase thyroid function; used to alleviate bloating (especially pre-menstrual); helpful postpartum energy restorer; increases lactation; to relieve hayfever.

NORI: *Porphyra umbilicalis* - **Part used**: leaves and stem. **Effective forms**: dry roasted food addition, broth, seaweed bath. **Therapeutic profile**: a sea vegetable with rich protein, carotene, vitamin E, B vitamins, and iron content. **Primary uses:** as part of a high mineral drink or broth. **Secondary uses:** externally as part of a mineral, tonifyg bath.

    🌿 **NOTOPTERYGIUM ROOT:** *Notopterygium incisum* (Chiang-huo) - **Part used:** root. **Effective forms:** tea. **Therapeutic profile:** a Chinese herb, noted for its bitter action, disperses cold out of the body. **Primary uses:** for cold and flu symptoms, including aches and chills, fever, headache, and pain. **Secondary uses:** alleviates back pain. **Contra-indications:** avoid in cases of blood deficiency; overdose may cause nausea and vomiting.

    🌿 **NUTMEG:** *Myristica fragrans* - **Part used:** kernel. **Effective forms:** decoction, capsules. **Therapeutic profile:** carminative, digestive stimulant, antispasmodic, prevents vomiting, appetite stimulant, anti-inflammatory. **Primary uses:** mainly used today as a digestive remedy for nausea, vomiting, indigestion, and also for diarrhea,especially if related to food poisoning. May be used to help treat Crohn's disease. **Secondary uses:** The Chinese use it to warm the stomach and regulate qi (energy) flow.

O**ATS & OATSTRAW:** *Avena sativa* - **Part used:** seeds and whole plant. **Effective forms:** tea, extract, food, capsules, decoction, poultice. **Therapeutic profile:** a strong nutritive nervine for depression, anxiety and insomnia; an effective herbal calcium and silica source. **Primary uses:** as a primary herbal source of calcium to strengthen nerves, and overcome debility; to help in withdrawal from nicotine, opiates and cocaine; as part of a formula for skin problems; apply as a poultice for eczema, cold sores and shingles; oatbran, derived from the course husks of the grains, helps lower cholesterol. **Secondary uses:** as part of a combination for improvement of the male regenerative system; as part of a formula to correct sugar use imbalances; helpful to strengthen weak or brittle fingernails, repair split ends, and fractures.

    🌿 **ONION:** *Allium cepa* - **Part used:** bulb. **Effective forms:** food, syrup, compress.**Therapeutic profile:** a sulphur-rich agent effective for anti-biotic, digestive and respiratory uses. **Primary uses:** as part of an stimulating anti-biotic syrup with garlic and honey for colds and flu; an expectorant for bronchitis. **Secondary uses:** as a digestive and circulatory stimulant; apply fresh slices on insect bites or rashes caused by food allergies; apply as a compress to sprains and bruises; may have application as a preventative for snakebites; hypoglycemic actions make it useful in diabetes treatment.

    🌿 **ORANGE PEEL & FLOWERS:** *Citrus aurantium* (Chu-hung) - **Part used:** peel and blossoms. **Effective forms:** tea, bath, extract, oil. **Therapeutic profile:** a digestive stimulant with plenty of natural vitamin C and bioflavonoids. **Primary uses:** a pleasant tasting vitamin C/bioflavonoid addition to a tea; helpful for food stagnation, abdominal pains with distention, indigestion and gas. **Secondary uses:** as part of an astringent toning skin bath; to stimulate blocked chi (Chinese medicine) energy.

    🌿 **OREGON GRAPE:** *Berberis aquifolium* - **Part used:** root. **Effective forms:** tea, capsules, extract. **Therapeutic profile:** a strong blood purifier; a liver/organ cleanser, with ability to release stored iron into the bloodstream for stronger blood and immune defense; preferred treatment for all chronic degenerative disease, especially cancer and arthritis. **Primary uses:** a specific in a liver, gallbladder or over all waste cleansing formula; helps improve blood chemistry in the treatment of syphilis, eczema and psoriasis, Crohn's disease, hepatitis, jaundice and mononucleosis. For the treatment of anemia, because of its ability to release stored iron in the liver; also has application in the treatment of cancer, and arthritis. **Secondary uses:** to improve poor digestion; as part of a formula for chronic constipation; to relieve nausea; to build reproductive ability; drink the tea to stimulate the menses. **Contra-indications:** avoid during pregnancy.

    🌿 **OSHA:** *Ligusticum porteri* - **Part used:** root. **Effective forms:** tea, tincture, smudge stick. **Therapeutic profile:** an important native American anti-viral, with broad spectrum immune-stimulating properties against pathogenic organisms; effective as a circulatory aid in lowering blood pressure; to loosen and expel mucous. **Primary uses:** as an important part of an immune-stimulating tea; as part of a combination to overcome flu, other viral infections, colds, coughs and fevers. **Secondary uses:** as part of a blood balancing formula for circulation; for ear infections in children; may also be used in a formula to treat gas, indigestion, rheumatic complaints and delayed menstruation. **Contra-indications:** Safe at half dosage for children and pregnant women.

P**APAYA:** *Carica papaya* - **Part used:** leaf, fruit, seed. **Effective forms:** tea, juice, fruit. **Therapeutic profile:** a nutritive protein and fat digestant with far reaching enzyme therapy properties for serious disease; stimulates pancreatic activity. **Primary uses:** as part of a gas, bloating, and flatulence relief formula; to relieve colic in

infants; as part of a cancer and degenerative disease control compound for enzyme therapy; very helpful in an enzyme therapy program for diabetes and diabetic obesity. **Secondary uses**: the ground seed as part of a vermifuge; externally, may be used for burns, corns, eczema, blemishes, freckles and warts. Eating the fruit, and applying the skin of the fruit directly, can assist in fading bruises and black eyes.

PARSLEY: *Petroselinum sativum* - **Part used**: root, seeds and leaf. **Effective forms**: tea, capsules, chlorophyll drink, extract. **Therapeutic profile**: a concentrated chlorophyll, B vitamin, potassium source, with broad healing activity; a strengthening diuretic and specific for liver, kidney and bladder problems; an effective gallstone dissolving agent, digestive aid, blood tonic, and immune enhancer. **Primary uses**: as a specific chlorophyll source in toxic blood and degenerative disease formulas; a key diuretic herb with balancing potassium for water retention; a specific for digestive improvement, gas and flatulence; in stomach ulcer combinations; as part of an herbal mineral combination; a blood and circulatory tonic; in many formulas for female menstrual problems; as a "breath refresher" to reduce mouth odor; a specific for cancer. **Secondary uses**: to dry up milk in lactation; for nervous system support; as part of a combination to expel intestinal worms; as a specific in a bedwetting formula. Parsley seeds have emmenagogue activity to stimulate menstruation; the root can be used for jaundice. **Contra-indications**: do not use during pregnancy in high doses; do not use if there is kidney inflammation.

PASSIONFLOWER: *Passiflora incarnata* - **Part used**: leaf. **Effective forms**: extract, tea, capsules. **Therapeutic profile**: a primary nervine, anti-spasmodic and sedative, high in flavonoids, effective for a broad range of nerve disorders, including Parkinson's disease, epilepsy, shingles, neuralgia, anxiety and severe depression. **Primary uses**: as a specific for almost every nerve, insomnia, and seizure condition, for rest and relief without the accompanying "narcotic hangover;" effective in a formula to overcome alcohol abuse and nicotine addiction; in the treatment of asthma spasms; as part of a formula to relieve the pain of shingles. **Secondary uses**: as part of menstrual cramping and relief formulas; to control hypertension in children. As part of tension headache combinations that also involve reducing hypertension. Used to relieve diarrhea; used to relieve nervous distress accompanying hormonal changes and pain associated with menstruation, menopause and parturition.

PAU D' ARCO: *Tabebuia impetiginosa* - **Part used**: inner bark. **Effective forms**: tea, capsules, extract, ointment, cream. **Therapeutic profile**: a primary antibiotic, anti-viral, antiparasitic and antifungal herb, effective against many kinds of virally caused cancers and tumorous malignancies; a primary agent for immune enhancement and overcoming opportunistic disease, such as *candida albicans* yeast overgrowth. An effective blood purifier against many toxic blood conditions, such as dermatitis and psoriasis. **Primary uses**: notably effective in the treatment of intestinal parasites; a specific in the treatment of candida albicans, and virally-caused, inflammatory tumors; a specific both externally and internally for inflammatory conditions, such as eczema, psoriasis and dermatitis; a blood purifier and builder for leukemia and pernicious anemia; a primary immune enhancer against viruses such as HPV, flu, herpes and hepatitis; part of treatment to overcome environmentally caused allergies and asthma. **Secondary uses**: in the treatment of most fungal diseases, including thrush, athlete's foot, nail fungus and ringworm; for digestive improvement in colitis, gastritis and stomach ulcers; as part of an anti-inflammatory prostate healing combination; externally as a cream or ointment in the healing of old sores and lesions, and for diaper rash in babies; used externally as an ointment for bee stings, spider bites, poison ivy, cuts and bruises; has application in a pain relief program associated with arthritis and chemotherapy. May be used as part of the treatment of diabetes.

PEACH: *Prunus persica* - **Part used**: leaves and bark. **Effective forms**: tea. **Therapeutic profile**: a bitters herb, helpful in urinary and kidney malfunction. **Primary uses**: as part of a kidney/blood purifying combination; as a female tonic and diuretic; excellent remedy for bladder problems; peach tree leaves are effective in the treatment of occasional constipation. **Secondary uses**: as an expectorant for whooping cough and bronchitis; tea of the leaves can be used for stomach problems, jaundice, and to expel worms

PENNYROYAL: *Mentha pulegium* - **Part used**: leaf. **Effective forms**: tea, oil. **Therapeutic profile**: an aromatic herb with strong emmenagogue activity to regulate and bring on menstruation. **Primary uses**: as part of a formula during the last five weeks of pregnancy to prepare the birth canal, etc. for delivery; for menstrual ease and regulation during menopause; to bring on suppressed menstruation; in large doses as an abortifacient. **Secondary uses**: a diuretic and diaphoretic to induce sweating during a cold or fever; a flea, tick and mosquito repellent oil; eliminates gas, relieves nausea and calms nervous tension; use the tea as an external wash for rashes, itching skin and various skin eruptions. **Contra-indications**: avoid during first eight months of pregnancy, and then take ONLY in combination with other appropriate herbs.

🌿 **PEONY:** *Paeonia albiflora*, (Bai Schao) - **Part used:** root. **Effective forms:** tea, extract, capsules. **Therapeutic profile:** a female liver tonic, blood purifyer and balancing herb. **Primary uses:** as part of a formula with licorice root for female problems, particularly for menstrual irregularity, pain and hormone imbalance. **Secondary uses:** as part of a female liver cleansing formula; to treat skin infections such as acne. Also used to treat functional and emotional nervous problems, including epilepsy and spasms.

🌿 **PEPPERCORNS:** (Black pepper) *Piper nigrum* - **Part used:** fruit. **Effective forms:** tea. **Therapeutic profile:** a digestive stimulant, effective where digestion is weak; not to be combined with astringents as it renders them inert. **Primary uses:** a stimulating catalyst for metabolism. **Secondary uses:** part of an ancient meditative formula to increase samadhi (inner) energies; use a poultice made from pepper, vinegar, and salt for corns; may correct flatulence and nausea.

🌿 **PEPPERMINT:** *Mentha piperita* - **Part used:** leaf. **Effective forms:** tea, oil, extract, capsules, aromatherapy, breath "mint." **Therapeutic profile:** a univerally liked aromatic, with antibacterial and viral healing properties for digestive and respiratory problems. An effective body cleanser and toner, promotes relaxation, and may be used for all kinds of aches and pains. **Primary uses:** a specific in digestive, colon cleansing/bowel combinations, to control gas, bloating, flatulence, nausea, diarrhea, ulcerative colitis and Crohn's disease; the oil is a specific for irritable bowel syndromes; as a nervine for migraine headaches, anxiety and tension; in a circulatory tonic; a specific for morning sickness. **Secondary uses:** for bad breath and mouth odor; a relaxing pain remedy for headache and menstrual cramping; a pick-me-up for fatigue; helpful for travel sickness; use the oil for skin problems, itching, ringworm, scabies, burns and to repel mosquitos; oil can be used as an inhalation for nasal congestion; can be used in a compress for rheumatism, neuralgia and inflamed joints. **Contra-indications:** Do not use the oil as an inhalation for an extended period of time; may reduce milk flow in lactating women; do not give any form of peppermint to babies as it is irritating to mucous membranes.

🌿 **PERILLA:** *Perilla frutescens* (zi su ye/su zi): **part used:** leaf and seed. **Effective forms:** capsules. **Therapeutic profile:** An acrid, aromatic and warm herb, perilla leaf is used in TCM to disperse cold and to promote the movement of ch'i through the body. Seeds are used in TCM to treat diseases of phlegm-cold and phelgm-dampness. **Primary uses:** indicated in the treatment of cold and flu symptoms such as fever, chills, headache, nasal congestion or cough. Seeds stop coughing and wheezing and dissolve phelgm. **Secondary uses:** used to treat nausea, vomiting and poor appetite; to be used during pregnancy for morning sickness and to calm the fetus; effective agent against food poisoning. Seed can be used to moisten the intestines in cases of constipation due to dry intestines. **Contra-indications:** not to be used when there is chronic diarrhea.

🌿 **PERIWINKLE:** *Vinca major* - **Part used:** dried herb. **Effective forms:** tea, fomentation. **Therapeutic profile:** an effective all-round astringent. **Primary uses:** for control of excessive menstrual flow, colitis, diarrhea, hemorrhoids, bleeding gums; improves blood flow in cerebral arteriosclerosis; this herb is useful to be taken after a stroke. **Secondary uses:** as a sugar balancing agent for diabetes; use as a fomentation for skin maladies. Contra-indications: This herb is considered toxic and is not available in the U.S. or Canada.

🌿 **PINEAPPLE:** *Ananas comusus* (source of the enzyme bromelain) - **Part used:** stem and fruit. **Effective forms:** bromelain capsules **Therapeutic profile:** contains a mixture of several proteases and small amounts of certain other enzymes as well as organically bound calcium, which exert a variety of pharmacological effects like digestion assistance, anti-inflammatory activity, enhancement of antibiotic absorption, prevention of swelling (edema), smooth muscle relaxation, etc. **Primary uses:** bromelain is effective as a substitute for trypsin or pepsin in cases of pancreatic insufficiency; helps reduce inflammation (sprains, strains, arthritis, etc.); has an antibiotic effect helpful for pneumonia, bronchitis, peri-rectal abscess, cutaneous staphylococcus infection and pyelonephritis. **Secondary uses:** helpful for respiratory tract diseases by enhanced resolution of respiratory congestion.

🌿 **PIPSISSEWA:** (Prince's Pine) *Chimaphilla umbellata* - **Part used:** leaf and stem. **Effective forms:** tea. **Therapeutic profile:** a diuretic for urinary tract infections; aids liver and kidney detoxification; eliminates excess water. **Primary uses:** to aid urinary/kidney problems in arthritic and other acid conditions where sediment has formed, and body chemistry balance is needed; for prostate irritation. **Secondary uses:** in combinations to lower high blood pressure, and relieve stress on the heart. **Contra-indications:** Avoid during pregnancy.

🌿 **PLANTAGO SEEDS** (che qian zi): **Part used:** seeds. **Effective forms:** decoction, compress. **Therapeutic profile:** a diuretic herb used in TCM to treat urinary complaints. **Primary uses:** to treat edema and painful urinary

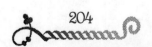

dysfunction; to clear up eye problems (redness, sensitivity to sunlight). **Secondary uses**: useful in treating diarrhea; also in combinations for coughs and excess phelgm. **Contra-indications**: do not use during pregnancy.

🌿 PLANTAIN: *Plantago lanceolata* - **Part used**: leaf. **Effective forms**: tea, capsules, ointment, tincture, douche. **Therapeutic profile**: a soothing astringent herb, ideal for relieving inflammation of lung and bronchial membranes, as well as burning hemorrhoid and bladder conditions; excellent for acute neuralgia. **Primary uses**: as a gentle expectorant for inflammatory lung and bronchial formulas; as a specific part of a kidney bladder healing combination in cystitis; as an astringent for hemorrhoids and diarrhea; as an antiseptic ointment for insect bites, scalds and skin abrasions. **Secondary uses**: as part of a lymphatic cleanser; as part of a mild diuretic formula; as a hemostat to help stop bleeding. Apply the tea in a douche for vaginal problems; use as a fomentation for skin problems including eczema, bee stings and boils; use as an infusion for constipation.

🌿 PLATYCODON ROOT (Jiengeng): *Platycodon grandiflorum*- **part used**: sliced, dried root. **effective forms**: tea, capsules. **Therapeutic profile**: Used in TCM to resolve phlegm and to expel pus. **Primary uses**: as an expectorant for coughs with profuse sputum, sore throat and hoarse voice; indicated for coughs with blood and yellow pus, especially in combination with the Chinese herbs *houttuynia, benicasa seed* and *trichosanthes fruit*.

🌿 PLEURISY ROOT: *Asclepias tuberosa* - **Part used**: rhizome. **Effective forms**: tea, capsules, extract. **Therapeutic profile**: a cleansing bitters herb, expectorant and anti-spasmodic, particularly effective in the treatment of lung, chest and respiratory infections. **Primary uses**: as a specific for pneumonia and pleurisy symptoms, acute bronchitis, and thick mucous chest congestion; as part of an anti-viral for flu. **Secondary uses**: to induce sweating for relief of fever and respiratory infection; for dry skin conditions, such as eczema or psoriasis. Helpful for stomach and bowel problems in children; use the tea for asthma.

🌿 POKEWEED: *Phytolacca americana* - **Part used**: fresh root and young shoots (should always be used fresh when taking internally - not dried). **Effective forms**: cut, powder (externally) and extract. **Therapeutic profile**: contains vitamins A and C, calcium, iron and phosphorus. Stimulates metabolism and reduces inflammation. It contains steroids resembling cortisone. **Primary uses**: excellent for enlarged glands (lymphatic, spleen and thyroid), hardening of the liver and reduced biliary flow. Helpful in stimulating a sluggish glandular system. Anti-inflammatory properties make it useful for rheumatism, tonsillitis, laryngitis and mumps. The steroids in pokeweed make it useful in treating psoriasis, rheumatism, and slow healing wounds. **Secondary uses**: Pokeweed applied as a powdered root poultice has been used for surface cancers and skin eruptions. The berry juice was used by the pioneers for skin cancers and wounds. **Contra-indications**: Pokeweed should be used sparingly and by someone trained in using herbs. Poke root contains toxic substances and should not be used in excess of one gram a day.

🌿 POPLAR BARK: *Populus tremuloides or P. candicans L.* - **Part used**: bark. **Effective forms**: bark. **Therapeutic profile**: harmonized urination, reduces fever and inflammation. **Uses**: urinary incontinence, mild urinary infections, neurogenic bladder, chronic clear leucorrhea, mucous cystitis, prostate hypertrophy, chrronic diarrhea

🌿 PORIA COCOS: *(Fu Ling)* - **Part used**: whole fungus. **Effective forms**: tablets, capsules. **Therapeutic profile**: a diuretic with organ-tonifying properties; calms the mind and emotions. **Primary uses**: to release excess fluid from the body, where extra kidney support is needed; useful for hepatitis and cancer. **Secondary uses**: for spleen, pancreas and liver support in a tonifying formula; for use in energy formulas combined with licorice.

🌿 PORTULACA (Machixian) - *Portulaca oleracea L.*- **part used**: entire plant. **effective forms**: decoction. **Therapeutic profile**: Acts on the large intestine and the liver to clear and release toxins and to cool the blood and stop dysentery. **Primary uses**: used in TCM alone or in combination with *scullteria root* and *coptis root* for dysentery symptoms such as fever, abdominal pain and blood and mucous in the stool.

🌿 PRICKLY ASH: *Zanthoxylum clavus herculis* - **Part used**: bark and berries. **Effective forms**: capsules, tea, linament; (prickly ash berries are Szechuan peppercorns used in cooking). **Therapeutic profile**: a central system stimulant to increase circulation and lymphatic activity; promotes sweating. **Primary uses**: increases circulation in the legs against cramping, varicose veins, etc.; esp. for rheumatism, stomach pain and skin diseases. **Secondary uses**: applied locally on toothaches, swellings and abrasions; to stop diarrhea; aids in warming extremities.

🌿 PROPOLIS: **Part used**: dry resinous secretion. **Effective forms**: capsules, lozenges, chewable gum. **Therapeutic profile**: a high bioflavonoid tonic and anti-biotic, anti-fungal and anti-oxidant bee secretion substance with antiseptic, soothing and healing properties. **Primary uses**: as part of an allergy control program; as an immune restorative substance particularly beneficial for colds, sore throat, tonsilitis, flu, fever and respiratory infections; as a male glandular tonic. **Secondary uses**: as part of a healing combination for skin lesions, gum disease, and tooth and mouth health; for diarrhea and intestinal infections; indicated for female ailments, painful menstruation, infections of the cervix, vagina and uterus. May have application in the treatment of ulcers. **Contra-indications**: do not use if allergic to bee stings or bee products.

PSYLLIUM: *Plantago psyllium* - **Part used**: seed *husk* or hulls. **Effective forms**: as an herbal fiber drink, capsules. **Therapeutic profile**: a soothing, lubricating, mucilagenous herb with drawing and cleansing laxative properties. **Primary uses**: in an herbal fiber complex as a "colon broom" for chronic constipation; effective for inflammatory diverticulitis; a balancer and regulatant for digestive and colon bacteria. **Secondary uses**: as a lubricant for ulcerous mucosal lining tissue; healing for wounds and skin infections. **Contra-indications**: not for use in cases where the colon is inflamed.

PULSATILLA ROOT (Baitouweng): *Pulsatilla chinensis* - **part used**: root. **effective forms**: tea. **Therapeutic profile**: used in TCM to clear heat and release toxins; to stop dysentery. **Primary uses**: Used in combination with *phyllodendron bark* and *coptis root* to treat dysentery symptoms such as fever, abdominal pain, and bloody stool.

PUMPKIN SEEDS: *Curcubita moschata* - **Part used**: seed. **Effective forms**: as a food, ground powder, or steeped tea. **Therapeutic profile**: a nutritive, high zinc vermifuge, effective against intestinal parasites. **Primary uses**: as part of a fasting and enema program to rid the body of tapeworm and roundworm; as a specific to reduce the swelling and inflammation of prostatitis. **Secondary uses**: as an aid against nausea and motion sickness; the seeds act as a tonic and rejuvenator to the male system.

PYGEUM AFRICANUM - **Part used**: bark. **Effective forms**: capsules, tea, extract. **Therapeutic profile**: an anti-inflammatory phytosterol with the ability to normalize male prostate prostaglandins. **Primary uses**: a specific in a formula for benign prostatic hypertrophy (BPH) to reduce inflammation and pain and normalize the passing of urine; as a specific to control and overcome prostate cancer. **Secondary uses**: as part of a combination to dissolve sedimentary formation in the prostate; to be used in many bladder problems.

QUASSIA: *Picrasma excelsa* - **Part used**: stem wood, stripped of the bark. **Effective forms**: tea, enema. **Therapeutic profile**: a bitters tonic effective as a liver cleanse and digestive stimulant and tonic. **Primary uses**: as part of a formula to stimulate the liver to increase fat metabolism; in a body balancing formula to overcome anorexia and bulemia; effective in a vermifuge combination and enema. **Secondary uses**: externally in a lotion to control head lice infestation or to repel flies and other pests.

QUEEN OF THE MEADOW: *Eupatorium purpureum* (See GRAVEL ROOT)

RADISH SEED (Laifuzi) - *Raphanus staivus L.*- **part used**: seed. **effective form**: tea, extract -**Therapeutic profile**: acts on the stomach, spleen and lung meridians to eliminate food retention and to descend ch'i and resolve phelgm. **Primary uses**: used in combination with *hawthorn*, medicated leaven and *tangerine peel* to aid in digestion to relieve abdominal distention and fullness, acid regurgitation, diarrhea and tenesmus; used for excess phelgm conditions such as cough with sputum and asthma.

RED CLOVER: *Trifolium pratense* - **Part used**: flowerheads. **Effective forms**: tea, capsules, extract. **Therapeutic profile**: a primary blood purifying herb, rich in minerals (particularly chromium), effective for many chronic and degenerative diseases. **Primary uses**: a specific in cancer and rheumatoid arthritis formulas; in the treatment of psoriasis and other inflammatory skin conditions such as childhood eczema; as part of a formula for bronchitis relief; an an effective relaxing nervine. **Secondary uses**: as an antispasmodic for whooping cough and inflamed lungs; an external wash for boils, bites, stings, sores and acne; for increased lactation in nursing mothers; soothing for ulcers; female tonic; effective against many bacteria, including the pathogen responsible for tuberculosis; relieves bladder complaints including mucous cystitis.

REDMOND CLAY: *Montmorillonite* - **Part used**: clay. **Effective forms**: powdered clay. **Therapeutic profile**: absorbs poisons internally and externally. **Primary uses**: used for skin problems, stings and bug bites; useful for muscle sprains and wounds, and for expelling worms from the intestinal tract. **Secondary uses**: may be used for fevers (forehead and back of neck). Can absorb poisons in the stomach quickly if taken with a glass of water.

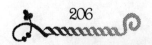

⚜ **RED PEONY** (Chishao): *Paeonia lactiflora pall.* **part used**: root. **effective forms**: tea, capsules. **Therapeutic profile**: Used to clear heat and cool the blood and to remove stagnant blood and reduce swelling, acting on the liver meridian. **Primary uses**: Used in combination with fresh *rehmannia root* and *moutan bark* for vomiting with blood and epistaxis; indicated for dysmenorrhea and amenorrhea. **Secondary uses**: has application for inflammation and swelling due to injury; can also be used to treat boils, carbuncles and furuncles. **Contra-Indications**: Do not combine this herb with *black false bellebore*.

⚜ **RED RASPBERRY**: *Rubus idaeus* - **Part used**: leaf, berries. **Effective forms**: extract, tea, capsules, gargle, wash. **Therapeutic profile**: a definitive high iron woman's tonic, with a long, effective history of strengthening and toning the female system and organs; especially helpful during the rigors of pregnancy and childbirth; a thyroid regulator, body balancer and aid during painful or excessive menstruation; soothing to the kidneys and urinary tract. **Primary uses**: a specific in all pregnancy, childbirth and lactation formulas to tone tissue, check hemorrhage, relieve nausea, increase milk production and balance gland activity; helps to prevent miscarriage; as a hemostat for irregular or excessive menstruation, diarrhea, and bleeding gums and mouth sores; for menopausal symptoms of low blood sugar and craving for sweets. **Secondary uses**: an accepted herb tea for children for stomach ache, diarrhea, and bowel problems; as a sore throat gargle; as an astringent for flu and vomiting; as an effective eyewash for swelling or inflammation; can be used to combat acid indigestion; can be used as a tonic for the prostate gland; use as an infusion to bath wounds; apply to varicose ulcers and sores; use the berries for indigestion and rheumatism.

⚜ **RED ROOT**: *Ceanothus Americanus* - **Part used**: root. **Effective forms**: capsules, tea, soap. **Therapeutic profile**: an anti-spasmodic and expectorant herb, effective for bronchitis, tonsillitis, lymphatic congestion and chest congestion. **Primary uses**: as part of a respiratory clearing combination; where there are fluid cysts or swollen lymph nodes. **Secondary uses**: to help reduce an enlarged, infected spleen; indicated for emotional despondency; use as a soap for sores. **Contra-Indications**: Avoid during pregnancy.

⚜ **RED SAGE** (Danshen): *Salvia miltiorrhiza Bge.* **part used**: root - **Therapeutic profile**: an herb used in TCM to invigorate the blood and move stagnation; to cool blood and reduce carbuncles; clears heat in the heart and soothes irritability. **Primary uses**: treats a variety of female ills such irregular menstruation, amenorrhea, abdominal pain and postpartum pain used in combination with *motherwort, peach seed, safflower* and *Chinese angelica root*; used for cardiac pain, abdominal pain, joint pain or epigastric pain; can help carbuncles, furuncles and swellings. **Secondary uses**: used for insomnia, irritability and palpitations due to a deficiency of nutritive blood with internal heat. **Contra-Indications**: Do not use in combination with *black false bellebore*.

⚜ **RED SAGE**: *Salvia officinalis* - **Part used**: leaf. **Effective forms**: tea, tincture, mouthwash and gargle. **Therapeutic profile**: a specific remedy for mucous membrane inflammation; as a specific to tonify the liver. **Primary uses**: a key part of a liver cleansing/toning tea; for inflammation of the mouth, throat and tonsils; a mouthwash for gingivitis or mouth ulcers; a gargle for sore throat, laryngitis and tonsilitis; to reduce the flow of breast milk; estrogenic properties make this herb helpful for menopausal ills. **Secondary uses**: part of a combination for indigestion; as a compress to aid in wound healing; reduces salivation in Parkinson's disease. **Contra-Indications**: Do not use during pregnancy.

⚜ **REHMANNIA**: *Rehmania glutinosa, (Shu Ti Huang)* - **Part used**: root. **Effective forms**: capsules, tea. **Therapeutic profile**: a blood building and balancing herb, effective in regulation against wasting diseases where there is anemia, dizziness and palpitations; particularly capable for the female system; an effective heart tonic. **Primary uses**: a hormonal precurser to treat hot flashes, night sweats, and excessive thirst; as part of a uterine and organ tonic to eliminate excess fluid and acids; useful in treating post-partum bleeding after childbirth; a regulant to the kidneys when there is chronic back pain and low adrenal function; as part of a sugar regulation formula for diabetes. **Secondary uses**: as part of a formula to relieve menstrual difficulties and infertility. **Contra-Indications**: Use with caution if digestion is weak.

⚜ **REISHI MUSHROOM**: *Ganoderma lucidum, (Ling Zhi)* - **Part used**: fungus cap. **Effective forms**: capsules, tea. **Therapeutic profile**: a powerful immune stimulating, antihistamine and antioxidant agent, with adaptogenic effectiveness against wasting and degenerative auto-immune diseases such as cancer and AIDS. **Primary uses**: as a specific in a formula to stimulate T-cell activity and inhibit replication of the HIV virus; as a strong anti-tumor agent; should be taken as part of a recovery program from chemotherapy and radiation. **Secondary uses**: as part of an immune system strengthening formula; effective in formulas addressing viral hepatits and liver dysfunction;

treats chronic bronchitis, peptic ulcer, hypertension, insomnia, sticky blood, and high cholesterol levels; useful in the treatment of allergies; may be helpful for altitude sickness and coldness of extremities.

RHUBARB ROOT: *Rheum officina, (Da Huang)* - **Part used:** root. **Effective forms:** capsules, tea. **Therapeutic profile:** a bitters cleanser for the stomach, liver and colon. **Primary uses:** a specific in a colon cleansing/toning formula; effective for chronic constipation and delayed menses; as part of a vermifuge combination for intestinal worms. **Secondary uses:** as an antiseptic healer for stomach and duodenal ulcers, and hemorrhoids; as an astringent agent in the control of diarrhea; use a strong decoction for boils and pustules. **Contra-Indications:** Avoid during pregnancy, arthritis and gout; never use the leaves.

ROSEBUDS & PETALS: *Rosa centifolia* - **Part used:** buds and petals. **Effective forms:** tea, oil for aromatherapy. **Therapeutic profile:** highly aromatic properties. **Primary uses:** for pollen and environmental allergy control. **Secondary uses:** in aromatherapy, as an aid in dispelling depression and exhaustion; use the oil in aromatherapy for dry or inflamed skin and acne.

ROSE HIPS: *Rosa canina* - **Part used:** fruit. **Effective forms:** tea, capsules, syrup, tincture. **Therapeutic profile:** a "spring cleaning" tonic and disease defense herb; an excellent source of non-acidic vitamin C and bioflavonoids. **Primary uses:** in all formulas where vitamin C is needed, especially colds, flu and respiratory infections; an effective cough syrup ingredient; in combinations to arrest arteriosclerosis, since natural bioflavonoids strengthen the arterial system. **Secondary uses:** in combinations for general debility and exhaustion; for gallbladder dysfunction; for kidney health, tone and balance; as a strengthening part of a diuretic formula; mild laxative for occasional constipation.

ROSEMARY: *Rosmarinus officinalis* - **Part used:** leaves. **Effective forms:** tea, capsules, wine, extract, healing oil, perfume, sleep pillow, wash, gargle, hair rinse, flea and moth repellent. **Therapeutic profile:** an anti-oxidant, circulatory toning agent, and strong nervine for stress and tension; effective for digestive problems. **Primary uses:** a specific in headache and tension relief formulas; to counteract depression; as a specific nervine to ease neuralgia, neuritis, tendonitis and muscle pain; as part of a formula for coughs, colds and flu. As part of a female system tonic; as part of high blood pressure formula. Used to improve memory and counteract the effects of aging; take as a tea for rheumatism pain. **Secondary uses:** a wash for mouth, gums and sore throat; a stimulant to hair follicles; a hair rinse to darken and retain original hair color; a shampoo or oil to control premature balding; as a part of a flea, moth and insect repellent combination. As part of a sleep pillow for insomnia and poor quality sleep; as a tonic wine; use the tea as a compress and apply to injuries. Use the oil in a bath to soothe aches and pains and to ease tension.

ROYAL JELLY: **part used:** jelly. **Effective forms:** jelly, capsules. **Therapeutic profile:** Possibly the most nutritious food produced by an animal, insect or plant, royal jelly is the food that the queen bee lives exclusively on. She lives 50 times longer than other bees and is much larger. In humans, royal jelly fights aging through its panthothenic acid content, a key B vitamin that stimulates the adrenal glands, increases resistance to infection and helps relieve stress. Modern French research shows that royal jelly acts like a natural hormone, stimulating both male and female sex glands and revitalizing endocrine gland function. **Primary uses:** Royal jelly is used to treat male impotence, sterility and female frigidity, acts as an antibiotic against viruses, especially those that cause flu and herpes; royal jelly balances the skin's acid mantle, improving skin tone and managing problems like eczema and neurodermatitis. **Secondary uses:** acetylcholine content in royal jelly make it useful in the prevention of Alzheimer's. Use topically for acne, especially adult acne.

RUE: *Ruta graveolens* - **Part used:** dried leaf. **Effective forms:** tea, gargle, poultice, homeopathic tincture, oil. **Therapeutic profile:** an emmenagogue herb with calming, anti-spasmodic activity. **Primary uses:** in small doses as part of formulas to regulate delayed menstruation; to ease stomach griping and bowel stress. **Secondary uses:** to relieve menstrual cramping, muscle spasms and rheumatic pain as an oil to relieve earache; helpful for relieving coughs, gas and poor digestion; use as a poultice to relieve headaches. **Contra-Indications:** Do not take in large doses. Avoid during pregnancy.

SAFFLOWER: *Carthamus tinctorius* - **Part used:** flowers. **Effective forms:** tea, capsules, liniment. **Therapeutic profile:** a bitters herb for digestive, colon and circulatory cleansing; provides glandular support. **Primary uses:** stimulates congested, obstructed blood flow, especially for women; an effective wash for measles rash; as part of a cholesterol lowering formula to remove arterial plaque; a mild, gentle bladder and bowel

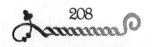

cleanser; as part of an arthritis, gout or kidney stone formula to neutralize and dissolve uric acid deposits. **Secondary uses:** a soothing digestive tract healant for heartburn, diverticulitis, and ulcer lesions; as part of a sports formula to reduce lactic acid build-up. The tea is useful during colds and flu to induce perspiration; also useful as a balancer in cases of hysteria.

🌿 **SAFFRON:** *Crocus sativus* - **Part used:** flower stigmas. **Effective forms:** medicated oils, capsules. **Therapeutic profile:** extremely expensive, but may be used interchangeably with safflowers (above) as a tonic catalyst; an excellent blood revitalizer and anti-inflammatory agent; a natural source of hydrochloric acid for improved blood sugar and fat metabolism. **Primary uses:** a specific in a blood and circulatory stimulant, with regulating benefits for the liver, spleen, and kidneys as well as the heart; a specific in arthritic, gout, bursitis and kidney stone formulas as an anti-inflammatory and to neutralize the uric acid which binds organic calcium in the joints; as part of a sugar regulating formula for hypoglycemia. **Secondary uses:** to reduce lactic acid build-up in the muscles; used for menstrual irregularities, impotence, anemia, and depression; assists the assimilation of food into the deeper tissues.

🌿 **SAGE:** *Salvia officinalis (white)* - **Part used:** leaf. **Effective forms:** tea, gargle, smudge stick, hair rinse, poultice. **Therapeutic profile:** a "spring cleaning," high mineral tonic herb, effective in improving weak digestion and drying up chronic winter mucous excess. (Especially effective as an aromatherapy herb for this purpose.) Estrogenic substances in sage make it a specific for most female disorders. **Primary uses:** as a specific in a blood cleansing formula; as part of an anti-infective formula for colds and flu; as a primary herb in teas for gas and indigestion; as an emmenagogue to regulate menses; as a specific in a deodorant formula; as a gargle for sore throat; as part of a treatment for chronic cystitis. **Secondary uses:** to help stop lactation during weaning; acts as a muscle relaxant for nerve conditions; trembling, vertigo and depression; as a hair rinse to return hair to its original color; as a poultice for tumors; improves circulation in the elderly. **Contra-indications:** epileptics should avoid this herb. Avoid during pregnancy.

🌿 **SANDLEWOOD:** *Santalum album* - **Part used:** heartwood. **Effective forms:** oil, capsules. **Therapeutic profile:** an aromatic wood used medicinally in aromatherapy for calming a "scattered" brain and to relieve indigestion; mild sedative effects. **Primary uses:** as part of a kidney or prostate formula to help in the passing of obstructive sediment deposits. **Secondary uses:** massage the oil on the forehead and between the eyes to center and calm the mind; oil is indicated in depressive conditions. **Contra-indications:** Do not use if there is serious degenerative disease such as cancer or AIDS.

🌿 **SARPAGANDHA:** (Indian snakeroot) *Rauwolfia serpentina* - **Part used:** root. **effective forms:** tea, decoction. **Therapeutic profile:** an Ayurvedic herb regarded as a vermifuge and a psychotropic. Soothing, potent tranquilizing effects make it very useful in the treatment of nervous disorders, and indeed many psychotropic drugs in the West are derived from sarpagandha. **Primary uses:** used to treat high blood pressure, hypertensive headaches, schizophrenia, severe anxiety and panic disorders, and all general psychoses. **Secondary uses:** In Ayurvedic medicine, sarpagandha is used to expel worms and as a wash for snakebites; Hindus use it for fevers and abdominal pains. **Contra-indications:** Do not take sarpagandha in large doses as it may cause hallucinations; avoid it in cases of congestive heart failure. Using this herb for any extended period of time may cause severe depression and a certain form of Parkinson's disease.

🌿 **SARSAPARILLA:** *Smilax aristolochaefolia* - **Part used:** root. **Effective forms:** capsules, extract, tea, root beer, oil (externally only). **Therapeutic profile:** a natural steroid and progesterone precursor with wide-ranging properties, from improving sports performance and scaling skin conditions, to tonifying the female system and relieving arthritic pain and stiffness. Cleans toxins in the blood: nourishes and tonifies the sexual glands and encourages the production of sexual hormones. **Primary uses:** as a specific in cases of hormone imbalance resulting in PMS and endometriosis; a definitive natural steroid for testosterone production in the body, particularly useful for body building as a source of muscle-increasing hormone; for prostate enlargement; to increase elimination of uric acid; as a specific for itching, scaling skin conditions, such as eczema, psoriasis and herpes. As a specific in a female or male hormone and gland balancing compound; as part of a treatment for rheumatoid arthritis; as a liver healant for chronic hepatitis; to be used in cases of impotence and sexual dysfunction. **Secondary uses:** in the treatment of venereal disease; as part of a douche for female leuchorrea; as part of a formula for petit mal; in the treatment of fungal infections, such as ringworm, skin eruptions, and athlete's foot. As a mild diuretic; as a hormone precursor to help counteract male pattern baldness; for gentle adrenal support; has application in the treatment of hypoglycemia.

 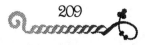

SASSAFRAS: *Sassafras albidum* - **Part used:** root bark. **Effective forms:** essential oil (externally only), tea, mouthwash, extract. **Therapeutic profile:** a highly aromatic diaphoretic and blood cleansing herb, useful against inflammatory skin diseases and arthritic conditions; stimulates and cleanses the liver of toxins. **Primary uses:** a warming diuretic to reduce the pain and congestion of arthritis, rheumatism and gout; for skin problems such as eczema and psoriasis; as part of a cold and flu compound to reduce fever and induce sweating; to be used during painful menses and for afterbirth pain. **Secondary uses:** as part of a mouthwash and tooth powder; the oil, externally to combat head lice and ringworm.

SAW PALMETTO: *Serenoa serrulata* - **Part used:** berries. **Effective forms:** tea, capsules, extract. **Therapeutic profile:** a strong natural steroid source with primary tissue building, gland stimulating properties to tone and strengthen the male reproductive system; effective in cases of prostatitis and pulmonary diseases; very supportive to the immune system. **Primary uses:** as a specific in formulas for male impotence, low libido, sterility and reproductive problems; to reduce inflammation and swelling of enlarged prostate (BPH) and dribbling of urine; as a general male toning agent; to help clear gastro-intestinal infection; to help rid the respiratory system of escess mucous. **Secondary uses:** helps increase female fertility, building stamina and endurance; an anti-adrogenic hormone stimulant to enlarge underdeveloped breasts in women, and testicle atrophy in men; use the berries to improve digestion and rebuild strength; useful for kidney problems and urethritis.

SCABIOUS ROOT & HERB: *Scabioa columbaria L.* - **Part used:** root, herb. **Effective forms:** decoction, tincture, swabs, compresses, ointments. **Therapeutic profile:** effective for bronchial conditions marked by heat, pain, coughing and asthmatic breathing. Addresses a large range of topical skin conditions. **Primary uses:** for bronchial conditions, wounds and skin infections, sores, skin blemishes and sunburn.

SCHIZANDRA: *Schizandrae chinensis, (Wu Wei Tza)* - **Part used:** berry. **Effective forms:** tea, capsules, wine infusion. **Therapeutic profile:** a very effective strong tonic and adaptogenic herb with circulation-stimulating activity. **Primary uses:** as part of a longevity and immune stimulation combination; to help in allergic skin reactions; used for asthma and dry cough. **Secondary uses:** as a tonic wine for wasting diseases, such as T.B. and diabetes; can be used to lessen chronic diarrhea, night sweats and seminal emissions. **Contra-indications:** avoid during pregnancy.

SCULLCAP: *Scutellaria latiflora* - **Part used:** whole herb. **Effective forms:** tea, extract, capsules. **Therapeutic profile:** a powerful nervine, with wide ranging sedative, anti-spasmodic and calming properties. **Primary uses:** as a specific for nervous system conditions, including DT's, insomnia, hysteria, convulsions, palsy, muscle tics, sciatica, neuralgia, Parkinson's disease, vertigo, and others. For nervous tension, exhaustion, anxiety and emotional upset; as part of formulas to break alcohol and drug addiction; as an antispasmodic for PMS, menopause symptoms, menstrual pain and cramping. As part of a formula for epilepsy, petit mal and seizures; as part of a high blood pressure combination. **Secondary uses:** as part of a treatment for bedwetting; as a gentle diuretic; as part of a brain tonic for promoting focused meditation; to relieve hiccups. Also useful for treating headaches due to stress and tense muscles; indicated for T.M.J.

SELF-HEAL: *Prunella vulgaris* - **Part used:** leaves, flower spikes, young shoots. **Effective forms:** tincture, infusion, poultice, ointment, eyewash, mouthwash/gargle. **Therapeutic profile:** leaves are antibacterial - reduce blood pressure, diuretic, astringent, heal wounds; flower spikes are a liver stimulant - reduce blood pressure, are antibacterial, and cooling. Constituents include flavonoids, vitamins A, B, C, K fatty acids, volatile oil, bitter principle. **Primary uses:** leaves and young shoots have been used by Western herbalists to stop bleeding. The fresh herb is used in poultices as emergency first aid on clean cuts. Flower spikes are used in China for the liver and gallbladder, because self heal is cooling in overheated conditions and soothing to the eyes, which the Chinese associate with the liver in traditional theory. **Secondary uses:** as a mouthwash/gargle for bleeding gums, mouth inflammations and sore throats.

SENECA: *Polygala tenuifolia* (Yuan Zhi) - **Part used:** root. **Effective forms:** tea, mouthwash. **Therapeutic profile:** a calming herb, partiularly useful as a heart tonic and anti-depressant. **Primary uses:** as an expectorant herb for bronchial asthma; as part of a heart tonic to counteract anxiety and mental instability. **Secondary uses:** as a mucous cleansing agent for the circulatory system; as a mouthwash for laryngitis and sore throat; helpful for problems related to congested emotions; promotes a feeling of well-being; also indicated for insomnia. **Contra-indications:** use sparingly for best results.

❧ SENNA: *Cassia angustifolia* - **Part used**: leaf, pods. **Effective forms**: tea, capsules. **Therapeutic profile**: a powerful cathartic that can cause laxative dependency, griping, cramping and stomach upset if over used. It is not for long term use. Senna is best used with other herbs, such as ginger, cardamom or fennel to reduce its strong cathartic effects and balance purgative activity. **Primary uses**: as a specific to relieve acute constipation; as part of vermifuge for intestinal worms or parasite. **Secondary uses**: as part of a formula to reduce fever. May be used in a formula for liver conditions. **Contra-indications**: Do not use during pregnancy, or if there is inflammation in the bowel or intestinal tract; overuse can cause laxative dependency.

❧ SHATAVARI: *Asparagus abscendens* - **Part used**: whole plant. **Effective forms**: decoction, powder, paste, medicated oil. **Therapeutic profile**: an Ayurvedic herb used to cleanse the blood. Considered a supplier of female hormones with similar properties to the Western asparagus but a stronger diuretic. Demulcent properties make shatavari useful for dry, inflamed membranes. **Primary uses**: used for hyperacidity (excess Pitta condition) anemia, and hemorrhoids; useful for a variety of hormone related problems including female reproductive debility, impotence, hysterectomies, menopause, PMS, and endometriosis. **Secondary uses**: useful in treating herpes, leucorrhea and inflamed membranes. May be used in cancer convalescence as a rebuilder; acts on the breasts to increase the flow of milk during lactation. **Contra-indications**: not to be used when there are excessive mucous conditions.

❧ SHAVEGRASS (See HORSETAIL HERB)

❧ SHEEP SORREL: **Part used**: seeds, leaves, stems, root. **Effective forms**: poultice, tea, capsule. **Therapeutic profile**: a very nutritive plant containing high amounts of vitamin A and B complex and minerals, including calcium, chlorine, iron, magnesium, silicon, sodium. High chlorophyll content make this herb useful in treating degenerative disease to stimulate regeneration, oxygenation, cleansing and purification of the body's systems. **Primary uses**: used mainly to treat cancer, tumorous growths, AIDS and other degenerative disease. **Secondary uses**: in relieving internal ulcers, jaundice and many skin diseases. Seeds can be used in an infusion to stop hemorrhaging and heavy menstrual flow; tonic to the urinary tract. Apply as a poultice to boils and tumors.

❧ SHEPHERD'S PURSE: *Capsella bursa pastrois* - **Part used**: leaf. **Effective forms**: tea, capsules, extract. **Therapeutic profile**: a very effective hemostatic to control bleeding, particularly in cases of excessive menstruation and in childbirth. **Primary uses**: as a specific for excessive menstrual and post-partum bleeding; as a specific to control excessive bleeding in the stomach, lungs, uterus and kidneys; as part of a formula to control bleeding ulcers; as a gentle diuretic to relieve water retention in kidney malfunction; as an astringent herb in a combination for diarrhea. **Secondary uses**: externally applied to bleeding sores, cuts, wounds, nosebleeds and bruises; as part of a formula for gout to control uric acid blood levels; as a mild diuretic; may be used as a decoction for bleeding hemorrhoids and chronic diarrhea.

❧ SHIITAKE MUSHROOM: *Lentinus edodes (Hsiang-ku)* - **Part used**: mushroom cap. **Effective forms**: capsules, soup or broth. **Therapeutic profile**: a powerful, revitalizing immune and T-cell stimulating agent; stimulates macrophage activity. Highly nutritious, rich in amino acids and B vitamins. **Primary uses**: as an interferon stimulant for major degenerative diseases such as AIDS, chronic fatigue syndrome and cancer; effective in the treatment of systemic conditions related to aging, immunity and sexual dysfunction. Lowers blood cholesterol, reduces blood pressure, and helps shrink tumors. **Secondary uses**: indicated for viral and bacterial infections; for liver dysfunction, including hepatitis B and cirrhosis. Helps prevent osteoporosis and Vitamin D deficiency.

❧ SLIPPERY ELM: *Ulmus fulva* - **Part used**: inner bark. **Effective forms**: tea, capsules, poultice, ointment, throat lozenges, suppositories. **Therapeutic profile**: a strengthening, soothing demulcent, ideal for sore, inflamed, ulcerated mucous membranes. **Primary uses**: a key part of combinations for stomach, bowel and colon ulcers and inflammation; a specific for stomach and lung cancer lesions; a throat coat and expectorant for dry sore throats and coughs; as part of a formula for indigestion, gastritis and duodenal ulcers; a soothing astringent for colitis and diarrhea. **Secondary uses**: a poultice or compress for bed sores, gangrene and abscesses; as part of an arthritis or gout formula; as a tea to settle the stomach from nausea; use in vaginal suppositories for vaginal inflammations and infections; use as rectal suppositories for alternating constipation and diarrhea. (Remove the slippery elm suppositories with a douche or enema).

❧ SOLOMON'S SEAL: *Polygonatum multiflorum* - **Part used**: root. **Effective forms**: tea. **Therapeutic profile**: a tonic herb used in control of wasting diseases; can be used to re-establish friendly flora in the intestines; acts as a tonic on the mucous membranes. **Primary uses:** as part of a bone building formula. **Secondary uses:** as part of a tonic against T.B. and diabetes fatigue; to be used as a poultice for inflammation, burns, poison ivy and bruises. **Contra-indications:** the berries are toxic, do not use.

SOUTHERNWOOD: *Artemisia abrotanum* - **Part used:** leaves. **Effective forms:** tea, and externally in a bath. **Therapeutic profile:** a bitters tonic effective as an abortifacient, febrifuge, and vermifuge; used to ward off infections. **Primary uses:** a specific to eliminate intestinal worms and parasites, and to counteract fevers; used in the treatment of anemia. **Secondary uses:** as a wash or bath to relieve skin itching, acne and rashes, and to repel moths. **Contra-indications:** southernwood has abortive properties - do not use during pregnancy.

SPEARMINT: *Mentha spicata* - **Part used:** leaf. **Effective forms:** tea, food flavoring, oil. **Therapeutic profile:** an aromatic almost identical in usage to peppermint for digestive problems, colds and fevers; however, it is not as strong as peppermint and can be used for children's complaints. **Primary uses:** as a digestive tea for gas and flatulence; as part of a warming colds and chills tea; as a flavoring herb in a myriad of combinations to overcome bitterness. **Secondary uses:** as an aromatic food flavoring to promote good digestion; used to prevent vomiting.

SPIKENARD: *Aralia racemosa* - **Part used:** root. **Effective forms:** capsules, fluid extract. **Therapeutic profile:** a lung and respiratory tonic, with diaphoretic blood purifying properties. Has many adaptogenic, ginseng-like properties. **Primary uses:** as part of a combination for chronic lung weakness. **Secondary uses:** as part of treatment for venereal disease; indicated for digestive weakness and pains associated with rheumatism. **Contra-indications:** not to be used for acute diseases or high fevers.

SPIRULINA: *Spirulina plantensis* - **Part used:** dried powder. **Effective forms:** capsules, tablets, food and drink supplement. **Therapeutic profile:** a highly nutritive, anti-oxidant micro-algae; an excellent source of protein, chlorophyll, vitamins, minerals (particularly calcium), and amino acids. A prime immuno-stimulant. **Primary uses:** important in many weight control formulas (especially those for over-eaters and sugar cravers); a protein source for high and low blood sugar support; indicated for rebuilding after acute diseases; as a tonic for goiter problems. May have use in combating AIDS, cancer, diabetes, allergies, cardiovascular problems, ulcers, and heavy metal poisoning. **Secondary uses:** as part of a blood building and liver support combination; in a formula for eyesight improvement in cases of glaucoma and cataracts. Used for hypotension to stimulate circulation.

SQUAWVINE: *Mitchella repens* - **Part used:** leaf and herb. **Effective forms:** tea, capsules. **Therapeutic profile:** a uterine tonic to prepare for childbirth, and for the relief of painful menstruation. **Primary uses:** in pre-delivery combinations to ease childbirth; in a formula to relieve menstrual pain by normalizing blood flow. **Secondary uses:** use as a tea for leucorrhea; used for bladder and kidney problems, including gravel and sediment formation. Also helps to insure proper lactation.

SQUILLS BULB: *Scilla maritima L.* - **Part used:** bulb. **Effective forms:** decoction, tincture, powder. **Therapeutic profile:** promotes urination, drains fluid congestion and relieves edema, stimulated heart, relieves urinary irritation, promotes expectoration, resolves viscous phlegm and relieves coughing, clears stasis and promotes menstruation. **Primary uses:** for edema, especially acute cardiac edema, chronic nephritis, urinary irritation, cardiac deficiency, dry cough, general plethora. **Contra-indications:** do not use during pregnancy as it promotes uterine contractions.

ST. JOHN'S WORT: *Hypericum perforatum* - **Part used:** flowers, buds, leaves. **Effective forms:** extract, capsules, tea, wine infusion, and ointment. **Therapeutic profile:** a strong anti-viral, analgesic, anti-inflammatory, and anti-depressant; Researchers theorize that St. John's wort anti-depressant action in the body is similar to that of an MAO inhibitor which works by interfering with the level of amines (e.g. serotonin, adrenaline, dopamine) in the brain. **Primary uses:** for control of viral infections, such as staph, strep, HPV and HIV viral strains; for reduction and control of tumor growths, both malignant and benign; for nerve pain control in conditions such as sciatica, neuralgia, and rheumatism; and for "mental burnout" conditions, such as chronic fatigue syndrome (EBV); effective for insomnia, depression and anxiety. **Secondary uses:** to help rebuild nerve structure, and mild immune stimulation; for topical trauma conditions, such as skin cancers, varicose veins, scrapes and burns; use as a tea for nervous disorders, cramping, and bedwetting. **Contra-indications:** avoid during pregnancy; may cause photosensitivity; toxic side effects have been encountered with St. John's wort ingested by sheep, cattle and mice.

STEVIA: *Stevia rebaudiana* - **Part used:** leaf. **Effective forms:** water solution for sweetening, extract, facial mask. **Therapeutic profile:** known as "sweet herb," stevia is a nutritive herb which contains the glycoside stevioside, thought to be over 200 times sweeter than sugar. Botanical composition and assimilation properties allow it to be acceptable to both hypoglycemics and diabetics in small quantities as a sweetener in cooking. **Primary uses:** as a tea, food and drink sweetener. Also useful in a weight loss and control program for sugar cravers, since it has no calories and significantly increases glucose tolerance and inhibits glucose absorption. Reported to decrease cravings for alcohol and tobacco as well. **Secondary uses:** a water-based extract of stevia in a facial mask helps smooth out wrinkles and heal blemishes, including adult acne.

STILLINGIA: *Stillingia sylvatica* - **Part used:** the fresh root. **Effective forms:** tea, tincture. **Therapeutic profile:** a specific for chronic skin diseases such as eczema and psoriasis. **Primary uses:** as a fresh tincture for skin disorders, syphilis and leuchorrhea. **Secondary uses:** stillingia is a folk remedy for bronchitis, cancer, croup, dysmennorrhea, and leucorrhea. May be used as a tea for some chronic liver disorders. **Contra-indications:** overdoses may cause vertigo, burning mouth, throat and gastrointestinal tract, nausea, vomiting, and diarrhea. In our experience, does not work well as a dried herb.

STONE ROOT: *Collinsonia canadensis* - **Part used:** root. **Effective forms:** tea, capsules, gargle, tincture, extract, decoction, poultice. **Therapeutic profile:** an astringent, diuretic and anti-spasmodic herb for the treatment and prevention of stones and sediment in the urinary, urethral, kidney and gallbladder systems. **Primary uses:** as a specific for hemorrhoids, varicose vein, and prostate inflammatory problems due to poor circulation. **Secondary uses:** as a strong diuretic in a bladder/kidney formula dealing with cystitis and inflammation; as a gargle for throat irritation from singing or shouting; strengthens the heart and improves circulation. Use the leaves in a poultice for wounds and sores.

STORAX (Suhexiang): **Part used:** resin. **Effective forms:** extract, aromatherapy. **Therapeutic profile:** This herb acts on the heart and spleen; opens the orifices and clears the mind; stops pain. **Primary uses:** indicated in TCM in combination with *cloves, musk* and *benzoin* for sudden coma caused by chi stagnation or unconsciousness due to windstroke; used for stifling sensation and pain in the chest.

STRAWBERRY: *Fragaria vesca* - **Part used:** fresh or dried leaves, fruit. **Effective forms:** tea, poultice **Therapeutic profile:** a blood purifying herb useful in skin cleansing; a cleansing diuretic for rheumatism, gout and arthritis. **Primary uses:** as part of an eczema/psoriasis healing combination; as part of a female balancing tea. **Secondary uses:** a balancing agent for the intestinal system, especially for diarrhea, and gastric inflammation. Useful for infections and jaundice. The tea is effective for nightsweats. The fruit may be used to whiten the complexion and remove freckles; the berries act as a liver tonic. Apply the crushed berries in a poultice for mild sunburns and other skin inflammations.

SUMA: *Pfaffia paniculata* - **Part used:** root. **Effective forms:** tea, capsules. **Therapeutic profile:** a South American herb, rich in germanium and allantoin, suma contains taurine and asparagine, two amino acids which are important in the conversion of protein and carbohydrates into ATP energy in the cells. Has ginseng-like adaptogenic properties, phytohormone constituents, and tonic activity on the endocrine system. **Primary uses:** as part of a combination to enhance both energy and immune strength; in a formula to reduce malignant tumor growth. A specific when used in formulas addressing chronic diseases such as CFS, EBV, mononucleuosis and candida; lowers blood cholesterol. **Secondary uses:** to help regulate blood sugar and provide energy, particularly for hypoglycemia; fortifies and balances hormones (esp. estrogen) and is used as an aphrodisiac in the Amazon; contains phytosterols of particular benefit for benign enlarged prostate. May have clinical applications for female estrogen therapy; promotes inter-cellular oxygenation, hormone regulation and acid/alkaline balance. **Contra-indications:** may cause mild nausea, not to be taken during fevers, oracute inflammatory stages of disease.

TAMARIND PULP: *Tamarindus Indica L.* - **Part used:** the fruit pulp. **Effective forms:** decoction, tincture. **Therapeutic profile:** promotes bowel movement, moistens the intestines, reduces infection and inflammation, reduces fever, stops urogenital discharges. **Uses:** constipation, fevers, inflammation/infection, discharges in venereal infections, premature ejaculation.

TANGERINE PEEL (Chenpi): *Citrus reticulata* - **Part used:** peel. **Effective forms:** extract, capsules, tea. **Therapeutic profile:** Tangerine peel is used to regulate ch'i in the spleen and stomach or to dry dampness and resolve phelgm. **Primary uses:** used in combination with *bitter orange* and *costus root* for epigastric and abdominal distention and fullness: indicated in combination with fresh ginger and bamboo shavings for nausea and vomiting. **Secondary uses**: also used with *pinellia tuber* and *poria* for coughing associated with phelgm blocking the lungs.

TANSY: *Tanacetum vulgare* - **Part used**: dried herb, seed and root. **Effective forms**: tea, infusion, tincture, extract, poultice, fomentation, enema. **Therapeutic profile**: an emmenagogue to promote delayed or suppressed menstruation. An effective vermifuge. **Primary uses**: in small doses as part of a menstrual regulant. **Secondary uses**: a digestive bitter to relieve indigestion; in an enema formula to rid the colon and digestive system of thread and round worms; externally as a wash or lotion for lice; valuable in treating hysteria and kidney weakness; a poultice made of fresh leaves is helpful for skin eruptions; use a hot fomentation for arthritic pain. **Contra-indications**: Use sparingly; avoid when pregnant.

TEA TREE: *Melaleuca alternafolia* - **Part used**: leaf. **Effective forms**: oil extraction. **Therapeutic profile**: an extremely effective Australian herb with anti-fungal, anti-biotic and antiseptic properties. A primary immuno-stimulant. **Primary uses**: internally as a dilute solution for mouth (esp. cold sores) and gum problems, and as a vaginal douche for yeast infections that does not irritate the vaginal membranes. Externally, undiluted, as an anti-fungal agent for warts, tumors, basal cell carcinomas, etc., dandruff, seborrhea, and psoriasis; potent antibacterial to be used topically for acne vulgaris and infectious skin diseases; antiseptic to be used for cuts and abrasions. **Secondary uses**: as an insect repellant and bite or sting healer, effective for both animals and people; also effective in killing the eggs of head lice in the hair.

THUJA: *Thuja occidentalis* - **Part used**: leaf, young twigs. **Effective forms**: tea, capsules, linament, tincture. **Therapeutic profile**: an oil rich blood cleansing, lung expectorant, hemostatic, anti-fungal herb, effective both internally and externally against rheumatic and inflamed skin conditions, diarrhea, ringworm and thrush. **Primary uses**: a specific against bronchial congestion especially when the phlegm is streaked with blood; alleviates coughs, externally and internally as an anti-fungal for ringworm, thrush and athlete's foot; an internal treatment for dysentery, especially where there is rectal bleeding; as part of a treatment for psoriasis. **Secondary uses**: used externally as a treatment for stubborn warts, corns and callouses; a soothing diuretic for urinary incontinence; to overcome side effects of vaccines and innoculations; as an aid in delayed menstruation. **Contra-indications**: Do not use when pregnant.

THYME: *Thymus vulgaris* - **Part used**: leaf, tops. **Effective forms**: tea, gargle, infusion. **Therapeutic profile**: a good children's all-purpose remedy, especially as an anti-spasmodic and aid to sluggish digestion, with anti-oxidant and antiseptic activity; expectorant properties make it a specific in throat and bronchial problems. **Primary uses**: as part of a digestive formula when there is weak HCl activity. As part of a remedy for childhood respiratory infections, asthma, bronchitis, diarrhea, lack of appetite, gas, colic, whooping cough, colds and flu. **Secondary uses**: taken before bed, thyme is a traditional remedy against bedwetting and nightmares; an infusion of the leaves helps relieve headaches. Externally, the tincture is a useful antiseptic for fungal and parasitic infections like ringworm, athlete's foot, scabies, crabs and lice. Internally, in capsules or a tea, it is helpful for candida albicans.

TILIA FLOWER: *Ternstroemia spp.* - **Part used**: dried flowers and bracts. **Effective forms**: tea. **Therapeutic profile**: an anti-spasmodic and sedative herb, effective for insomnia and spasmodic coughs. **Primary uses**: as part of a sleep aid formula. **Secondary uses**: in small amounts, as part of a cough control combination.

TORMENTIL ROOT: *Potentilla tormentilla* - **Part used**: root. **Effective forms**: capsules, extract, gargle. **Therapeutic profile**: the root is an excllent astringent, a hemostatic, styptic; anticatarrhal. **Primary uses**: its astringent properties are used for dysentery, diarrhea and jaundice. **Secondary uses**: the extract diluted in water can be used as a gargle for tonsillitis, laryngitis and canker sores.

TREE PEONY CORTEX: *Moutan radicis, (Mu Dan Pi) (root bark), (Bai Shao Yao), (white peony root) (Chi Shao Yao) (red peony root)* - **Part used**: root, root bark. **Effective forms**: tea, decoction, compress, capsules. **Therapeutic profile**: a strong circulatory balancing herb with anti-inflammatory activity; excellent women's tonic. **Primary uses**: as part of a menstrual formula where there is congestion and pain. **Secondary uses**: to help strengthen against internal bleeding, nose bleeds, heavy bruising, etc; root bark is an antibacterial used for boils and abcesses. Red peony is useful in treating childhood eczema when combined with certain other Chinese herbs; white peony is more specific for liver function than the red.

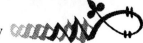

❧ **TRIKATU: Therapeutic profile**: Ayurvedic formula containing black pepper (*piper nigrum*), long pepper (*piper longum*) and ginger (*zingiber officinale*) used to enhance digestive wellness. **Primary uses**: used to treat heartburn, gas, constipation and poor nutrient absorption.

❧ **TRIPHALA: Effective forms**: tablets. **Therapeutic profile**: Ayurvedic formula composed of tropical almond fruit (*Terminalia chebula*), belleric myrobalan (*Terminalia bellerica*) and emblic (*Emblica officinale*) which is most often noted for its ability to restore tone of the colon and treat psychosomatic conditions affecting the digestive tract; less likely to cause laxative dependence than other formulas. **Primary uses**: used to cleanse and tone the digestive tract. **Secondary uses**: protects the heart; useful in the treatment of liver damage and liver dysfunction.

❧ **TURMERIC**: *Curcuma longa (Chiang-huang)* - **Part used**: rhizome. **Effective forms**: capsules, externally as a compress. **Therapeutic profile**: an aromatic liver stimulent to alkalize, cleanse the blood and help dissolve sediment. Turmeric has antibacterial and antifungal, anti-inflammatory, anti-oxidant, antiallergic and wound healing properties. **Primary uses**: a specific to reduce uterine tumors; a specific in the reduction and clearing of skin cancers; part of a menstrual pain relief formula; a remedy for jaundice and gall bladder problems. **Secondary uses**: applied externally to injuries and skin tumors; reduces pain when applied topically in post-hepetic neuralgia and arthritis, particulary when combined with capsicum ssp. **Contra-indications**: not to be used in cases of irritable stomach or hyperacidity because turmeric's yellow pigment has an irritant effect on the gastric mucosa.

UNA DE GATO: *Uncaria tomentosa* (Cat's Claw) - **part used**: bark, root. **effective forms**: extract, tablets, capsules, tea, topical cream or gel. **Therapeutic profile**: a Peruvian rainforest herb which has gained much popularity in recent times as an immuno-stimulant, anti-tumor, and anti-inflammatory agent against many chronic degenerative diseases. Acts an effective anti-viral and antibiotic which shows much promise in fighting stress, fatigue and illness. **Primary uses**: used to treat cancer (particularly urinary tract), diabetes, herpes, Parkinson's disease and AIDS. Cat's claw is also used to fight inflammatory bowel diseases, fibromyalgia, and all forms of arthritis. **Secondary uses**: can be used in the treatment of environmental sensitivities, allergies, candidiasis, PMS, and asthma. Use topically on Kaposi's sarcoma lesions and other skin disorders; use the tea as a wash for wounds, hemorrhoids and infections.

❧ **USNEA**: *Usnea barbata* - **Part used**: lichen. **Effective forms**: extract, decoction, tea, oil, commercial creams and salves. **Therapeutic profile**: the *usnea* species contains usnic which is more effective against some bacterial strains than penicillin. Usnic acid inhibits the growth of different strains of human tuberculosis and has been found to be effective against Staphylococcus, Streptococcus and Pneumonococcus. These lichen acids are effective against gram postive bacteria but have little effect on gram negative bacteria. U. longissima also has expectorant properties. **Primary uses**: for fungus infection, acute bacterial infection, colds and flu, bronchitis, pleurisy, pneumonia, tuberculosis, and sinus infection. **Secondary uses**: against cases of vaginal trichomonas, and urinary tract infections.

❧ **UVA URSI**: *Arctostaphylos uva ursi* - **Part used**: leaf. **Effective forms**: tea, capsules, douche, extract. **Therapeutic profile**: a definitive urinary antiseptic for bladder and kidney infections; a broad range remedy for diabetes, liver and spleen problems, hemorrhoids, kidney stones, bedwetting and mucous discharges. **Primary uses**: a specific in all formulas for cystitis, nephritis, bladder and kidney infection and irritation; in a formula to dissolve kidney stones; as a major component in a prostate inflammation compound; a diuretic in treating female disorders and diabetes; to cleanse and strengthen the liver and spleen; to control excess mucous discharge in urine (particularly highly acidic urine) and bowels; externally and internally for hemorrhoids and piles. **Secondary uses**: as a treatment for bedwetting; as a douche for vaginal sores and infection; as part of a combination for venereal disease; to control post-partum kidney/bladder infection. **Contra-indications**: avoid during pregnancy.

VALERIAN: *Valeriana officinalis* - **Part used**: root. **Effective forms**: tea, capsules, extract. **Therapeutic profile**: a strong pain relieving safe sedative herb for insomnia, anxiety, and emotional depression, without narcotic side effects. An effective anti-spasmodic and healer for the nervous system. **Primary uses**: a specific in combinations for nervous tension, PMS, stress, insomnia, nerve and arthritic pain, menstrual cramping and muscle spasms. A specific with feverfew to relieve migraine and cluster headaches; as a cardio-tonic agent to normalize heart palpitations while strengthening circulatory activity. As part of a safe calming formula for hyperactivity and restlessness in children, and as a sedative for childhood diseases, so that natural rest and sleep can promote healing; to counteract epileptic fits and petit mal. As part of a combination for hypertension and high blood pressure. **Secondary uses**: as a brain tonic from mental exhaustion; as a calmative for hysteria and manic-depression where the cause is emotional or mental trauma; to overcome hypochondria; for the treatment of colic, gas and flatulence in infants; in a formula for indigestion from nervous stomach; useful for low fevers, colds and gravel in the bladder; mild brain stimulant. **Contra-indications**: extended use may cause depression.

✻ VANILLA: *Vanilla planifolia*- **Part used**: pod. **Effective forms**: extract, essential oil. **Therapeutic profile**: pods are the source for commercial vanilla, a culinary ingredient that therapeutically helps curb a sweet tooth; used also as a popular fragrance ingredient in perfumes. **Primary uses**: the extract is sometimes used as an aphrodisiac or to satisfy sugar cravings. The essential oil is calming and soothing and reported to have aphrodisiac effects - especially for women.

✻ VERVAIN, BLUE: *Verbena hastata* - **Part used**: leaves and tops. **Effective forms**: tea, infusion. **Therapeutic profile**: a nervine tonic to relax and relieve tension, especially during a cold or flu. Also effective in controlling fever by encouraging sweating. **Primary uses**: as part of a nervous tension control formula, particularly where there is stress headache; drink the tea to aid in relief of menstrual cramping and stomach upset; as part of a liver cleanse when there is inflammation and jaundice. **Secondary uses**: as part of a detoxifying combination for fever, colds or flu; for throat and lung congestion; as a sedative nervine in seizures and hysteria; as part of a combination to expel intestinal worms.

✻ VIDARI: *Pomoea digitali,* (Indian Ginseng) - **Part used**: root. **Effective forms**: confection, juice, powdered root. **Therapeutic profile**: A tonic, galactogogue, alterative herb used frequently in Ayurveda in combination with other herbs or by itself; useful in liver complaints; considred a nutritive aphrodisiac. **Primary uses**: used to increase milk flow when there is poor lactation; useful in spermatorrhea, impotence, infertility and menorrhagia. **Secondary uses**: indicated for debility and emaciation; may have application in treating enlarged spleen and liver.

✻ VIOLET: *Viola odorata* - **Part used**: flowers and leaves. **Effective forms**: extract, syrup, mouthwash. **Therapeutic profile**: contains vitamins A and C. Properties in violet flowers and leaves seem to have abilities to reach places only the flood and lymphatic fluids penetrate. **Primary uses**: effective in helping to heal internal ulcers. Used internally and externally for tumors, boils, abscesses, pimples, swollen glands and malignant growths. **Secondary uses**: Useful for difficult breathing when the causes are from morbid accumulation of material in the stomach and bowels which cause gas, distention and pressure. Used for coughs, bronchitis, and phlegm.

✻ VITEX: (See CHASTE TREE BERRIES)

WAKAME: (Pacific Coast and San Riku) *Undaria pinnatifida* - **Part used**: dried plant. **Effective forms**: broth, food addition for flavor and seasoning, bath. **Therapeutic profile**: a sea vegetable rich in protein and minerals. **Primary uses**: as part of an iodine therapy or mineral combination. **Secondary uses**: as a bath for electrolyte and mineral balance. An alkalizer and blood purifier for the body, aiding in nutrient absorption and the elimination of toxic metals and environmental pollutants; wakame strengthens the body against disease

✻ WALNUT: *Juglans spp.* - **Part used**: leaves, nut, outer nut rind, inner bark. **Effective forms**: extract, homeopathic preparation. **Therapeutic profile**: astringent, expels intestinal worms, antispasmodic, digestive tonic; the nut rind is anti-inflammatory. Constituents include quinones, oils, tannins; nuts contain essential fatty acids. **Primary uses**: the tree is cultivated for its nuts which yield an important oil containing essential fatty acids that are vital for healthy cell function and prostaglandin development. Walnut leaves have been used as a remedy for both eczema and blepharitis (eyelid inflammation), especially in children. Both traditional usage and recent research show strong antifungal and antiseptic action. Hulls and leaves are a specific for intestinal worms and as a bitters type digestive tonic.

✻ WATERCRESS: *Nasturtium officinale* - **Part used**: flower and leaf. **Effective forms**: tea, capsules. **Therapeutic profile**: a mineral-rich diuretic herb effective as part of a liver and organ cleanse. **Primary uses**: in a liver formula to stimulate metabolic activity, increase bile production and dispel gas. **Secondary uses**: as a specific in an herbal mineral combination. Also used to treat fluid retention, mucous in the lungs and indigestion. A light herbal tonic used to rebuild the system from acute disease.

✻ WATERMELON SEED: *Cucurbita sativus* - **Part used**: seed and juice. **Effective forms**: tea, decoction and as a juice drink. **Therapeutic profile**: a mild flushing diuretic. **Primary uses**: as a morning flush to relieve excess fluid retention. **Secondary uses**: used to treat urinary inflammations, dysentary, fever, dry heaves, and thirst.

✻ **WHITE ATRACYLODES** (Baizhu): *Atracylodes macrocephala Koidz*- **Part used**: rhizome. **Effective forms**: capsules. **Therapeutic profile**: used in TCM to replenish ch'i and strengthen the spleen; to resolve dampness, promoting water metabolism: to calm the fetus and to arrest profuse sweating. **Primary uses**: used with *ginseng* and *poria cocos* for lack of appetite, diarrhea and epigastric and abdominal distention and fullness; has application in treating edema and excess phelgm conditions such as asthma and coughing with sputum. **Secondary uses**: Indicated for spontaneous sweating due to a chi deficiency; also used to calm the fetus during pregnancy.

✻ **WHITE OAK**: *Quercus alba* - **Part used**: bark and gall. **Effective forms**: tea, extract, fomentation, capsules, compress, wash, gargle, bath, enema, douche. **Therapeutic profile**: a strong astringent/antiseptic effective for strengthening capillaries in inflammatory swelling problems, such as hemorrhoids, varicose veins, gums, goiter, and internal tumors; normalizes liver, kidney and spleen functions. **Primary uses**: a specific for hemorrhoid inflammations; a specific in the treatment of diarrhea, leucorrhea and dysentery; tones prolapsed organs; to dissolve kidney stones and other bleeding kidney bladder problems; to help prevent the clumping of tumor cell platelets, and thus the spread of cancer. **Secondary uses**: in a formula to dissolve gallstones and kidney stones by increasing the flow of urine; as a gargle for sore throat; as a wash for gum and vein inflammations; used topically for ringworm, and fungal sores; as a douche for vaginal infection; as a part of a combination to decrease menstrual flow; as part of a formula to expel pin and thread worms. Externally, the tea is good for washing scabs, poison oak, sores and insect bites; the tea can also be taken for bleeding of the rectum, stomach and lungs. Or apply as a fomentation to swollen glands, mumps and other lymphatic swellings.

✻ **WHITE PINE**: *Pinus strobus* - **Part used**: inner bark, sprigs, resin. **Effective forms**: tea, capsules, extract, resin. **Therapeutic profile**: as a primary anti-oxidant; a warming, circulation stimulant, expectorant. **Primary uses**: as an anti-oxidant to enhance oxygen uptake by the respiratory system; particularly effective in cases of pneumonia and/or pleurisy; as an expectorant to facilitate the removal of mucous in bronchial and catarrhal trouble. **Secondary uses**: in combinations to overcome or prevent colds and flu by raising circulatory action; the heated resin can be used as a dressing to draw out splinters or bring boils to a head; also effective for most sores, cuts, swellings and insect bites; can be used on a hot cloth and applied for sciatic pain and muscular soreness.

✻ **WHITE PEONY ROOT** (Baishao): *Paeonia lactiflora pall.*- **Part used**: root. **Effective forms**: capsules, extract, tea. **Therapeutic profile**: Used in TCM to nourish the blood; to soothe liver yang and stop pain. **Primary uses**: used in TCM for irregular menstruation, dysmenorrhea and uterine bleeding; helpful for spontaneous sweating and night sweating; indicated for liver ch'i stagnation manifested by hypochondriac pain, breast distention and irregular menstruation in combination with Bupleurum root and *Chinese angelica root*. **Secondary uses**: helps in the treatment of muscle spasms and abdominal pain; may have use for fighting headache pain and dizziness.

✻ **WHITE WILLOW**: *Salix alba* - **Part used**: bark. **Effective forms**: tea, tincture, capsules, decoction, eyewash. **Therapeutic profile**: a bitters tonic herb generally used to treat headache pain and nervous disorders without the stomach irritation of aspirin. (Aspirin is a synthetic extraction of white willow.) A high immune response herb that inhibits Prostaglandin production, and kills cancerous cells. **Primary uses**: as an anti-inflammatory specific in headache combinations; as an analgesic for the pain of arthritis, neuralgia, bursitis and gout; for sore muscles and tendons; to lower fever through increased blood flow and sweating. **Secondary uses**: as a natural, safe treatment for earache and toothache; as a relaxant in a vermifuge; as part of a strengthening eyewash compound. The tea is effective for kidney, urethra and bladder problems, acting as an analgesic to those tissues. The tea can also be used as a snuff to stop nose bleeds and other surface bleeding. Used as a decoction, white willow is an excellent gargle for tonsil and throat infections.

✻ **WILD CHERRY**: *Prunus serotina* - **Part used**: bark, dried inner bark. **Effective forms**: tea, extract, capsules, eyewash. **Therapeutic profile**: one of the best herbs for respiratory complaints, coughs and lowered immune defenses. (Makes a good spring tonic). **Primary uses**: as a specific in a throat coat for irritating coughs, whooping cough, and bronchial congestion cough; as part of a formula for asthma. **Secondary uses**: as a tonic for a sluggish digestive and elimination system; it is a tonic for the stomach, improving digestion by stimulating the gastric glands; remedy for heart palpitations when caused by a stomach disorder; as an eyewash for inflammation.

✻ **WILD GINGER**: (See CANADA SNAKEROOT)

✻ **WILD LETTUCE**: *Lactuca virosa* - **Part used**: leaf, seed oil. **Effective forms**: tea, extract. **Therapeutic profile**: an anti-spasmodic and calming nervine/sedative herb for relaxation and sleep. **Primary uses**: in combinations to relieve insomnia and hyperactivity (particularly effective for children); as part of a menstrual relief formula. **Secondary uses:** for spasmodic coughs, and colic; as a muscle relaxant to relieve body aches and strain; the seed oil is used for arteriosclerosis; also used in home remedies for asthma, cancer, dropsy, gout and jaundice

WILD YAM: *Dioscorea villosa* - **Part used:** root. **Effective forms:** tea, capsules, extract. **Therapeutic profile:** a contraceptive herb with hormone precursors of progesterone and other steroids. As a female hormone balancer for fatigue and menstrual problems. **Primary uses:** as a specific for female toning combinations, for PMS, water retention, breast tenderness and headaches; as a soothing digestive herb for diverticulitis and gallbladder problems; a natural steroid for arthritic and rheumatic relief; valuable as an antispasmodic for abdominal cramping, menstrual cramps and bowel spasms. **Secondary uses:** as a blood sugar regulant for hypoglycemia; for morning sickness, stomach irritation and cramping; will aid in the removal of wastes from the body, relieving stiff and sore muscles; will aid in the prevention of miscarriage; also indicated as a tincture for afterbirth pain.

WINTERGREEN: *Gaultheria procumbens* - **Part used:** leaves, oil, root. **Effective forms:** tea, oil, gargle, liniment. **Therapeutic profile:** an aromatic analgesic herb with aspirin family qualities, used both externally and internally for pain relief. **Primary uses:** externally as an analgesic in a variety of pain relief formulas, from headaches to muscle and sciatic pain, to rheumatic/arthritic pain; as a gargle for sore throat. **Secondary uses:** as an anti-inflammatory in urinary problems; leaves are used to treat asthma; root can be chewed to prevent tooth decay; can also be used in a douche for leukorhea.

WINTER SAVORY: *Satureia montana L.* - **Part used:** the herb. **Effective froms:** essential oil, tincture. **Therapeutic profile:** has antibacterial and antifungal properties. Has been shown to have pituitary-stimulant actions. **Uses:** a specific for Candida albicans, C. tropicalis and other intestinal yeast variants. Antimicrobial strength is on the same level as oil of thyme. Useful for a variety of disorders caused by hormonal deficiencies. Traditionally drunk as a supportive tea for diabetes.

WITCH HAZEL: *Hamamelis virginiana* - **Part used:** bark, leaf. **Effective forms:** tea, tincture, ointment, poultice, liniment and wash. **Therapeutic profile:** a strong astringent herb effective in stopping bleeding (especially menstrual and hemorrhages from the lungs, stomach, uterus and bowels) both internally and externally, and in reducing swelling and inflammation from bruises, hemorrhoids and varicose veins. **Primary uses:** as part of a formula to stop hemorrhage; as an aid in controlling vaginal discharge in leucorrhea. **Secondary uses:** externally to reduce swelling of hemorrhoids and varicose veins; internally to reduce diarrhea. Externally as a fomentation or poultice for bed sores, wounds, sore and inflamed eyes and oozing skin diseases. Use the tincture diluted in water in a mouthwash or gargle for infection and, like cider vinegar in a healthy mouth maintenance program.

WOOD BETONY: *Betonica officinalis* - **Part used:** whole herb, tops. **Effective forms:** tea, capsules, infusions, extract, poultice and powder. **Therapeutic profile:** a sedative and analgesic herb with particular effectiveness for face, head and nerve pain. **Primary uses:** as part of a headache, migraine or nervous tension pain formula; in the treatment of neuralgia. **Secondary uses:** as a relaxant in a stress combination. When taken three to four times daily in three ounce dosages, helps kill worms and open up obstructions of the liver and gall bladder. The fresh herb used as a poultice helps draw out splinters and heal open wounds. Infusion and powder may be used to treat jaundice, convulsions, gout and colds.

WORMWOOD: *Artemisia absinthium* - **Part used:** leaves, stems, oil and tops. **Effective forms:** tincture, tablets or capsules, tea, wash. **Therapeutic profile:** a bitters herb generally used to expel intestinal worms and parasites. **Primary uses:** as a specific for all intestinal parasite and worm infestations. **Secondary uses:** as a bitters digestive stimulant; to reduce fever; as a wash to relieve skin itching and rashes. Oil is used to repel house flies, moths and fleas. **Contra-indications:** Has abortive properties - do not take while pregnant.

YARROW: *Achillea millefolium* - **Part used:** flower, leaf, whole herb. **Effective forms:** tea, extract, poultice, shampoo, hair rinse and herbal tobacco. **Therapeutic profile:** a thyroid regulant; a powerful diaphoretic and antiseptic used for fevers, cold and flu. **Primary uses:** as a specific in a formula for cold and flu to induce sweating and lower fever; as a urinary antiseptic for cystitis; for inter-menstrual spotting because of uterine cramping or spasms. **Secondary uses:** as a diuretic in a combination to lower blood pressure; as a poultice to stop bleeding wounds; as part of a skin formula for acne where an imbalanced thyroid is the cause. Useful for spastic conditions in the pelvis. Bitters action make it useful for sluggish stomach conditions. Used for earches, for alleviating epilepsy attacks, fever, fistulas of various kinds (such as anal), hemorrhoids.

❧ YELLOW DOCK: *Rumex crispus* - **Part used:** root. **Effective forms:** tincture, tea, capsules. **Therapeutic profile:** a rich source of herbal iron, particular effective for liver, gallbladder, spleen and skin disorders; a hormone regulant. **Primary uses:** as a specific in treating anemia, and in blood building formulas in general; a specific in liver, gallbladder, spleen and other iron deficiency disorders; as an effective lymphatic cleanser and mild blood purifier; as a mild astringent in a combination for hemorrhoids and other internal bleeding problems; as part of a formula for eczema and psoriasis; as a treatment for jaundice due to congestion; as part of a combination to dissolve cancerous growths and tumors. As part of a strengthening formula in the elimination of intestinal parasites; for hormone regulation after discontinuing the birth control pill. **Secondary uses:** as part of a mild purgative for constipation; used to treat diarrhea, fever, itch, and rheumatism. Used to help promote production of bile; as part of a blood-building iron and vitamin C compound. As part of a building male system combination for bad breath and skin eruptions (acne, eczema, psoriasis) due to blood composition imbalance. **Contra-indications:** Toxic to animals, Overdoses of the root extract may cause diarrhea, nausea and polyuria in humans.

❧ YERBA MATE: *Ilex paraguariensis* - **Part used:** leaf. **Effective forms:** tea. **Therapeutic profile:** a South American nervine used as a refreshing tonic drink. **Primary uses:** as a tonic, energizing tea without undesirable stimulant effects. **Secondary uses:** recommended for people suffering from debility and neurasthenia. A folk remedy for rheumatism and scurvy. **Contra-indications:** contains 2.5g caffeine per kilogram of leaves.

❧ YERBA SANTA: *Eriodictyon californicum* - **Part used:** leaf. **Effective forms:** tea, externally as a skin wash. **Therapeutic profile:** an expectorant with digestive cleansing properties. **Primary uses:** in a "spring cleaning" combination. **Secondary uses:** externally as an antidote for poison oak. Yerba santa reduces infections, promotes astriction and opens the sinuses. It is able to treat mild bladder conditions with antiseptic, diuretic properties. It also is a mild appetite stimulant. Contains a mild amount of caffeine.

❧ YOHIMBE: *Coryanthe yohimbe* - **Part used:** bark. **Effective forms:** capsules, powdered extract. **Therapeutic profile:** a hormone stimulant, particularly effective in the production of testosterone. **Primary uses:** as an aphrodisiac affecting both the male impotence and female frigidity. **Secondary uses:** in bodybuilding, athletic formulas where more testosterone production is desired. Note: Avoid if there is high blood pressure, schizophrenia, heart arrythmia or if taking nasal decongestants or diet aids containing phenylpropanolamine. Side effects include tremors, agitation, insomnia, anxiety, hypertension, tachycardia, vomiting and nausea.

❧ YUCCA: *Yucca spp.* - **Part used:** root, stems, leaves. **Effective forms:** capsules, extracts. **Therapeutic profile:** an anti-inflammatory phytosterol with the ability to break up inorganic mineral obstructions and deposits. **Primary uses:** in pain-relieving combinations for arthritic and joint pain, and sediment-caused inflammation as in gout, rheumatism, and cystitis or prostatitis. **Secondary uses:** as an aid to establishing stable friendly flora balance in the G.I. tract, and for asthmatic symptom relief. Yucca steroidal saponins may indirectly stimulate the absorption of nutrients and decrease the amounts of toxins available for absorption in the digestive tract, thus, improving the efficacy of the elimination systems (kidney, liver, lymph and blood).

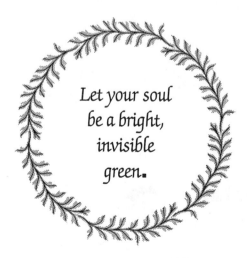

Let your soul
be a bright,
invisible
green.

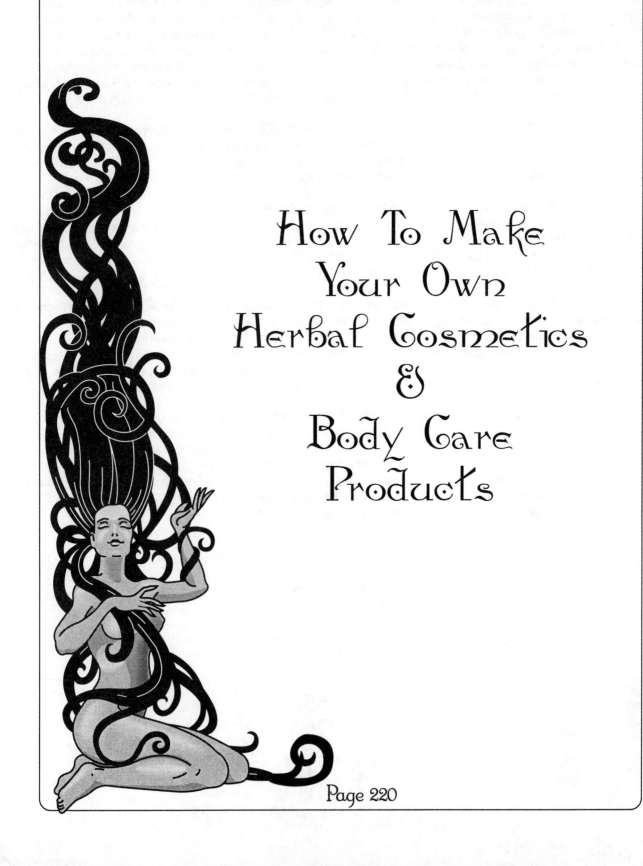

How To Make Your Own Herbal Cosmetics & Body Care Products

Making Your Own Herbal Cosmetics

hy make your own cosmetics?
Multiple chemical sensitivities and allergic contaminant reactions are multiplying in every area of our lives today. Over 2 million synthetic substances are known, over 25,000 are added each year, and 30,000 are produced on a commercial scale. Only a tiny fraction are ever tested for toxicity, and many come to us from countries that have few safeguards in place. It's no wonder that our bodies have trouble staying normal in the face of $2\frac{1}{2}$ billion pounds of pesticides used in America every year, or the 300 million pounds of chemicals that are part of American household products. An abundance of the allergy/sensitivity generating chemical substances are found in today's cosmetics and beauty products. Although heredity plays a role in determining our potential predisposition to cosmetic problems, the daily onslaughts from environmental toxins, and free radical damage from both chemicals and the aging process impact cosmetic beauty far more. For people whose systems can't tolerate this chemical overload or those with sensitive skin, taking care of their bodies extends to making all-natural, non-chemical health and beauty products.

What can we do to stay healthy on the inside and beautiful on the outside in a seemingly destructive world? While we have a measure of control over our diets, our lifestyle and how we manage the stress in our lives, I believe that herbal therapy and herbally based cosmetics can go a long way toward minimizing problems and maximizing potential.

Herbs are Nature's quintessential body balancers and normalizers. They work at the deepest levels of the body, from the inside out to address gland, hormone and digestive problems, those most involved with our beauty elements. Herbs are also Nature's most effective medicinal foods, working with the body's own enzyme activity, from the inside out, so they are gentle and long-lasting.

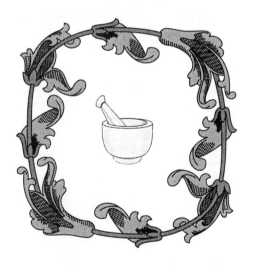

How do free radicals affect cosmetic problems?
Free radical cell damage to connective tissue results in loss of skin tone and elasticity and contributes to other cosmetic problems. Although the body normally produces some free radicals in its ordinary metabolic breakdown of organic compounds (indeed some are released to fight bacteria during immune response), free radicals play a key role in the body's deterioration. However, as always in Nature, the body also produces the necessary substances (in this case, the enzymes superoxide dismutase, catalase, and glutathione peroxidase) to deactivate them.

So, lower the fat in your diet, add antioxidant rich foods like broccoli and salads, and plenty of vegetables like leafy greens and garlic that have free-radical de-activating enzymes; avoid exposure to radiation, rancid oils, food additives and colors, tobacco smoke, heavy metal pollutants, UV sunlight, and fast foods to reduce free-radical attacks on your body.

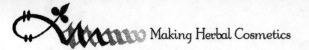

Can you really make your own herbal cosmetics?

Yes, you can .... and it's easy! If you experience sensitivities like redness, itchiness or breakouts to drugstore or department store cosmetics, you may be reacting to their chemical irritants, hidden substances or other ingredients (sometimes even when they're called natural).

If you make your own herbal cosmetics, you're in control. You'll know everything they contain, you'll know each ingredient is pure and natural and whether it's something good for your body. In addition, you can personalize your cosmetic recipes for your own individual needs.

Making your own cosmetics is like trying out a new recipe; these are essentially "kitchen cosmetics." We'll address herbal compounds for your eyes, nails, skin, hair, smile and feet in this section. You'll need a little patience and a little trial and error as you get the hang of it. But their simplicity is part of their charm. There are no harsh chemicals to irritate the body or the environment, and their subtle effects can bring out a more naturally beautiful you!

It's wonderful to be able to use freshly picked herbs in your cosmetics. You might even want to plant a small herb garden as your own personal beauty aid! However, the herbal compounds in this section can be made with both dried or fresh herbs. Dried herbs equal about one-half the volume of fresh herbs. One cup fresh equals $^1/_4$ to $^1/_2$ cup dry. Try to use distilled water or bottled water rather than highly fluoridated tap water.

Here are some of the basics: (refer to herbal preparations and delivery methods on pg. 11 for other delivery mediums.)

A cosmetic ointment, cream or salve is an herbal combination crisped in a solid fat, strained, beaten until cold and stored away for use.

An unguent is a type of healing ointment made with a liquid fat source and solidified with wax. About an ounce of finely crushed herbs is simmered with an ounce of white wine until the wine boils off. The mixture is then cooled, the herbal solids are strained off, and 1 oz. of melted wax is added. Beat with a wooden spoon until the mixture is cold.

A mellite is a cosmetic infusion made with honey. Mix 1 oz. of herbs and about 10 oz. of honey for 15 to 20 minutes in tepid water. Then, strain out the herbs and store the mellite away in a cool, dark, dry place.

Here are some of the tools and supplies you'll need.

> beeswax
> funnels
> enamel pots and bowls
> measuring cups, spoons
> jars
> containers for creams and liquids
> wire sieve
> small food scale
> apple cider vinegar
> witch hazel
> eggs
> tincture of benzoin (purchase from the drug store)
> cheesecloth
> wooden spoon
> wire whip or egg beater
> herbs from a garden or the health food store

For Beautiful, Healthy Eyes

Your eyes can become a victim of pollutants and chemical contaminants quicker and with more unhappy consequences than almost any other part of your body. At the very least, they react with redness, and irritation in an unhealthy environment. I believe the most natural, gentlest way is the best way for "looking" at eye problems.

❧Herbal compounds can make your eyes clear and bright.
• A mild, strained rosemary leaf tea is gentle, works right away, and makes your eyes clear and sparkly. (I find it far more effective than Visine.)
• Use strained eyebright tea as an eyewash, or an eyebright tea combination that includes plantain leaves, bilberry leaves, passionflowers, rosemary and goldenseal leaves. These herbs are available loose from a good health food store - use about 2 pinches of eyebright to 1 pinch of each of the other herbs. Steep in 2 cups of water for 10 minutes, strain and cool before using. Makes enough for 6 or 7 eyewashes. Store covered in the fridge.
• Use an elderberry tea on a warm compress and apply to closed eyelids to brighten.

❧Herbal compounds can relieve red, tired, puffy eyes.
• Place wet black tea bags over closed eyes for 10 minutes, or put a few drops of witch hazel on cotton pads, chill in the fridge for about 20 minutes and place over closed eyes.
• Use strained red raspberry tea or Japanese green tea for bloodshot eyes.
• Drop 10 to 15 drops of passionflower extract into warm water; then dip cotton balls in the liquid and use on closed eyelids to relieve fatigue.
• Make a rosebud/rose petal tea and use as an eyewash.

❧Herbs can relieve "computor eyes" that are strained, jumpy and irritated:
• Apply wet green tea bags or cucumber slices to closed eyelids for 10 minutes.
• Use a diluted, plain aloe vera juice eyewash.
• Strain chamomile tea; then dip a clean cloth in the liquid and place as a compress on closes eyelids to ease strain..

❧For eye stress (sparks of light or colors when your eyes are closed indicate stressed eyes):
• Soak dried sea vegetables like kelp, kombu or wakame in hot water for 20 minutes, then saturate cotton balls with strained liquid and press gently on closed eyes (especially if vision is blurred).
• Bathe eyes in cool witch hazel or chamomile tea.
• Bathe eyes in ice water.
• Take ginkgo biloba to support healthy circulation to the eye area.
• Squeeze eyes tight shut for a few seconds to increase circulation to the area.
• Press points under the eyebrows; then points under the

❧Herbs can help relieve red, infected eyelids:
• Soak goldenseal root powder and crushed fennel seed in boric acid for 24 hours. Strain and use as an eye bath twice a day.
• Drop 10 to 15 drops of a goldenseal/echinacea extract into warm water. Let cool for 5 minutes and use as an eye bath.
• Soak chamomile and elder flowers in rosewater; then dip cotton balls in the liquid and use on closed eyelids to reduce inflammation.
• Use a diluted, plain aloe vera juice eyewash.

❧Herbs can help relieve eye inflammation, swelling and styes:
• Use tansy tea as a compress to relieve irritation.
• Use wormwood tea on a cloth compress applied to closed eyelids.

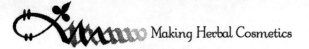

◈}Herbs can help dry eyes:
  • Use a diluted, plain aloe vera juice eyewash.

◈}Herbs can help watering eyes:
  • Use cotton balls dipped in strained fennel tea as an eyewash.

◈}For ongoing eye health:
  • Liver health is critical to eyesight health - use milk thistle seed extract for long term liver health; use weekly dandelion root tea for gallbladder, spleen and fat digestion help.

  Eyebrow beauty tip.....
  • Make a thick tea of fresh sage leaves from your herb garden. Rub onto your eyebrows as often as as needed to darken brows without a "pencilled" look.

For A Beautiful Smile

Plaque-causing bacteria begins to form, and damage teeth and gums within 12 hours after a meal. (Sugary foods cause plaque formation much quicker.) Brush at least twice a day and floss or water-pik before going to bed. (Floss after every meal if you have tooth tartar build-up.) Fluoride build-up in areas with highly fluoridated water and fluoride toothpaste has been linked to skin eruptions and thyroid problems in some fluoride-sensitive people. Natural mouth care should be considered for these people.

◈}For clean sweet breath:
• Use to keep breath sweet and clean, drink a cool infusion of rosemary petals in distilled water in the morning and evening.

◈}For abscessed, infected teeth:
  • Rub anti-bacterial tea tree oil on teeth and gums daily, and use as a daily gargle.
  • Use garlic compresses to draw out the infection.
  • Use clove oil compresses on infected area.
  • Apply myrrh extract drops twice daily directly on infected area.
  • Use sage tea as a mouthwash morning and evening to reduce inflammation.
  • Rinse mouth daily with acidophilus powder dissolved in water.

◈}For dull, dingy teeth:
  • Use a peelu herb (Ayurvedic) toothpaste with natural chlorine and vitamin C to whiten teeth, remove tartar and control plaque.
  • Mix equal parts cream of tartar (or baking soda) and sea salt to remove tooth tarter.

◈}For mouth (canker/cold) sores:
  • Rinse mouth regularly during the day with red raspberry, white oak or camomile tea to help heal mouth sores.
  • If sores are menstrual cycle related, drink 2 cups of burdock tea daily during pre-period days to balance hormones.

◈}For salivary duct stones:
  • Rinse mouth with equal parts goldenseal root tea and white oak bark tea to reduce pain, swelling and bleeding.
  • Rinse mouth with a solution of ginger root and water, and apply ginger root compresses to affected area.

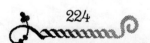

Make your own natural, non-abrasive toothpaste:
- Soak 1 tsp. dried Irish moss in a cup of water til soft in a saucepan, then bring to a gentle boil and let simmer for about 10 minutes. Add a teaspoon of sea salt, a teaspoon of baking soda or papain powder and blend well. Blend in 3 drops of liquid chlorophyll, and 3 drops of essential peppermint or cinnamon oil (from the health food store) for flavor. A little on your brush goes a long way.

Make your own natural cinnamon, anise or mint mouthwash concentrate:
- Steep 4 heaping tsp. anise seed, 2 heaping tsp. star anise, 2 heaping tsp. licorice root pieces, 1 heaping tsp. whole cloves, 1 heaping tsp. chopped cinnamon bark in 8-oz. vodka for 2 weeks. Add 3 drops essential cinnamon, mint or anise oil (from the health food store). Add 1 tsp. of the concentrate to a small glass of water and rinse the mouth to freshen breath. No need to refrigerate.
- Or add 3 to 4 drops tea tree oil to a small glass of water and rinse mouth.

Out to lunch (or breakfast or dinner) without a toothbrush or mouthwash?
- Order strawberries at the end of the meal, cut them in half and rub the halves on your teeth and gums - then swallow the strawberries. Your mouth will look and feel fresh for hours.
- Or order your water with a lemon twist, and use the twist to scrub your teeth after a meal - a sure-fire natural breath and mouth freshener.

For ongoing tooth and mouth health:
- Use horsetail herb extract drops in water as a mouthwash to build tooth enamel.
- Use ginseng/licorice extract drops in water as a daily mouthwash to inhibit bacteria formation that cause cavities, and to better handle harmful sugars in the body so cavities don't form.
- Dandelion root tea or parsley/sage tea are specific teas for tooth health.

Lips and smile beauty tip.....
- Make your own natural, moisturizing lip gloss. Gently heat 6 tablespoons of sweet almond or sesame oil with 1 tablespoon of beeswax til just melted. Remove from heat and whisk in 2 teaspoons of honey, and 12 drops of your favorite essential oil for flavor (cinnamon, peppermint or anise oil are good choices). I use this gloss without color as a good lip conditioner *under* my lipstick, or as a moisturizing finisher on top of lipstick. If you want a colored gloss, blend in about $\frac{1}{2}$ tube of your favorite all natural, lipstick from the health food store, or add a few drops of beet juice while gloss is still hot. Whisk until cool to prevent separation. Add flavor oil after the gloss has cooled.
- Use the same method to make a healing lip balm for dry, chapped lips. Reduce the amount of almond or sesame oil to 5 tablespoons, and add healing agents of $1\frac{1}{2}$ teaspoons *each* St. John's wort oil and calendula oil mixture, and 2 teaspoons aloe vera gel. I like essential oil of vanilla for flavor.

For Shiny, Healthy Beautiful Hair

Herbal hair care products are being enthusiastically rediscovered all over America. Herbs are ane excellent choice for hair problems, because hair problems are never isolated conditions, and always the result of more basic body imbalances.Herbs can act as both nourishment and toners for healthy hair. Nutrition is the real secret to healthy hair. In fact, changes in hair are often the first indication of nutritional (especially mineral) deficiencies. Herbs are good sources of absorbable minerals. Your hair itself can tell you its state of health. In damaged or dry hair, the cuticle shingles are broken and create gaps that make hair porous and dull. In healthy hair, the cell walls of the hair cuticle lie flat like shingles, leaving hair soft and shiny.

Regardless of your hair type, wash hair in warm, not hot water. Rinse in cool water for scalp circulation. Condition regularly. Use alcohol-free gels as style holders, not hair sprays that damage hair and pollute the atmosphere. Remember that sunlight helps hair grow, but too much dries and damages. Be careful.

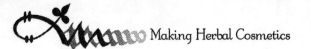

❧Herbal compounds can add luster, thickness and sheen to all types of hair and all hair shades:
- Natural silica is a source of hair strength. Consider horsetail extract drops daily.
- Adrenal gland health is involved with hair color retention - especially in preventing graying. Consider herbal combination capsules or extracts that include licorice root, sarsaparilla root, sea plants and ginger root.
- Sea plants, with their wealth of iodine and potassium, are excellent both internally and externally for hair health. Take kelp tablets daily, and rinse hair with a kelp tea infusion after shampooing.
- Take 2 TBS. daily of fresh rosemary sprigs steeped in wine for enhanced uptake of minerals.
- Essential fatty acids are imperative to hair health and growth. Consider evening primrose oil or borage oil capsules, about 500mg. daily.
- Drink burdock tea regularly to cleanse the system and to give the hair more shine.
- Rinse the hair with fresh nettles tea to add more luster to hair.

❧Herbal compounds can intensify and enhance hair color:
- To add sheen to dark hair, apply a simple tea of sage or rosemary to hair after shampooing.
- Use a chamomile/lemon tea rinse to lighten and add golden highlights to mousy, brown hair.
- Add strong rosemary tea to hair rinses, to strengthen hair, add shine and prevent dandruff.
- Use apple cider vinegar to clean hair product build-up from hair and for pH balance.
- Use nettles/sage/rosemary to darken and shine brown hair.
- To darken graying hair that hasn't been chemically treated with commercial hair color, add one handful **each** dried sage, dried nettles, dried rosemary, cut black walnut hulls, chopped dry dulse and black loose tea (any kind) to 2 qts. boiling water. Immediately remove from heat, cover and let steep for 4 hours. Add 1 tablespoon wheat germ oil. Refrigerate for three weeks. Strain and put liquid into bottles.
- A marigold/lemon rinse for summer blonde highlights: Mix 1 cup of marigold flowers, 1 cup of chamomile flowers, $^1/_2$ cup lemon peel, $^1/_2$ cup cut burdock root. Heat two quarts apple cider vinegar for body and shine and pour over herbs in a gallon jar. Store in a cool garage or basement, shaking every 24 hours for 7 days. Place a double piece of cheesecloth on top of the jar and strain off vinegar. Put luiquid in bottles, and use 2 to 3 tablespoons in a cup of warm water as a hair rinse several times a week during the summer. Leave on 2 minutes, then rinse. I have used this rinse for many years; it looks best (blonde, not brassy) on non-chemically treated hair.

What about henna? Is it a good choice for hair coloring? Henna is a natural non-carcinogenic plant used for centuries for nail, body and hair coloring. It offers hair extra body while it colors - often dramatically. Henna works best on thin, light porous hair.
- To add gold highlights to darker hair, add chamomile powder to henna hair color.

What about hair treatments for dry, damaged hair, or dandruff? Pityriasis (simple dandruff) is a dry skin problem, and can usually be controlled with a better diet, cleansing and brushing. Seborrheic dandruff appears as dry, flaky particles of skin in the hair. While it looks like a dry skin condition, it is actually the opposite - too much oil is being produced, clogging the highly active sebaceous glands. It can result from a variety of conditions, both physical and emotional, appearing when skin cells turn over at a faster rate than normal and break away in large flakes into the hair. It tends to occur more in the winter and fall months. Diet improvement and herbal balancers are the key to long term dandruff control for either kind of dandruff. Avoid commercial ointments that often do more harm than good by clogging sebaceous glands.
- Use jojoba oil for damaged, brittle and overprocessed hair (men)
- Use wheat germ oil as a hot oil treatment for overprocessed hair. (women)
- Wet hair and blot; mix 2 TBS. mayonnaise and 2 TBS. olive oil - apply to hair and wrap in a towel for 30 minutes, rinse and shampoo.
- Mix 2 TBS. yogurt and 1 egg, apply to hair, wrap in a towel for 30 minutes, rinse and shampoo, or mix an egg yolk in your second shampoo to add bounce.

 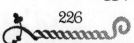

• *Essential fatty acids help your body fight dandruff.* Take evening primrose oil capsules 1000mg daily and rub your scalp with flax oil before you shampoo for 1 month.

• *Effective herbal oil scalp treatments work for dandruff:* Mix the juice from fresh grated ginger with an equal amount of sesame oil. Rub on scalp at night. rinse in the morning. Use for 1 week.

• Or steep bay leaves, rosemary sprigs in olive oil until fragrant. Rub on scalp before shampooing. Leave on 30 minutes as an effective hot oil treatment and shampoo out. (women)

• Or massage jojoba or rosemary oil into scalp. Leave on 1 hour. Shampoo out. (men)

• *Boost your shampoo or conditioner with herbal dandruff fighters:* Add a few drops of grapefruit seed extract to shampoo and use daily.

• Add a few drops of tea tree oil to shampoo.

• Use olive oil or aloe vera based shampoos (women), jojoba shampoo (men)

• Rinse the hair with cider vinegar and water after every shampoo to keep sebum deposits from clogging pores. Or use a natural shampoo specifically designed to remove build-up.

• Rinse hair in nettles or red clover tea.

• Rinse hair in chamomile or comfrey tea if there is also scalp irritation.

What about hair loss and thinning hair? Over 30 million men and 20 million women have thinning or falling hair. Although androgenic alopecia is hereditary and not easily reversible, there are other factors, both internal and external, involved in most hair loss that can indeed result in hair improvement, thickness and regrowth. Hair health depends on blood supply, circulation and nutrition. Your therapy choice must be vigorously followed. Occasional therapy has little or no effect. Two months is usually the minimum for really noticeable growth. External factors that cause hair loss are tight hairstyles and curlers, hot rollers, and chemicals for perming and straightening. Discontinue commercial hair coloring and hair dryers.

• Drink white sage or horsetail tea to stimulate hair growth when hair is thin.

• Take fo-ti root tea daily for 3 months.

• Rinse hair with sea water or apple cider vinegar to thicken thinning hair.

• Use sage, cedarwood, rosemary, or thyme aromatherapy oils for falling hair.

What about male pattern baldness? Male pattern baldness is a condition emanating from testosterone production; treat your prostate to treat your hair loss; herbal prostate remedies include saw palmetto, potency wood, panax ginseng and pygeum africanum.

• Phyto-estrogen and hormone balancing can help hair loss in women: an internal capsule combination with herbs like Black cohosh, dong quai, or burdock rt. has shown promise.

Head circulation is a big key to hair growth.

• Massage the scalp every morning for 3 minutes.

• Brush dry hair well for 5 minutes daily.

• Rinse for several minutes with alternating hot and cold shower water.

• Use a slant board once a week for 15 minutes.

• Use herbal scalp rubs: apply warm ginger tea to scalp and rub, leave on 15 minutes.

• Rub scalp with cayenne extract before shampooing; leave on for 30 minutes.

• Drink Japanese green tea to keep your system metabolically active.

For Beautiful nails:

Nails can be very useful as an "early warning system" in diagnosing illness and evaluating health. If the eyes are the "windows of the soul", the nails are considered the "windows of the body". They are one of the last body areas to receive the nutrients carried by the blood, and show signs of trouble before other better-nourished tissues do. Healthy nails are pink, smooth and shiny. Changes in their shape, color and texture signal the presence of disease in the body. Disorders of the blood, glands, circulation and organs as well as nutritional deficiencies all show up in nail conditions. Good nutrition and a well-balanced diet are the keys for nail health. Give your program at least a month to show improvement. We have found that nothing seems to happen for 3 weeks, and then noticeable changes appear in the 4th week.If your problem is a mineral deficiency; herb and plant minerals are the best choice for supplementation. Note: nail enamels and supplies are among the most toxic environmental polluters. Fake nails or tips add weight to the nails and prevent them from thickening naturally. Nail color dyes penetrate the skin, often causing allergic reactions. If you do polish your nails, don't keep them constantly polished. Allow them to breathe at least 1 day a week.

❧Herbal compounds can strengthen nails:
• Soak nails in a dulse/oatstraw infusion, or pau d'arco tea and take an herbal calcium combination that includes oatstraw, watercress, dandelion and rosemary internally for a month.
• Mix a mud face mask in water and use as a nail soak.
• Silica is a key nail strengthener, drink horsetail tea or take horsetail extract 3x daily.

What about toenail or fingernail fungus infection? Can herbs help?
• Apply a honey/garlic paste to impede bacterial growth.
• Make an antifungal footbath or fingernail soak with tea tree oil, marshmallow root and black walnut extract; soak for 20 minutes daily. Also apply tea tree oil to infected areas 3 to 4x daily.
• Use a grapefruit seed extract solution - 3 to 4 drops in 8 oz. water until fungus clears.
• Use a topical myrrh and goldenseal fungus extract spray.
• *On cleaned nails,* use 1 part diluted DMSO solution mixed with $\frac{1}{2}$ part oregano oil and $\frac{1}{2}$ part olive oil. Use daily for 2 weeks.
• For nail infection, use a poultice of green clay to draw out harmful bacteria.

❧Herbal compounds can improve the color and texture of your nails:
• For brittle nails, massage castor oil onto your nails regularly for a month.
• For discolored nails, rub fresh lemon juice on nail base. Take extra chewable papaya enzymes.
• For weak nails, soak daily for 5 minutes in warm olive oil or cider vinegar.
• For splitting nails: take 2 TBS. brewer's yeast, or 2 teasp. wheat germ oil daily for a month.
• To improve color and texture, mix honey, avocado, egg yolk and a pinch of salt, rub onto nails and leave on for 30 minutes. Rinse.
• To relieve inflammation and pain from ingrown nails or hangnails, use a mixture of cranesbill and water into a paste and apply.

Natural Nail Beauty tips......
• For a manicured look without polish: apply a beeswax spread on the nails and buff to a shine, leaves nails naturally beautiful.
• To tint nails naturally: make a thin paste of red henna powder and water. Paint on and let dry in the sun. Rinse off for pretty pink nails without chipping.

For Softer, Healthier Feet
Our feet reflect the story of our physical lives..... active, barefoot, outdoors, temperate climate, or sedentary, indoors, well-shod, cold climate, young, middle or elder years, etc. Your feet have to deal with our environment first, and they take a lot of abuse and they have to work hard. Taking good care of your feet naturally can help your life from the "ground up."

(For best results, soak your feet in warm water before using any of the recommended topical applications)

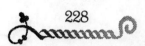

❧Herbal compounds can effectively address foot problems:
- **For bunions,** thickened layers old skin on the sides of the big toe, apply a raw garlic poultice.
- **For callouses,** thickening of the foot skin formed at the site of continual pressure, rub green papaya skins or dandelion stem juice directly on area; also try castor oil packs.
- **For corns,** thickening of the skin, hard or soft, on the feet, apply olive oil compresses.
- **For heel pain** (usually a thyroid-related problem), take essential fatty acids from evening primrose oil or Omega-3 rich flax oil, horsetail extract twice daily, sprinkle 2 tablespoons of dry sea vegetables over your daily soup or salad.
- **For plantar warts,** painful, sometimes ingrowing, warts on the sole of the foot, soak feet in the hottest water you can stand for as long as you can, then spray grapefruit seed extract spray directly on a wart twice daily. Removal takes about 2 months.
- **For bone spurs,** a horny out growth, usually on the heel, often the result of acid/alkaline imbalance in the body. Spurs may accompany rheumatoid arthritis, because individuals with this disease are deficient in stomach acid and normal enzyme production. Apply DMSO for pain and to help dissolve crystalline deposits. Or mix a solution of vitamin C crystals and water to a paste. Apply to spur and secure with tape. Leave on all day for several weeks to see improvement.

❧Herbal compounds can effectively address athlete's foot and foot fungus:
- Bathe the feet in a black tea/ pau d'arco combination.
- Apply diluted oregano oil directly to affected areas.
- Use tea tree oil (diluted) as a potent antifungal to combat foot fungus.
- Apply a honey/garlic poultice to impede bacterial growth or make an antifungal footbath with tea tree oil, marshmallow root and black walnut extract and soak feet for 20 minutes daily.
- Apply a flaxseed/garlic powder paste and leave on overnight for a week. (men)
- Soak feet in goldenseal tea every night for a week.

❧Herbal compounds can make your feet more beautiful:
- To soften cracked, dry feet, apply pure aloe vera gel regularly.
- Make a footbath with 2 handfuls of comfrey root to 1 gal. warm water. Soak feet 15 minutes.
- For chapped feet, infuse a handful of calendula flowers into a cup of aloe gel. Apply nightly.
- To rub off dead skin, use a mix of lemon juice and sea salt, and use a pumice stone in your daily shower to remove dead skin. Rub your feet as you dry off before applying your cream.
- To soothe tired feet, use a sage, chamomile or peppermint foot bath.
- For swollen feet, apply a *capsaicin* ointment or bathe them in potato water.
- To improve circulation in the feet and legs, take ginkgo biloba extract drops twice daily, and make a mix of 6 TBS. sesame oil, add a pinch each of dry mustard, cinnamon and cayenne pepper, two chili pods, and three pinches of peppercorns in a small pan. Simmer on low for about an hour, then strain and apply.

For Healthy, Beautiful Soft Skin:

Beautiful skin is more than skin deep. Our skin is the essence of renewable nature...it sloughs off old, dying cells every day, and gives a chance for a new start. The skin is the body's largest organ of nourishment and elimination. The skin's protective acid mantle inhibits the growth of disease - causing bacteria. Skin mirrors our emotional state and our hormone balance, too, and it's a sure sign of poor nutrition. (Allergies show up first on the skin.) Skin problems reflect a stressed lifestyle almost immediately. Relaxation and improved food nutrition show quickly in skin health and beauty. Herbs are great for the skin - packed with absorbable minerals, anti-oxidants, essential fatty acids and bioflavonoids, to cleanse, hydrate, heal, alkalize and balance glands and hormones. Herbal nutrients nourish feed the skin and improve nutrition deficiencies that show up in the skin.

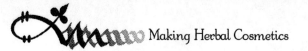
Herbal compounds can help your skin look younger, softer or more beautiful:
- To open the pores and release blackheads and dirt, use a warm chamomile flower steam.
- To clean clogged pores of make up and environmental pollutant residues, and balance skin pH make a steam tea of yarrow flowers, sage leaves, rosemary sprigs and peppermint.
- To soften a rough complexion, apply aloe vera gel regularly.
- To activate a sallow complexion, add rosemary as a stimulating tonic to a facial steam.
- For skin inflammations, apply a chickweed poultice and leave on for 20 minutes.
- To control oily skin, use witch hazel as a face splash.
- Lavender reduces puffiness.
- Rose hips tea/ lemon juice blend cleanse and balance pH..
- Sandalwood or rose essential aromatherapy oils and chamomile tea can smooth and hydrate.
- Apply a drop of lavender or lemon grass to spotty skin several times daily.
- For skin clarity, make a skin wash with 1-oz. *each* licorice root, burdock root, rosemary, rose hips, fennel seed, chamomile, sage, dandelion leaf and sarsaparilla root; use nightly for a month.
- To neutralize over acid skin, rub the face with the insides of papaya and cucumber skins.
- For unsightly warts, cover the wart with a small section of a very soft, black/brown banana (inside down). Leave on for 24 hours. Repeat the process until wart is gone. Or make a mix of lemon juice, sea salt, onion juice and wheat germ oil to the wart regularly for 1 month. Or apply papaya skin to the wart for enzyme therapy. Or apply tea tree oil or a paste of garlic cloves directly to wart and cover with a bandaid.

Herbal compounds can give you a natural face lift. Apply, leave on 30 minutes and rinse off.
- Yogurt/lemon juice to balance skin pH.
- Oatmeal to exfoliate dead skin cells gently.
- To tighten wrinkles, rub the face with the insides of fresh papaya skins for enzyme therapy.
- Or pat on a mix of whipped egg white and cream. Let dry 20 minutes. Rinse off.

Make your own nourishing make-up removers: Use plain sesame oil, especially for eye make-up. (Your eyes will look soft and dewy in the morning.) Or mix in a dark bottle, apricot, avocado, almond and sesame oils in a dark bottle. It's good for all skin types and makes your skin feel wonderful.

Feed your skin essential fatty acids; take evening primrose oil, two 500mg capsules daily, eat salmon once a week, and use flax seed oil to clean face and neck of make-up and residues each night.

Make a gentle, balancing herbal mask once a week. Blend 1 teaspoon *each* of the following herbal powders into French white clay (available at your health food store) - chamomile, calendula, lemon peel, eucalyptus, rosemary, spearmint and fennel. Mix 1 TB. masque powder to a paste with water; leave on for 15 minutes until dry; follow with a blend of aloe vera gel and wheat germ oil.

Make your own exfoliating skin treatments for glowing skin:
- Use aloofa sponge, ayate cloth, or dry skin brush.
- Rub your face with the insides of cucumber or papaya skins.
- Blend honey, crushed almonds and oatmeal into a scrub.
- Make a body glow with sea salt, lemon peel powder, aloe vera powder and almond oil.

Herbal compounds can help control and prevent acne outbreaks:
Teenage acne, a hormone-related problem of the action of male testosterone on the sebaceous skin glands, is extremely common (4 out of 5 teenagers develope it). Adult acne is now more prevalent - a clear sign of our modern poor diet. Whiteheads (comedones) are plugs of oil and dead skin cells under the surface of the skin that block oil from flowing freely to the skin surface. They can either turn into blackheads (open comedones) when they reach the surface of the skin and are exposed to the air, or in a more severe condition, can spread under the skin, rupture and expand the inflammation.

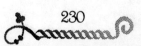

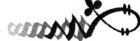

• To help control acne and blackheads, rub lemon juice on affected areas.

• To stop the spread of infected acne pustules, apply diluted tea tree oil directly to blemishes or apply a goldenseal /myrrh solution; or a propolis tincture; or *stevia extract* drops; or calendula gel to the affected area. Pat high-sulfur aloe vera juice directly on acne blemishes.

• To reduce acne scarring, place fresh pineapple slices on the affected area for enzyme therapy.

• To bring acne pustules to a head, apply a white clay toning mask, and let dry 2x daily then use once a week until pustules are clear.

• Prick open 4 evening primrose oil capsules. Blend with a little licorice root powder and a little siberian ginseng powder. Pat on acne areas.

• Relieve inflammation and infection from acne with a face wash of 15 drops goldenseal root/ echinacea root extract in water, 4x daily for one week.

⛶Herbal compounds can make aging skin look younger:

Age spots are an external sign of harmful waste accumulation (particularly in the liver, which shows up as sallow skin), and a result of free radical damage in skin cells. Lipofuscin is the age-related skin pigment that oxidizes to actually appear as the brown age spots. Wrinkles, lines and rough skin texture are a sign of poor dermal collagen health. The look of aging skin occurs when collagen becomes hard and crosslinked with neighboring collagen fibers, preventing it from holding water and maintaining elasticity. It collapses on itself, forming a kind of fish net below the surface of the skin, seen as wrinkles. The cause of the crosslinking is free radical formation. Free radical attack the skin cell membranes, collagen and elastin proteins, resulting in wrinkles, dry skin and sagging skin contours. Smoking is the worst skin wrinkler. Tar and nicotine deprive skin of oxygen, causing shriveling and wrinkling.

• **For anti-wrinkle effects**, estrogen is a key to tissue building, working with collagen to renew skin elasticity. **Effective phyto-estrogen herbs** include dong quai, licorice root, ashwagandha, damiana, sarsaparilla root, suma and panax ginseng.

• Egg whites can tighten wrinkled, sagging skin.

• Make your own AHA wrinkle treatment with a mix of honey and red wine. Smooth on; leave on 20 minutes. Rinse off.

• Apply evening primrose oil, 4 pricked open capsules daily for wrinkled eye skin.

• Steam face with a mix of hydrating aromatherapy herbs - chamomile flowers, eucalyptus leaves, rosemary and nettles.

• Make your own anti-wrinkle facial. Use one teasp. *each*, vegetable glycerine, rosewater and witch hazel with 3 TBS. honey. Leave on 15-20 minutes.

• Use sunscreen regularly - SPF 15 or greater. Even minimal sun exposure is enough to sustain spots. **Sunscreens help prevent age spots from darkening.**

• To reduce spider veins on the face, use a calendula flower infusion gel.

• For varicose veins, apply hot sage/ calendula compresses, use an oak bark decoction as a compress to relieve pain. For extended veins, apply fresh wood sorrel leaves to the affected area; for large, knotted veins, use hot compresses of tansy tea.

• **A seaweed bath can detoxify and cleanse your skin, and release cellulite deposits.** Dry brush the body before and brush during the bath for greatest release of wastes. You can use any mix of kelps, seaweeds and sea grasses to total 8 to 10 cups. All sea plants stimulate circulation, potentiate lipolysis and release toxins in the skin.

There are two ways to take a seaweed bath:

1) Draw very hot water in a tub to half full. Put seaweed into the tub and steep for 5-10 minutes and the water is cool enough to enter. or 2) Make a strong infusion in a large pot on the stove, soak the seaweeds for 10-15 minutes before straining and adding to hot bathwater.

Soak in the deep bath, covering the body for 30-45 minutes. Rub the body with the seaweed solids. If overheated, sit on the edge of the tub for a couple of minutes. The seaweed's gel mantle will often times be attracted to and adhere to the body. When the gel coating disappears, the therapeutic process of the bath is finished. Rub the body with the rough seaweeds to exfoliate skin for best results.

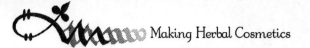

❧Herbal compounds can help skin infections:

Dermatitis is an external skin condition caused by a systemic reaction to an allergen - usually in cosmetics, jewelry metals, drugs or topical medications. It can also be the body's reaction to emotional stress, or to a severe deficiency of essential fatty acids. Its systemic nature means that it can and does spread, and can become quite severe. Inflamed skin with itch and rash symptoms can come from a variety of causes, ranging from systemic to emotional stress, from food allergies to an infective reaction to cosmetics. Investigate the cause of your symptoms thoroughly. Rashes are often symptoms of common food allergens, so avoid foods such as milk and wheat products, eggs, meats (that usually have nitrates), refined grains and sugars, and fried foods.

• For skin infections, apply una da gato tea or a topical gel with una da gato. Anti-Bio™ gel, especially if skin is infected (especially good for ringworm type infections).

• For skin rashes and redness, apply a tea of 1-oz. *each* licorice root, burdock root, rosemary, rose hips, fennel seed, chamomile, sage, dandelion leaf and sarsaparilla root; use nightly for a week as a skin wash.

• For histamine-type rashes on the stomach, chest or arms, take an herbal anti-histamine formula with herbs like ephedra, marshmallow root, bee pollen. white pine bark, goldenseal root, mullein and parsley root. Dip cotton balls in the tea and apply as well.

• For rough skin, itchiness, sores and inflammation, apply an oatmeal paste to the skin to neutralize topical irritants, then apply an itchy skin tea made from equal parts dandelion root, nettles, burdock root, echinacea root, kelp, yellow dock root, and chamomile. Avoid detergents on the skin. Use mild castile soap. Avoid perfumed cosmetics

• For abrasions,mix lavender essential oil and aloe vera gel and apply, or apply fresh comfrey leaf compresses.

• Use a papaya peel to smooth skin after inflammation is gone.

❧Herbal compounds can help damaged skin (scars, sunburn, stretch marks):

For every sunburn you get that blisters, you double your risk of skin cancer. Even on a cloudy day, 80% of the sun's harmful rays come through. Sun damage is cumulative over a lifetime. Moderation is the key. Sunlight can help you avoid breast and prostate cancer (new research shows that a lack of protective vitamin D provided by sunlight may be involved). People who get almost no sun exposure are at a higher risk for melanoma than those who get regular, moderate early morning sunshine. Practice good sun sense so that you don't fry now and pay later.

• For sun damaged skin: apply cold compresses, or take a cool bath immediately (do not use soap or hot water) Effective herbal topicals for sunburns include chamomile, tea tree oil, a green clay poultice, calendula gel.

• Apply yogurt, honey, black tea, or vinegar to burned areas. Apply grated apple to eyelids for immediate relief.

• Use a ginseng based skin repair gel, especially for burned or scarred skin.

• For scars, massage the scar well when rubbing in any topical applications, to bring up healthy circulation and skin tone. Effective herbal topicals for scarring include: aloe vera gel, calendula gel, gotu kola, and echinacea cream.

• Phyto-estrogen herbs like dong quai, vitex, black cohosh help stimulate better estrogen supply for scar skin healing.

• Try a massage with sesame oil, wheat germ oil or avocado oil. Eat avocados for skin elasticity.

• For stretch marks, massage aloe vera gel mixed with vitamin E oil on stomach. Some women have had success with AHAs. Or use a wheat germ, vitamin E, comfrey leaf and honey poultice.

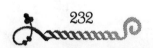

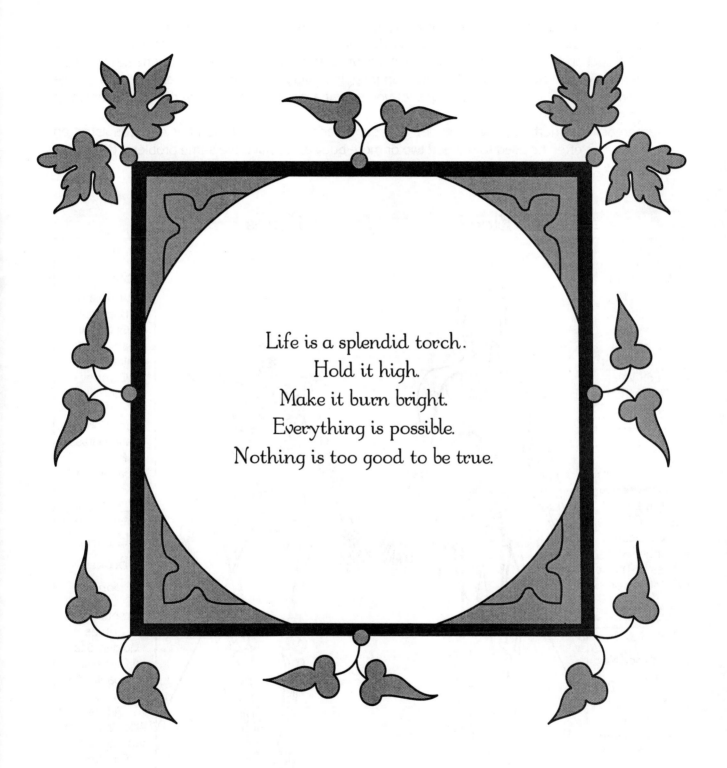

Life is a splendid torch.
Hold it high.
Make it burn bright.
Everything is possible.
Nothing is too good to be true.

HERBS & ANATOMY

Which Part Of Your Body Do You Want To Work On?

Herbal medicines can work for every body system, every body function and every body structure. There are even herbs for the mind and spirit. The ANATOMY & HERB CHARTS in this section graphically show just how all-encompassing herbs can be for your health and well-being. Herbs can also be quite specific; you can pinpoint a very small body area as easily as a large one to work on. The charts on these pages let you see at a glance just which herbs to use for which body part or system.

Remember that herbs are very gentle, very subtle and very safe. A number of herbs listed on these charts can often be used together if two or more body areas have the same problem. Keep your combinations simple and direct if you decide to use more than one herb.

Blood

Bones

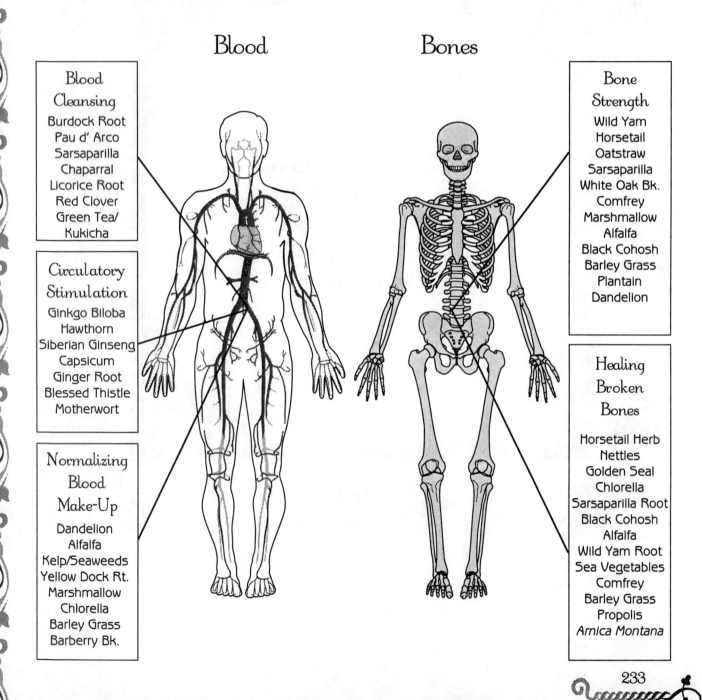

Blood
Cleansing
Burdock Root
Pau d' Arco
Sarsaparilla
Chaparral
Licorice Root
Red Clover
Green Tea/
Kukicha

Circulatory
Stimulation
Ginkgo Biloba
Hawthorn
Siberian Ginseng
Capsicum
Ginger Root
Blessed Thistle
Motherwort

Normalizing
Blood
Make-Up
Dandelion
Alfalfa
Kelp/Seaweeds
Yellow Dock Rt.
Marshmallow
Chlorella
Barley Grass
Barberry Bk.

Bone
Strength
Wild Yam
Horsetail
Oatstraw
Sarsaparilla
White Oak Bk.
Comfrey
Marshmallow
Alfalfa
Black Cohosh
Barley Grass
Plantain
Dandelion

Healing
Broken
Bones
Horsetail Herb
Nettles
Golden Seal
Chlorella
Sarsaparilla Root
Black Cohosh
Alfalfa
Wild Yam Root
Sea Vegetables
Comfrey
Barley Grass
Propolis
Arnica Montana

Muscles & Tendons

Nerves

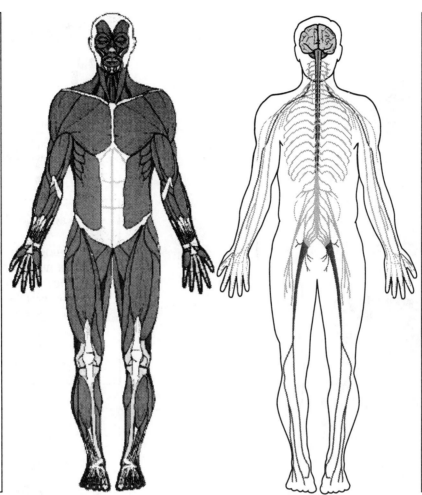

Muscle Tone

Sarsaparilla Root
Siberian Ginseng
Bee Pollen
Royal Jelly
Barley Grass
Suma
Sea Vegetables
Rosemary
Saw Palmetto
Damiana
Licorice Root
Alfalfa
Gotu Kola
Fo-Ti
Panax Ginseng
Scullcap
Horsetail Herb
Rose hips
Spirulina
Evening Primrose
Chlorella
Bilberry
Wild Yam
Yarrow
Ginger Root
Capsicum

Nerve Health

Gotu Kola
Scullcap
Oatstraw
Lady Slipper
Kava Kava
Black Cohosh
Chamomile
Rosemary
Siberian Ginseng
Barley Grass
Catnip
Eur. Mistletoe
Lobelia
Barley Grass
Dandelion
Pau d'Arco
Evening Primrose
Peppermint
Reishi Mushroom
Wood Betony
Black Haw
Nettles
Parsley Rt. & Lf.
Bee Pollen
Valerian Root
Watercress

CardioPulmonary System

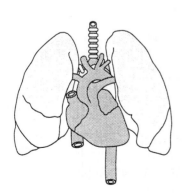

Cardio-Pulmonary Health

Hawthorn
Siberian Ginseng
Garlic
Capsicum
Sea Vegetables
Barley Grass
Chlorella
Bilberry
Ginger Root
Ginkgo Biloba
Motherwort
Evening Primrose
Scullcap

Respiratory System

Respiratory & Breathing Health

Marshmallow
Mullein
Ephedra
Fenugreek
Sarsaparilla Root
Pau d' Arco
Echinacea
Aloe Vera Juice
Royal Jelly
Lobelia
Barley Grass
Pleurisy Root
Comfrey

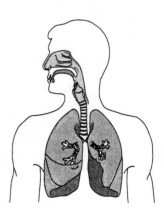

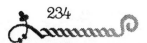

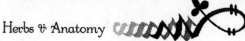

Digestive System

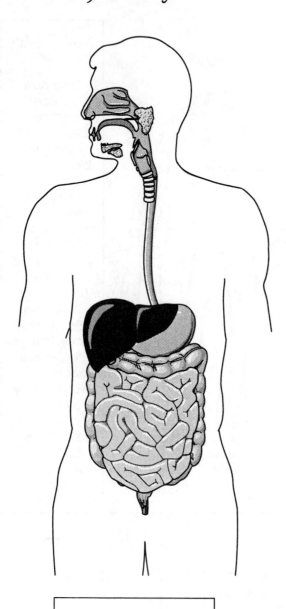

Digestive Health

Ginkgo Biloba
Fenugreek Seed
Barley Grass
Golden Seal Root
Garlic
Ginger Root
Alfalfa
Licorice Root
Fennel Seed
Catnip
Capsicum
Kelp/Sea Vegetables
Slippery Elm

Elimination Systems

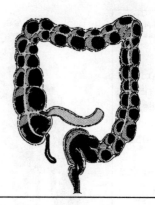

Colon Health

Aloe Vera
Fennel Seed
Kelp/Sea Vegetables
Marshmallow
High Chlorophyll Herbs
Licorice Root
Butternut Bark
Flax Seed

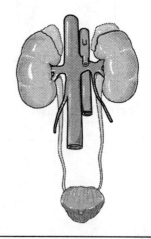

Urinary Health

Dandelion
Uva Ursi
Parsley
Cornsilk
Watermelon Seed
Cleavers
Barley Grass
Alfalfa
Oregon Grape Root

Liver & Gallbladder

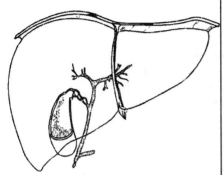

Liver Health

Chlorella
Milk Thistle Seed
Licorice Root
Gotu Kola
Sea Vegetables
Barley Grass
Goldenseal Root
Garlic
Dandelion
Yellow Dock
Siberian Ginseng
Panax Ginseng
Alfalfa
Barberry Bark
Astragalus
Royal Jelly
Reishi Mushroom
Evening Primrose
Fennel Seed

Heart & Arteries

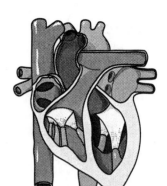

Heart Health

Ginkgo Biloba
Hawthorn
Cayenne
Barley Grass
Panax Ginseng
Siberian Ginseng
Garlic
Ginger Root
Bee Pollen
Licorice Root
Wild Cherry Bk.

Kidney System

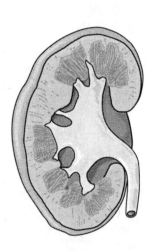

Kidney Health

Dandelion
Uva Ursi
Parsley
Cornsilk
Nettles
Juniper Berry
Barley Grass
Alfalfa
Burdock Root
Garlic
Goldenseal Root
St. John's Wort
Green Tea
Ginger Root

Lung System

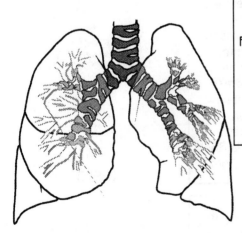

Lung Health

Ginkgo Biloba
Sea Vegetables
Rosemary
Chlorella
Fenugreek Seed
Comfrey
Bee Pollen
Chaparral
Pau d' Arco
Marshmallow

Spleen System

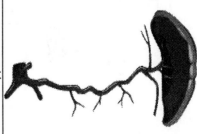

Spleen Health

Licorice Root
Panax Ginseng
Siberian Ginseng
Yellow Dock Root
Burdock Root
Oregon Grape
Root
Dandelion

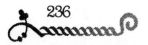

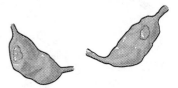

THE ENDOCRINE SYSTEM
Herbs For Your Glands

Adrenals

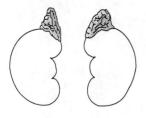

Adrenal Health

Royal Jelly
Bee Pollen
Licorice Root
Hawthorn
Astragalus
Sea Vegetables
Siberian Ginseng
Gotu Kola
Sarsaparilla Root

Ovaries

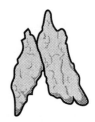

Ovary Health

Dong Quai Root
Damiana
Ashwagandha
Wild Yam Root
Burdock Root
Sea Vegetables
Evening Primrose
Vitex
Sarsaparilla Root

Pituitary

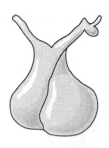

Pituitary Health

Royal Jelly
Sarsaparilla
Damiana
Dong Quai
Barley Grass
Horsetail Herb
Alfalfa
Oatstraw
Burdock Root
Licorice Root

Thymus

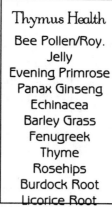

Thymus Health

Bee Pollen/Roy.
Jelly
Evening Primrose
Panax Ginseng
Echinacea
Barley Grass
Fenugreek
Thyme
Rosehips
Burdock Root
Licorice Root

Lymph

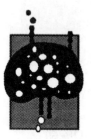

Lymph Health

Chaparral
Echinacea
Astragalus
Barberry Bark
Goldenseal Root
Yellow Dock Root
Garlic
Panax Ginseng
Burdock Root
Licorice Root
Green Tea

Thyroid

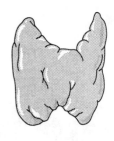

Thyroid Health

Sea Vegetables
Chlorella
Siberian Ginseng
Evening Primrose
Cayenne
Barley Grass
Mullein
Lobelia
Parsley
Sarsaparilla Root
Licorice Root

Pancreas

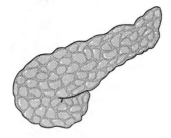

Pancreas Health

Juniper Berries
Dandelion
Licorice Root
Horseradish Root
Garlic

Testes

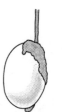
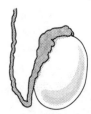

Testicle Health

Panax Ginseng
Damiana
Licorice Root
Dandelion Root
Sarsaparilla

Mind & Spirit

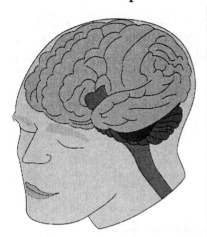

Mind/Spirit Balance

Ginkgo Biloba
Gotu Kola
Panax Ginseng
Sea Vegetables
Chlorella
Evening Primrose
Royal Jelly
Bee Pollen
Siberian Ginseng
Alfalfa
Rosemary
Sage

Skin System

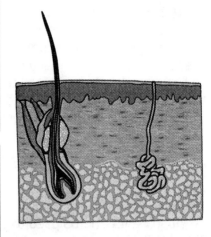

Skin Health

Evening Primrose
Dandelion
Rosehips
Chamomile
Royal Jelly

Skin Healing

Bee Pollen
Barley Grass
Horsetail
Panax Ginseng

Vision System

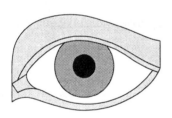

Eye Health

Eyebright
Bilberry
Parsley Root
Aloe Vera
Calendula
Chaparral
Ginkgo Biloba
Burdock Root
Hawthorn
Yellow Dock Root
Barley Grass
Sea Vegetables

Hair Health

Rosemary
Jojoba Oil
Reishi Mushroom
Sea Vegetables
Sage

Hair Growth

Horsetail
Oatstraw
Cayenne

Hair Health

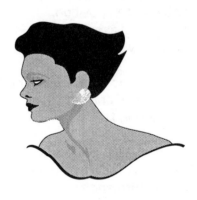

Hearing System

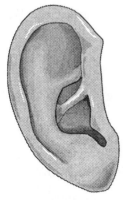

Ear Health

Mullein
Ginkgo Biloba
Turmeric
Yellow Dock Rt.
Garlic
Sea Vegetables
Spirulina
Echinacea Root
Yarrow
Bayberry Bark
Lobelia

Nail Health

Horsetail
Nettles
Rosemary
Sage
Sea Vegetables
Oatstraw
Pau d' Arco
Evening Primrose
Garlic
Chamomile
Royal Jelly

Nail Health

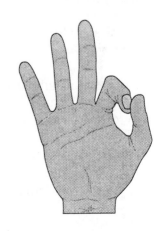

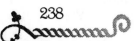

Medicinal Herb Glossary

The glossary in this chapter is a ready reference of common terms for herbal activity that are used in herbology and herbal formulating. It is important for anyone who works with harbal healing to become familiar with these terms. Medicinal herbs, unlike drugs, have broad spectrum activity with many layers of healing properties Understanding the attributes and abilities of an herb through its herbology terms is essential to recognizing not only how to use the herb itself for a particular problem, but how to best combine it with other herbs for synergistic healing effects.

Examples of herbs that represent each category are listed along with the definition.

Abortifacient - an herb used to induce abortion.
Examples of abortifacients include Pennyroyal, Canada snake root, lovage, angelica, tansy, rue, and wormwood.

Absorbents - herbs used to produce absorption of exudates or diseased tissues.
Examples of absorbents include Black Elm, Mullein and Slippery Elm.

Adaptogens - herbs that help normalize body chemistry and increase resistance to stress.
Examples of adaptogen herbs include Siberian Ginseng, Panax Ginseng, Chlorella, Astragalus, Suma and Hawthorn.

Alteratives - tonifying herbs that restore proper body function and vitality by correcting and improving blood composition.
Examples of alteratives include Echinacea, Burdock, Garlic, Red Clover, Sarsaparilla, Golden Seal, Nettles and Yellow Dock.

Analgesic - orally taken herbs that relieve pain.
Examples of analgesics include St. John's Wort, Valerian, Scullcap, Devil's Claw Root, Lady's Slipper and Passion Flower.

Anodynes - externally applied pain relieving herbs.
Examples of anodynes include St. John's Wort, Comfrey Rt., Calendula, Arnica, Marshmallow, Cayenne, Ginger, Turmeric and Mullein.

Antacids - agents which correct acidic conditions in the stomach, blood and bowels.
Examples of antacid herbs include Comfrey, Flax Seed, Hops, Mullein, Red Raspberry, Slippery Elm and Wood Betony.

Anthelmintics - herbs that help destroy or expel intestinal worms and parasites from the digestive system. (see also Vermifuge)
Examples of anthelmintics include Wormwood, Pumpkin Seed, Tansy, Aloe Vera, Rue, Black Walnut Hulls, and Garlic.

Anti-arthritics - herbs used to relieve and heal arthritic-type conditions.
Examples of anti-arthritic herbs include Yucca, Black Cohosh, Burdock, Cayenne, Chapparral, Dandelion, Irish Moss, Sarsaparilla, Scullcap, Wintergreen and Yellow Dock.

Anti-asthmatics - herbs that are used to relieve asthma.
Examples of these anti-asthmatic herbs include Agrimony, Black Cohosh, Blue Cohosh, Cajuput Oil, Cayenne, Chaparral, Comfrey Root, Eucalyptus, Flax Seed, Ginger, Garlic, Licorice and Wild Yam.

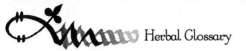

Anti-bilious - herbs that help neutralize and remove excess bile, and overcome jaundice conditions.
Examples of antibilious herbs include Barberry, Dandelion Root, Golden Seal, Wild Yam and Gentian.

Anti-biotics (anti-bacterial) - herbs that kill and arrest the growth of harmful micro-organisms. (see Anti-microbial)
Examples of antibiotic herbs includes Goldenseal root, Echinacea, Myrrh, Marshmallow, St. John's Wort, Lomatium, and Garlic.

Anti-catarrhal - herbs that help remove excess mucous and congestion, particularly from the sinus, bronchial and chest areas.
Examples of anti-catarrhal herbs include Boneset, Echinacea Root, Garlic, Golden Seal, Elecampane, Marshmallow, Mullein, Sage, Boneset and Yarrow.

Anti-emetic - herbs that relieve nausea and upset stomach, and help prevent vomiting.
Examples of anti-emetic herbs include Ginger Root, Cayenne, Cloves, Peppermint and Spearmint, Fennel, Lemon Balm, Wild Yam, Alfalfa and Dill.

Anti-fungal - an herb that destroys or prevents the growth of fungal infections.
Examples of anti-fungal herbs include Black Walnut Hulls, Tea Tree Oil, Propolis, Maitake Mushroom, Wormwood and Garlic.

Anti-hydropics - herbs used to eliminate excess body fluids or dropsy.
Examples of anti-hydropic herbs include Anise, Asparagus, Barberry, Black Cohosh, Burdock Seeds and Root, Camomile, Carrot, Celery, Chaparral, Dandelion, Fennel, Flaxseed, Mullein and Rosemary.

Anti-inflammatory - an herb that helps reduce and overcome inflammation. Effective both externally and internally.
Examples of anti-inflammatory herbs include Calendula, Chamomile, Devil's Claw Root, St. John's Wort, Feverfew and White Willow.

Anti-lithics - herbs to help remove and prevent the formation of sediment, gravel and stones in the urinary/urethral area.
Examples of anti-lithic herbs include Gravel Root, Hydrangea, Stone Root, Cornsilk, Buchu, Uva Ursi, and Parsley Root.

Anti-microbials - herbs that help overcome and destroy pathogenic bacteria, and strengthens the immune system.
Examples of anti-microbials include Myrrh, Garlic, Echinacea, Calendula, Elecampane, Golden Seal, and Astragalus.

Anti-neoplastic - herbs to help combat tumorous growth.
Examples of anti-neoplastic herbs include Calendula, Red Clover, Burdock, Dandelion, Cleavers, Mistletoe, Guaicum and Echinacea.

Anti-oxidant - herbs that increase the uptake of tissue oxygen and scavange free radicals.
Examples of anti-oxidant herbs include White Pine Bark and Grapeseed, Ginkgo Biloba, Chaparral, Rosemary, Mullein, Ephedra, Ginkgo Biloba Lf., Wild Cherry, Wheat Germ, and Chlorella.

Anti-periodics - herbs used to relieve malarial-type fevers and chills.
Examples of anti-periodic herbs include Alstonia Bark (powerful), Black Walnut, Bladderwrack, Chamomile, Eucalyptus, Horseradish, Lemon and Red Raspberry.

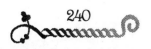

Anti-phlogistics - herbs used to reduce inflammation or swelling. (see Anti-inflammatory)
Examples of anti-phlogistic herbs include Arnica (external), Balm of Gilead, Bayberry, Black Cohosh (nerves), Blue Cohosh (uterus), Burdock Root (external), Cayenne, Comfrey and Licorice.

Anti-pyretic - herbs that help reduce fevers. (See Febrifuge)

Anti-septic - herbs to combat and neutralize pathogenic bacteria, and prevent infection. (see Anti-microbial and Anti-biotic)

Anti-spasmodic - muscle relaxant herbs that relieve cramping and spasms in a wide variety of uses, from hiatal hernias to lower back pain.
Examples of anti-spasmodic herbs include Cramp Bark, Black Haw, Lady's Slipper, Motherwort, Lobelia, Scullcap, Wild Yam, Chamomile and Valerian.

Anti-syphilitic - herbs that help overcome venereal diseases.
Examples of anti-syphilitic herbs include Sarsaparilla, Black Walnut, Burdock, Lobelia, White Oak Bark, Golden Seal and Myrrh.

Anti-tussive - herbs to prevent and relieve coughing and sore throat.
Examples of anti-tussive herbs include Licorice, Horehound, Comfrey Rt., Mullien, Plantain, Coltsfoot, Wild Cherry Bark, and Valerian.

Anti-venomous - herbs used as antidotes to animal, vegetable, and mineral poisons.
Examples of anti-venomous herbs include Plantain (powerful), Black Cohosh, Cornflower, Fennel, Garlic, Juniper Berry, Lobelia, Marigold, Olive Oil, Parsley, Slippery Elm, and Wormwood.

Anti-viral - herbs that combat and neutralize pathogenic viruses.
Examples of anti-viral herbs include Echinacea Root, St. John's Wort, Lomatium Dissectum, Myrrh, Goldenseal Root, Astragalus and Propolis.

Aperient - herbs with mild laxative activity.
Examples of aperients include Rhubarb Root, Flax Seed, Barberry, Butternut Root Bark, and Cleavors.

Aphrodisiacs - herbs that help impotency problems and strengthen sexual desire and vitality.
Examples of aphrodisiacs include Yohimbe, Gotu Kola, Kola Nut, all the Ginsengs, Damiana, Saw Palmetto, Muira Pauma (potency wood) and Dong Quai.

Aromatic - herbs with strong, pleasant odors, that can stimulate digestion and well-being through both carminitive activity and smell.
Examples of aromatic herbs include Anise Seed, Basil, Peppermint, Fennel, Cinnamon, Dill, Rosemary, Ginger, Cloves, Chamomile, and Coriander.

Astringent - herbs that tighten and contract tissue, and reduce irritation, secretions and discharges.
Examples of astringent herbs include Bayberry, St. John's Wort, Red Raspberry, Witch Hazel, Cranes-bill, Plantain, White Oak Bark, and Red Sage.

Balsamic - herbs that mitigate, soothe and heal inflamed parts.
Examples of balsamic herbs include Avocado Leaves, Balm of Gilead Buds, Clary, Larch, Ox-eye Daisy Flowers, Poplar Buds and Spikenard.

Bitters - herbs with a bitter taste that stimulate and tone the digestive system to produce healthful counteractive juices and secretions, such as bile.

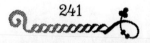

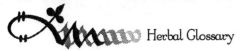

Examples of bitters herbs include Gentian, Tansy, Angelica, Wormwood, Chamomile, Barberry, Goldenseal, Dandelion Rt. and Oregon Grape.

Calmative - herbs used to calm stress and nervous tension.
Examples of calmatives include Peppermint, Chamomile, Scullcap, Catnip, Rosemary, Hops, Lady's Slipper, Garlic and Siberian Ginseng.

Cardio-tonics - herbs that strengthen and tonify heart and circulatory activity.
Examples of cardiotonic herbs include Hawthorn, Cayenne, Motherwort, and Siberian Ginseng.

Carminatives - herbs that normalize digestive system peristalsis to relieve gas.
Examples of carminatives include Anise Seed, Cayenne, Licorice, Peppermint, Ginger Root, Cinnamon, Caraway, Ginger and Thyme.

Cathartic - herbs to stimulate purging from the bowel. (see also Purgative)
Examples of cathartic herbs include Cascara Sagrada, Senna, Butternut Bark, Barberry, Aloe Vera, Psyllium Husks, Flax Seed and Bentonite.

Caustics - herbs that burn or destroy living tissues.
Examples of caustics include Celandine Juice, Lesser Celandine Leaves and Yellow Anemone Herb.

Cell Proliferant - herbs to promote rapid new cell growth.
Examples of cell proliferant herbs include Chlorella, Spirulina, Barley Grass, Horsetail, Evening Primrose oil, Sea Vegetables, and Ginsengs of all kinds.

Cholagogue - herbs that stimulate bile secretion from the gall-bladder, engendering natural laxative activity and digestive improvement.
Examples of cholagogues include Barberry Bark, Wild Yam, Dandelion Rt., Oregon Grape, Calendula, Golden Seal, Garlic and Gentian Root.

Contra-indicated - a term denoting conditions not to use a certain herb or formula.
Examples of contra-indicated herbs might be Tansy and Rue during pregnancy, or Yohimbe if there is high blood pressure.

Cordials - tonic herbs that warm the stomach and stimulate cardiac activity.
Examples of these herbs include Ginger, Ginsengs, Cardamon, Cinnamon, Cloves and Coriander.

Demulcent - soothing coating mucilaginous herbs that protect irritated and inflamed tissue.
Examples of demulcent herbs include Comfrey, Marshmallow, Milk Thistle, Slippery Elm, Flax Seed, Parsley Root, Irish Moss, Aloe Vera and Mullein.

Dental Anodynes - herbs used locally to relieve pain from an exposed tooth nerve (toothache).
Examples of anodyne herbs include Oils of Cloves, Peppermint, Capsicum, Cajuput, Mullein and Rosemary, Chamomile, Hops and Ginger.

Deobstruents - herbs that remove obstructions. (See also Aperients and Laxatives)
Examples of deobstruent herbs include Barberry (liver, gall bladder), Culvers root (bowel), Goldenseal (glands), Gravel Root (kidneys), Hydrangea Root (kidneys), and Plantain (blood, kidneys).

Dessicants - herbs that dry surfaces by absorbing moisture.
Examples of dessicant herbs include Agar, Bladderwrack, Marshmallow Rt. and Slippery Elm.

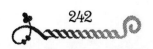

Depurant - blood purifying herbs that stimulate the elimination of toxins.
Examples of depurants include Garlic, Goldenseal, Chlorella, Barley Grass, Cranberry, and Sea Plants.

Diaphoretics - herbs that induce sweating, releasing body toxins through perspiration.
Examples of diaphoretic herbs include Cayenne, Elder Flowers, Garlic, Ginger, Chamomile, Boneset, Angelica, Bayberry, Prickly Ash Bark, Spikenard and Buchu.

Digestant - amino acid, enzyme-containing herbs that promote digestion and nutrient assimilation.
Examples of digestant herbs include Ginseng, Chlorella, Barley Grass, Spirulina, Yellow Dock, Sea Vegetables, Papaya and Garlic.

Discutients - herbs that dissolve and remove tumors and abnormal growths. They may be used in poultices and fomentations or taken internally as teas.
Examples of discutients include Aloe Vera, Ginseng, Pau d' Arco, Calendula, Echinacea and Sea Plants.

Diuretics - herbs that stimulate kidney and bladder activity, and increase the flow of urine.
Examples of diuretic herbs include Uva Ursi, Cleavers, Dandelion Leaf, Buchu, Couchgrass, Juniper, Yarrow, Corn Silk and Gravel Root.

Electuary - a sweet paste, food or drink that is used to mask bitter or medicine-tasting herbs so they may be taken by children.
Examples of electuaries include peanut butter, fruit juices, honey/butter pastes, bread, or cream cheese.

Emetic - herbs that in high doses cause vomiting to rid the body of toxic substances or excess mucous congestion.
Examples of emetic herbs include Lobelia, Senega, Elder Flowers, Boneset, and Ipecacuanha.

Emmenagogues - herbs that stimulate and normalize menstrual flow.
Examples of emmenagogues include Pennyroyal, Blue Cohosh, Blessed Thistle, Motherwort, Lovage, Angelica, Tansy, and Shepherd's Purse.

Emollient - externally applied, soothing herbs that smooth and soften the skin and reduce inflammatory skin conditions.
Examples of these herbs include Slippery Elm, Marshmallow, Plantain, Comfrey, Irish Moss, Chickweed, Borage, Mullein and Aloe Vera.

Expectorants - herbs to help remove mucous congestion from the chest and respiratory system.
Examples of expectorant herbs include Licorice Root, Horehound, Pleurisy Root, Coltsfoot, Comfrey, Anise Seed, Marshmallow, and Thyme.

Febrifuge - herbs that help reduce fevers.
Examples of febrifuge herbs include Boneset, Lobelia, Peppermint, Prickly Ash Bark, Elder Flower, Thyme, Calendula, Vervain, and Plantain.

Galactagogue - herbs that increase the flow of Mother's milk.
Examples of galactogogues include Blessed Thistle, Nettles, Red Raspberry, Marshmallow, Fennel, Anise Seed and Vervain.

Hemostatic - herbs that help stop bleeding. (see Styptic).
Examples of hemostatic herbs include Shepherd's Purse, Comfrey Rt., Turmeric, Plantain, Witch Hazel, Cayenne, Buckthorn, and Cranesbill.

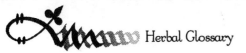

Hepatics - herbs that support and stimulate the liver, gall bladder and spleen and increase bile flow.
Examples of hepatics include Barberry, Oregon Grape, Beet Root, Dandelion, Goldenseal, Hyssop, Wild Yam, Fennel, and Cleavers.

Hormonal - an herb that promotes hormone secretion and formation in the body.
Examples of hormonal herbs include Black Cohosh, Sarsaparilla, Dong Quai, Ginseng, Licorice, Dandelion, Burdock and Damiana.

Hypnotic - herbs that help induce normal natural sleep. (see Sedatives and Soporifics)

Hypotensive - an herb that lowers blood pressure.
Examples of hypotensive herbs include Garlic, Hawthorn, Valerian, Yarrow and European Mistletoe.

Laxative - herbs that promote evacuation of the bowels.
Examples of laxative herbs include Cascara Sagrada, Senna, Cleavers, Oregon Grape, Rhubarb Rt., Butternut Bark, Buckthorn and Barberry.

Lithotriptics - herbs that dissolve and discharge urinary and gall bladder stones and gravel.
Examples of lithotropics include Barberry, Buchu, Cascara Ssgrada, Chaparral, Corn Silk, Dandelion, Horsetail, Juniper Berries and Parsley.

Lymphatics - herbs used to stimulate and cleanse the lymphatic system.
Examples of lymphatics include Black Walnut, Garlic, Chaparral, Dandelion, Echinacea Root, Oregon Grape Root, Yellow Dock.

Mucilaginous - herbs with high mucilage content that have soothing, demulcent action.
Examples of mucilaginous herbs include Comfrey, Slippery Elm, Irish Moss, Iceland Moss, Flax Seed, Psyllium, Aloe Vera, and Marshmallow Root.

Nervines - herbs that tone, relax and have a strengthening effect on the nervous system.
Examples of nervines include Lady's Slipper, Passionflower, Mistletoe, Chamomile, Oatstraw, Lobelia, Cramp Bark, Valerian and Scullcap.

Nutritives - food supplement herbs, rich in minerals, that nourish and promote physical growth.
Examples of nutritive herbs include Chlorella, Spirulina, Barley Grass, Ginseng, Wheat Grass, Sea Vegetables, Suma, Astragalus and Bee Pollen.

Ophthalmic - herbs that heal and relieve eye disorders.
Examples of ophthalmic herbs include Eyebright, Passionflower, Aloe Vera, Goldenseal, Red Raspberry, and Capsicum.

Oxytocic/Parturient- herbs that aid uterine contractions in childbirth.
Examples of parturient herbs include Blue Cohosh, Pennyroyal, Rue, and Squaw Vine.

Parasiticides - herbs that kill and remove parasites from the skin.
Examples of paraciticide herbs include Black Walnut, Cinnamon and Cajuput Oils, Chaparral, Garlic, Echinacea, Rue, Thyme, Gentian and Wood Betony.

Pectoral - an herb that helps heal and strengthen the lung and respiratory system.
Examples of these herbs include Comfrey, Coltsfoot, Goldenseal, Elecampane, Mullein, Licorice, Marshmallow, Pleurisy Root, and Hyssop.

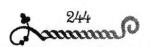

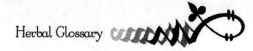

Prophylactics - herbs which help ward off and prevent disease.
Examples of prophylactic herbs include Chlorella, Goldenseal, Echinacea, Siberian Ginseng, and Garlic.

Purgative - herbs which promote watery evacuation of the bowels. (see Laxative)

Rubefacient - herbs that increase circulation and stimulate dilation of the capillaries.
Examples of rubefacient herbs include Cayenne, Ginger, Horseradish, Nettles, Rosemary, Peppermint oil, Cloves, Black Pepper and Garlic.

Sedative - herbs that calm the nervous system, and reduce stress and tension.
Exampes of sedative herbs include Valerian, Wild Lettuce, Scullcap, Lady's Slipper, Hops, Black Cohosh, Black Haw, and Passionflower.

Sialagogue - an herb that stimulates salivary secretions.
Examples of sialogogues include Cayenne, Gentian, Ginger, Prickly Ash, Black Pepper and Cinnamon.

Soporifics - herbs that help induce sleep. (see Hypnotics)
Examples of soporifics include Valerian, Wild Lettuce, Passionflower, Scullcap, Mistletoe, and Hops.

Stimulants - herbs that accelerate, enliven and vitalize body functions.
Examples of stimulant herbs include Bayberry, Cayenne, Ginger Root, Horseradish, Cardamom, Peppermint, Wild Yam, and Ginsengs of all kinds.

Stomachic - herbs to strengthen and tone the stomach and its function, and stimulate appetite.
Examples of stomachics include Dandelion, Wild Yam, Hibiscus, Chlorophyll-rich herbs, Catnip, Fennel, Peppermint and Spearmint.

Styptic - herbs to reduce and stop external bleeding. (see Hemostatics and Astringents)
Examples of styptics include Plantain, St. John's Wort, Witch Hazel, Yarrow, Bayberry Bk., Cranesbill, White Oak Bark, and Cayenne.

Sudorific - herbs that stimulate and increase perspiration. (see Diaphoretic)

Tonic - herbs that strengthen and tone specific organs and body parts.
Examples of these herbs include the Ginsengs of all types, Hawthorn, Black Cohosh, Dandelion, Garlic, Gotu Kola, Licorice Rt. and Damiana.

Vaso-dilator - herbs that cause relaxation and expansion of the blood vessels.
Examples of vasodilators include Ephedra, Hawthorn, Ginkgo Biloba, Feverfew, and Siberian Ginseng.

Vermifuge - an herb that helps expel and/or destroy intestinal parasites. (see Anthelmintic)
Examples of vermifuge herbs include Thyme, Black Walnut Hulls, Chaparral, Garlic, Barberry, Psyllium Husks, Tea Tree oil, Tansy and Wormwood.

Vulnerary - externally applied herbs that aid in healing cuts and wounds.
Examples of these herbs include Aloe Vera, Calendula, Arnica, Comfrey, Marshmallow, Goldenseal, Garlic, St. John's Wort, and Mullein.

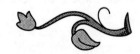

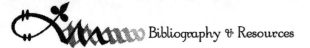
Bibliography & Resources

The bibliography listings in this section reflect a small part of the wealth of documentation available today about medicinal herbs and their uses. They are intended for you to use for corraborative as well as expanded information. In addition, the RESOURCES files at the end of the BIBLIOGRAPHY are intended as herbal ingredient pathways for you to access if you cannot find some of the herbs or other ingredients in order to make up a formula. Besides herb shops, many natural food stores today carry a wide selection of bulk and packaged herbs; but if you need something they don't have, the resources in this section have both stock and information.

Mowrey, Daniel B., Ph. D. *The Scientific Validation of Herbal Medicine.* 1986

Werbach, Melvyn R., M.D. *Nutritional Influences On Illness - A Sourcebook Of Clinical Research.* 1988

Mowrey, Daniel B., Ph.D. *Next Generation Herbal Medicine.* 1990

Rodger, Katie. "Back To Our Roots: Pharmacists Explore the Potential of Phytomedicinals" *Drug Topics* 1995

Murray, Michael T., N.D. *Healing Power of Herbs.* 1992

Hobbs, Christopher. *Ginkgo - Elixir of Youth.* 1995

Brown, Donald J., N.D. *Herbal Prescriptions for Better Health.* 1995

Tierra, Lesley, L. Ac. *The Herbs of Life.* 1992

Ody, Penelope. *The Complete Medicinal Herbal,* 1993

Duke, James Alan & Rodolfo Vasquez. *Amazonian Ethnobotanical Dictionary.* 1994

Thomas, Clayton L., M.D., M.P.H. *Taber's Cyclopedic Medical Dictionary.* 1989

Hobbs, Christopher. "Herbs For Health - Losing Addictions Naturally." *Let's Live.* April 1993

Zand, Janet, L.Ac., O.M.D. "Nutrients and Herbs for the Recovering Addict." *Health World.* July 1992

Gaia Herbal Research Institute, *Gaia Symposium Proceedings-Naturopatic Herbal Wisdom,* 1994

Stein, Diane. *The Natural Remedy Book For Women,* 1995

Herbal Research Publications. *The Protocol Journal Of Botanical Medicine,* 1995

Chen, Ze-lin M.D. & Mei-fang Chen, M.D. *Comprehensive Guide to Chinese Herbal Medicine.* 1992

Yen-Hsu, Hong. *How to Treat Yourself with Chinese Herbs.* 1993

Frawley, David, O. M.D. "Ayurveda, the Science of Life." *Let's Live.* 1993

Zucker, Martin. "Women's Health - Ayurveda Offers Ancient Solutions for Modern Times." *Let's Live.* 1995

Valnet, Jean, M.D. *The Practice of Aromatherapy.* 1990

Tisserand, Robert. *Aromatherapy to Heal and Tend the Body.* 1988

Price, Shirley. *Practical Aromatherapy, How to Use Essential Oil to Restore Vitality.* 1987

Wolfson, Evelyn. *From the Earth To Beyond the Sky Native American Medicine.* 1993

Laux, Marcus. *Cures from the Rainforest Pharmacy.* 1995

Schwontkowski, Donna. *Herbal Treasures from the Amazon.* 1995

Mendelsohn, Robert & Michael J. Balick. "More Drugs Await Discovery in Rainforests." *ABC.* 1995

Baar, Karen. "Grow Your Own Pharmacy." *Natural Health.* 1995

Foster, Steven. "Memory Power: Don't Forget Rosemary, Gotu kola, Ginkgo," *Herbs For Health,* March 1996

Santillo, Humbart, B.S., M.H. *Natural Healing With Herbs.* 1984

Tierra, Michael, C.A., N. D. *Planetary Herbology.* 1988

Duke, James A. *Handbook of Medicinal Herbs.* 1985

Murray, Michael T., N.D. *Natural Alternatives to Prozac.* 1996

Mills, Simon Y. *The Dictionary of Modern Herbalism.* 1988

Tyler, Varro E., PhD, ScD. *Herbs of Choice - The Therapeutic Use of Phytomedicinals.* 1994

Tourles, Stephanie. *The Herbal Body Book.* 1994

Sanderson, Liz. *How To Make Your Own Herbal Cosmetics.* 1979

Rose, Jeanne. *The Herbal Body Book.* 1982

Rose, Jeanne. *Kitchen Cosmetics.* 1978

Wesley-Hosford, Zia. *The Beautiful Body Book.* 1989

Nadkarni, Dr. A. K. *Indian Materia Medica.* 1976

Software:

Blake, Steve. *Global Herb v.5.1.* 1995

Hoffmann, David. *The Herbalist v.2, Hopkins Technology.* 1992-1996

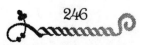

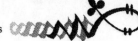

Traditional Chinese Medicine and Pharmacology. Hopkins Technology. 1995

Websites:
Ayurveda Holistic Center - http://www.holistic.com/listings/11709acl.html
Moore, Michael. S.W. School of Botanical Medicine - http://chili.rt66.com/hrbmoore/HOMEPAGE/
Phytochemical and Ethnobotanial Databases - http://www.ars-grin.gov/~ngrlsb/
Medline (The Physician's National Medical Research Database). *Physical Conditions Affected By A Deficiency Of The Metabolic Catalysts*. Hawaii Medical Library, Inc.

Ingredients Resources

Most of the herbs and nutrient ingredients (like brewer's yeast, miso powder or acidophilus) may be obtained through a good herb or health food store, who generally stock a wide selection of bulk herbs. Bulk herbs are usually fresher and fuller potency than packaged herbs. But, if you live in an area where good stock is not available, or you cannot find the herbal materials you wish to use, the following listing contains the names, addresses and phone numbers of high quality suppliers of herbs. Many are wholesalers, but sometimes sell herbs in one pound sizes for individual use.

Aloe Life International, 4822 Santa Monica Ave. #231, San Diego, CA 92107, 800-414-2563
American Health & Herbs, P.O. Box 940, Philomath, OR 97370, 800-345-4152
Beehive Botanicals, Route 8, Box 8257, Hayward, WI 54843, 800-233-4483
Body Ecology, 295 King Road, Atlanta, GA 30342, 800-478-3842
Burt's Bees, P.O. Box 90157, Raleigh, NC, 27675-0157, 919-510-8720
Desert Essence, 9510 Vassar Ave., Unit A, Chatsworth, CA 91311, 800-645-5768
Diamond Herpanacine Assocs., P.O. Box 544, Ambler, PA 19002, 215-542-2981
Ecco Bella Botanicals, Inc., 1133 Route 23 South, Wayne, NJ 07470, 201-696-7766
Educated Beauty Inc., 77 Digital Drive, Novato, CA 94949, 888-323-8423
Elizabeth Van Buren, Inc., 303 Potrero Street #33, Santa Cruz, CA 95060, 800-710-7759
Herbal Products/Development, P.O. Box 1084, Aptos, CA 95001, 408-688-8706
Herbs for Kids, 151 Evergreen Dr. Suite D, Bozeman, MT 59715, 406-587-0180
In Life Energy Systems, Red Marine Algae, 107 California Ave., Mill Valley, CA 94941, 415-389-1738
Innovative Natural Products, 640 Alpine Way, Escondido, CA 92029, 800-266-4447
Jarrow Formulas, 1824 South Robertson Blvd., Los Angeles, CA 90035, 310-204-6936
Live Food Products, Inc., Box 7, Santa Barbara, CA 93102, 800-446-1990
Maine Coast Sea Vegetables, RR1 Box 78, Franklin, Maine 04634, 207-565-2907
McZand Herbal Inc., P.O. Box 5312, Santa Monica, CA 90409, 310-822-0500
Mendocino Sea Vegetable Co., P.O. Box 1265, Mendocino, CA 95460, 707-937-2050
Motherlove Herbal Co., P.O. Box 101, Laporte, CO 80535, 970-493-2892
Nature's Alchemy / Lotus Brands, Inc., Box 325, Twin Lakes, WI 53181, 800-824-6396
New Chapter, 99 Main Street Brattleboro, VT 05301, 800-543-7279
NutriCology, P.O. Box 489, 400 Preda Street, San Leandro, CA 94577-0489, 800-545-9960
Oshadhi Essential Oils, 32422 Alipaz, Ste C, San Juan Capistrano, CA 92675, 800-933-1008
Premier Labs, 27475 Ynez Road, Suite 305, Temecula, CA 92591, 909-699-8801
Prevail Corporation, 2204-8 NW Birdsdale, Gresham, Or 97030, 800-248-0885
Source Naturals, 19 Janis Way, Scotts Valley, CA 95066, 800-815-2333
Starwest Botanicals, 11253 Trade Center Dr., Rancho Cordova, CA 95742, 800-800-4372
Trout Lake Farm Co., 149 Little Mountain Road, Trout Lake, WA 98650, 800-395-6093
Vagosang Skin Care system, 55 West Sunset Way, Issaquah, WA 98027, 206-557-4605
Waddell Creek Organic Bee Farm, 654 Swanton Road, Davenport, CA 95017
Wakunaga of America Co., Ltd., 23501 Madero, Mission Viejo, CA 92691-2764, 714-855-2776
Y.S. Royal Jelly & Organic Bee Farm, RT. 1, Box 91-A, Sheridan IL 60551, 800-654-4593

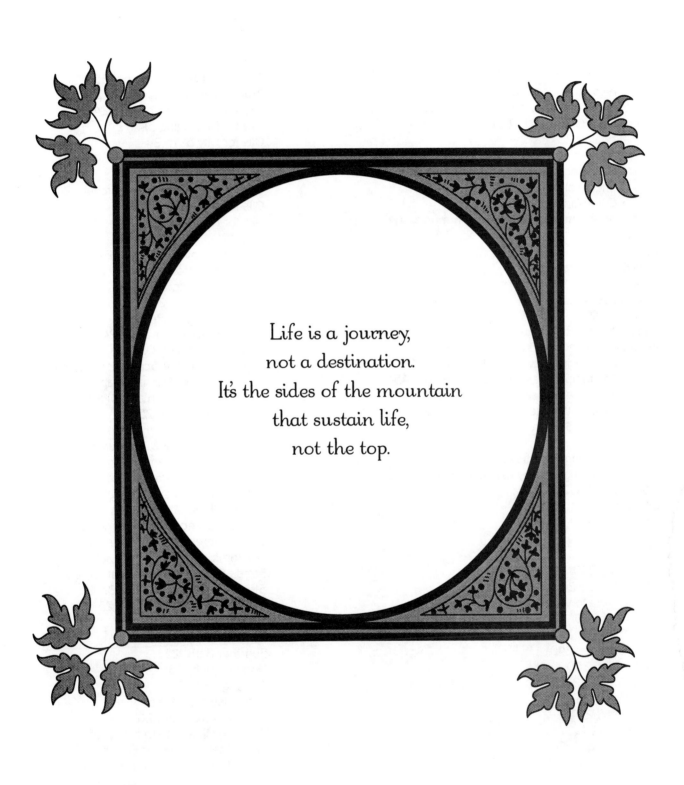

Life is a journey,
not a destination.
It's the sides of the mountain
that sustain life,
not the top.

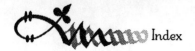

Index

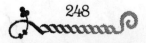

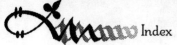

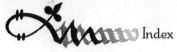

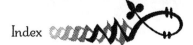

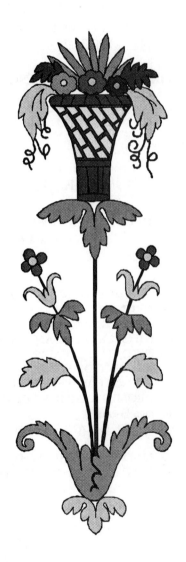

HEALTHY HEALING PUBLICATIONS
Books

HEALTHY HEALING - *Tenth Edition, A Guide to Self Healing for Everyone* - by Dr. Linda Rector Page, N.D., Ph.D. - A 500 page alternative healing reference used by professors, students, health care professionals and private individuals. $28.95 - S&H $4.50 - ISBN# 1-884334-85-7

HOW TO BE YOUR OWN HERBAL PHARMACIST - *Herbal Traditions, Expert Formulations* - by Dr. Linda Rector Page, N.D., Ph.D. A complete reference guide for herbal formulations and preparations. $18.95 S&H $4.50 - ISBN# 1-884334-77-6

COOKING FOR HEALTHY HEALING - *Diets and Recipes for Alternative Healing* - by Dr. Linda Rector Page, N.D., Ph.D. - Over 900 recipes and 33 separate diet and healing programs. $29.95-S&H $4.50 ISBN# 1-884334-56-3

PARTY LIGHTS - *Healthy Party Foods & Earthwise Entertaining* - by Dr. Linda Rector Page. N.D., Ph.D., and Doug Vanderberg - A party reference book with over 70 parties and more than 500 original recipes you can prepare at home. $19.95 - S&H $4.50 - ISBN# 1-884334-53-9

THE BODY SMART SYSTEM - *The Complete Guide to Cleansing & Rejuvenation* - by Helene Silver - A complete 21 day regimen and guide that includes diet, relaxation techniques, massage and bath, exercise programs and recipes. $19.95 - S&H $4.50 - ISBN# 1-884334-60-1

30-X **RENEWING MALE HEALTH & ENERGY**
32-6 **THE ENERGY CRUNCH & YOU**
35-0 **ALLERGY CONTROL & MANAGEMENT**
13-X **REVEALING THE SECRETS OF ANTI-AGING**
27-X **DO YOU WANT TO HAVE A BABY?**
33-4 **STRESS MANAGEMENT, DEPRESSION & OVERCOMING ADDICTIONS**
37-7 **A FIGHTING CHANCE FOR WEIGHT LOSS & CELLULITE CONTROL**
14-8 **FATIGUE SYNDROMES & IMMUNE DISORDERS** - New - 46 Page Book - $3.95
New Expanded 48 Page Format:
64-4 **RENEWING FEMALE BALANCE** - $4.50

49-0 **DETOXIFICATION & BODY CLEANSING**
34-2 **BOOSTING IMMUNITY WITH POWER PLANTS**
47-4 **COLDS, FLU & YOU** - Building Optimum Immunity
29-6 **FIGHTING INFECTIONS WITH HERBS**

NEW SERIES - DR. LINDA PAGE'S HEALTHY HEALING GUIDES
90-3 **MENOPAUSE & OSTEOPOROSIS** - 64 Pages - $5.95
36-9 **CANCER** - 96 Pages - $8.95
15-6 **SEXUALITY** - 96 Pages - $8.95

(S&H $1.00 on all small books.)

Mail to: Healthy Healing Publications, P.O. Box 436, Carmel Valley, CA 93924.
Or, fax your order to: 408-659-4044.
Or, order online - www.healthyhealing.com.
(California residents add 7.25% sales tax)
For infomation about *Dr. Linda Page's Natural Healing Report*, call 1-800-811-8725.

Natural Health Questions? Get help. Have a private consultation with a professional.
Call 1-900-903-5885 M-F, 9 to 5 Pacific Time
$2.29 per minute - ave. call 5 min. - must be 18